Urinary Tract Infections: Pathophysiology and Clinical Management

Urinary Tract Infections: Pathophysiology and Clinical Management

Editor: Hayley Atkins

MURPHY & MOORE
www.murphy-moorepublishing.com

www.murphy-moorepublishing.com

MURPHY & MOORE

Cataloging-in-Publication Data

Urinary tract infections : pathophysiology and clinical management / edited by Hayley Atkins.
p. cm.
Includes bibliographical references and index.
ISBN 978-1-63987-562-7
1. Urinary tract infections. 2. Urinary tract infections--Pathophysiology. 3. Urinary tract infections--Treatment.
4. Urinary organs--Diseases. 5. Infection. I. Atkins, Hayley.
RC901.8 .U75 2021
616.6--dc23

Murphy & Moore Publishing,
1 Rockefeller Plaza,
New York City, NY 10020, USA

ISBN 978-1-63987-562-7 (Hardback)

Contents

Preface

The purpose of the book is to provide a glimpse into the dynamics and to present opinions and studies of some of the scientists engaged in the development of new ideas in the field from very different standpoints. This book will prove useful to students and researchers owing to its high content quality.

The infections that affect the urinary tract are termed as urinary tract infections (UTIs). These include bladder infections and kidney infections. Bladder infections or cystitis are the infections that affect the lower part of the urinary tract. Kidney infections or pyelonephritis are the infections that affect the upper part of the urinary tract. Symptoms of cystitis include frequent urination, pain with urination and feeling the need to urinate despite having an empty bladder. Symptoms associated with pyelonephritis are fever and flank pain along with the symptoms of cystitis. In some cases, urine may appear bloody. A few of the risk factors of UTIs are diabetes, family history, obesity, female anatomy and sexual intercourse. From theories to research, case studies related to all contemporary topics of relevance to this field have been included in this book. Its aim is to give a general view of the pathophysiology and clinical management of urinary tract infections. This book will help new researchers by foregrounding their knowledge in this branch.

At the end, I would like to appreciate all the efforts made by the authors in completing their chapters professionally. I express my deepest gratitude to all of them for contributing to this book by sharing their valuable works. A special thanks to my family and friends for their constant support in this journey.

Editor

1

Urinary Tract Infection in Diabetics

Ajay Kumar Prajapati

Abstract

Diabetes is a metabolic disease with increase blood sugar level. A large population of world is affected by diabetes. The patients suffering from diabetes have many other complications like cardiovascular disease, kidney disease, retinopathy, diabetic foot, diabetic neuropathy, urinary tract infection, etc. The patients with diabetes are more prone to get urinary tract infection due to frequent urination and high blood sugar level. The high sugar level gives favorable growth environment to the pathogens. Early diagnosis and proper medication are necessary for management of urinary tract infection in diabetic patients. The diagnosis of urinary tract infection is dependent on urine culture reports. The treatment should preferably be started after antimicrobial susceptibility reports. The misuse or overuse of antibiotics may lead to antimicrobial resistance. The antimicrobial resistance is another challenge in management of urinary tract infection.

Keywords: diabetes mellitus, urinary tract infection, Gram-negative bacilli, antibiotic, antimicrobial resistance

1. Introduction

Diabetes is a global threat that affects the quality of life, and it is estimated that it will affect 220 million people by the year 2020 worldwide. Morbidity and mortality in diabetic patients are caused by infections. Evidence suggests that, urinary tract infection (UTI) is the most common bacterial infections among diabetic patients. According to American Diabetes Association (ADA) report, patients suffering from type 2 diabetes are more likely to have a urinary tract infection (UTI) and repeat UTI than patients without diabetes. Symptomatic bacteriuria in patients with diabetes is serious and warrants proper clinical attention for diagnosis and treatment. High glucose concentration in the urine can provide a rich source of nutrients for bacteria. Therefore, bacteria can multiply and make foundation for infection also.

High glucose concentration in the urine can allow urinary colonization by microorganisms. Moreover, multiple mechanisms were involved in UTI patients with diabetes. Diabetic female, diabetic overweight, and diabetic obese patients are having the highest risk of UTI. In general diabetic population, other risk factors associated with urinary tract infection were found to be diabetic nephropathy, diabetes with hypertension, and insulin therapy. Emphysematous pyelonephritis, emphysematous cystitis, renal and perinephric abscesses, urosepsis, and bacteremia are the complications of diabetes-associated UTI. Longer hospitalization, recurrence of UTI, relapse and re-infection, bacteremia, azotemia, and septic shock are the outcomes of diabetes-associated UTI [1].

2. Diabetes

Diabetes is a persistent disease. This disease is characterized by increase of blood glucose level. The reasons of increase of blood glucose level may be either insufficient production of insulin, a hormone that regulates the blood glucose level, or the insulin produced cannot be used properly. Frequent urination, increased thirst, and increased hunger are the common symptoms of diabetes. Uncontrolled blood sugar level can cause many complications. These complications include cardiovascular disease, stroke, chronic kidney disease, foot ulcers, damage to the eyes, diabetic ketoacidosis, etc. Diabetes mellitus can be described as group of metabolic disorders causing increase in blood sugar level due to defect in insulin secretion, insulin action, or both [2]. The digestive system breaks carbohydrates, sugars, and starches found in many foods into glucose, which is a type of sugar that enters the bloodstream [3]. By the action of the hormone insulin, cells throughout the body absorb glucose and use it for energy. Diabetes develops when the body does not produce enough insulin or is unable to use insulin effectively or both. Insulin is produced in the pancreas. Clusters of cells found in the pancreas are called islets. Pancreas having islets, which contain beta cells, produces insulin and releases it into the blood.

3. Types of diabetes

- Type 1 diabetes also called as insulin-dependent diabetes mellitus (type I diabetes occurs due to β-cell destruction, usually leading to absolute insulin deficiency).
- Type 2 diabetes also called as noninsulin-dependent diabetes mellitus (type II diabetes occurs due to a progressive loss of insulin secretion).
- Gestational diabetes mellitus (GDM) (diabetes detected in the second or third trimester of pregnancy that is not clearly overt diabetes).
- Specific types of diabetes due to other reasons, for example, monogenic diabetes syndromes (such as maturity-onset diabetes of the young [MODY] and neonatal diabetes),

diseases associated with exocrine pancreas (such as cystic fibrosis), and drug- or chemical-induced diabetes (such as use of glucocorticoid, in the treatment of HIV/AIDS or after organ transplantation).

Type 1 diabetes occurs in childhood, mainly due to destruction of pancreatic β-cell islets through autoimmune-mediated, causing complete insulin deficiency. Type 2 is more associated with adults and elderly people, which are mainly due to insulin resistance or abnormal insulin production. The exact reason of pancreatic failure and insulin resistance is unknown, but they are associated with disease condition, food habit, and environmental impact. Diabetic patients are more susceptible to various type of infection such as skin diseases and carbuncles [4].

Gestational diabetes is other type of diabetes, which is mainly associated with pregnancy. It occurs in the 4% of pregnancies in US, usually during the third trimester. It causes increased perinatal morbidity and mortality unless properly diagnosed or managed. Genetic defects of β-cell function or insulin action is also a type of diabetes mellitus commonly called maturity onset diabetes. Neonatal diabetes mellitus is also a type of diabetes, in which first 3 months of life insulin is required for the maintenance of blood glucose level in. It may be caused by intrauterine growth retardation and defects of chromosome. The heart, blood vessels, eyes, kidneys, and nerves can be damaged by diabetes, leading to disability and premature death.

4. Urinary tract infection in diabetics

Infections are frequent causes of morbidity and mortality in diabetic patients. Evidence suggesting that urinary tract infection (UTI) is the most common bacterial infections among diabetic patients. High glucose concentration in the urine can provide a rich source of nutrients for bacteria [5, 6]. Therefore, bacteria can multiply and make foundation for infection; also, high glucose concentration in the urine can allow urinary colonization by microorganisms. Moreover, some of the immunological defects like impaired neutrophil function, reduced T cell-mediated immune response, low levels of prostaglandin E, thromboxane B2, and leukotriene B4 may contribute to the increased risk for infection. Other conditions such as bladder dysfunction (incomplete bladder emptying) caused by autonomic neuropathy also may contribute to the increased risk for infection [7, 8]. UTI in diabetes can lead to severe complications including bacteremia, renal abscess, and renal papillary necrosis. In some cases, diabetes modifies the genitourinary system and may cause damage to the organ, which leads to pyelonephritis. This type of UTI occurs 15 times more frequently in diabetic patients. Therefore, early diagnosis and correct treatment are very important for diabetes patients with UTI [9, 10]. Molecular reasons for an increased frequency of UTI in diabetic patients include depression in the function of polymorphonuclear leucocytes especially during acidosis, dysfunction of chemotaxis, and phagocytosis [10]. High blood glucose levels may cause nerve damage, affecting the ability of the bladder to sense the presence of urine and thus allowing urine to stay for a long time in the bladder and increasing probability of infection [11].

Various types of UTI in patients with diabetes include

- Asymptomatic bacteriuria
- Acute cystitis
- Complicated lower UTI (including catheter-associated UTI)
- Uncomplicated pyelonephritis
- Complicated pyelonephritis/urosepsis

5. Pathogenesis of UTI in diabetics

The chance of occurrence of UTIs in diabetic patients used to increase many folds due to several factors. Multiple potential mechanisms unique to diabetes may cause increased risk of UTI in diabetic patients. Elevated renal parenchymal glucose levels create a positive environment for the growth and multiplication of microorganisms, which is one of the precipitating factors of pyelonephritis and renal problem such as emphysematous pyelonephritis. Several problems in the immune system, including humoral, cellular, and innate immunity, may help in the pathogenesis of UTI in diabetic patients [12–14]. Lower urinary interleukin-6 and interleukin-8 levels were found in diabetic patients with UTI. An outline of process involved in pathogenesis of urinary tract infection in diabetic patients is mentioned in **Figure 1**.

Some suggested host related mechanisms include [15]:

i. Presence of glycosuria

ii. Increased adherence to uroepithelial cells

iii. Immune dysfunction

5.1. Presence of glycosuria

The presence of glycosuria is responsible for the growth of different microbial strains. Among all *E. coli* is the major cause for the condition of UTI [15]. The bacteria isolated from diabetic patients with a UTI are similar to the bacteria found in nondiabetic patients with a complicated UTI. As in uncomplicated UTIs, *E. coli* causes the majority of infections. For example, one study reported *E. coli* to be the causative uropathogen in 47% of the UTIs in diabetic patients and in 68% of the UTIs in nondiabetic patients. Non-*E. coli* uropathogens found in patients with diabetes, include *Enterobacter* spp., *Klebsiella* spp., *Proteus* spp., Group B *Streptococci,* and *Enterococcus faecalis* [16].

Geerlings et al. [17] in their study reported that urine samples with glucose concentrations between 100 and 1000 mg/dL, which comes in the range of moderate to severe glucosuria, were responsible for enhanced bacterial growth after 6 h, compared with normal urine.

E. coli gain access to the urinary tract by the mechanism which reflects an exceptional ability to adapt to an environment very different from the gut. They need to alter their metabolism [18],

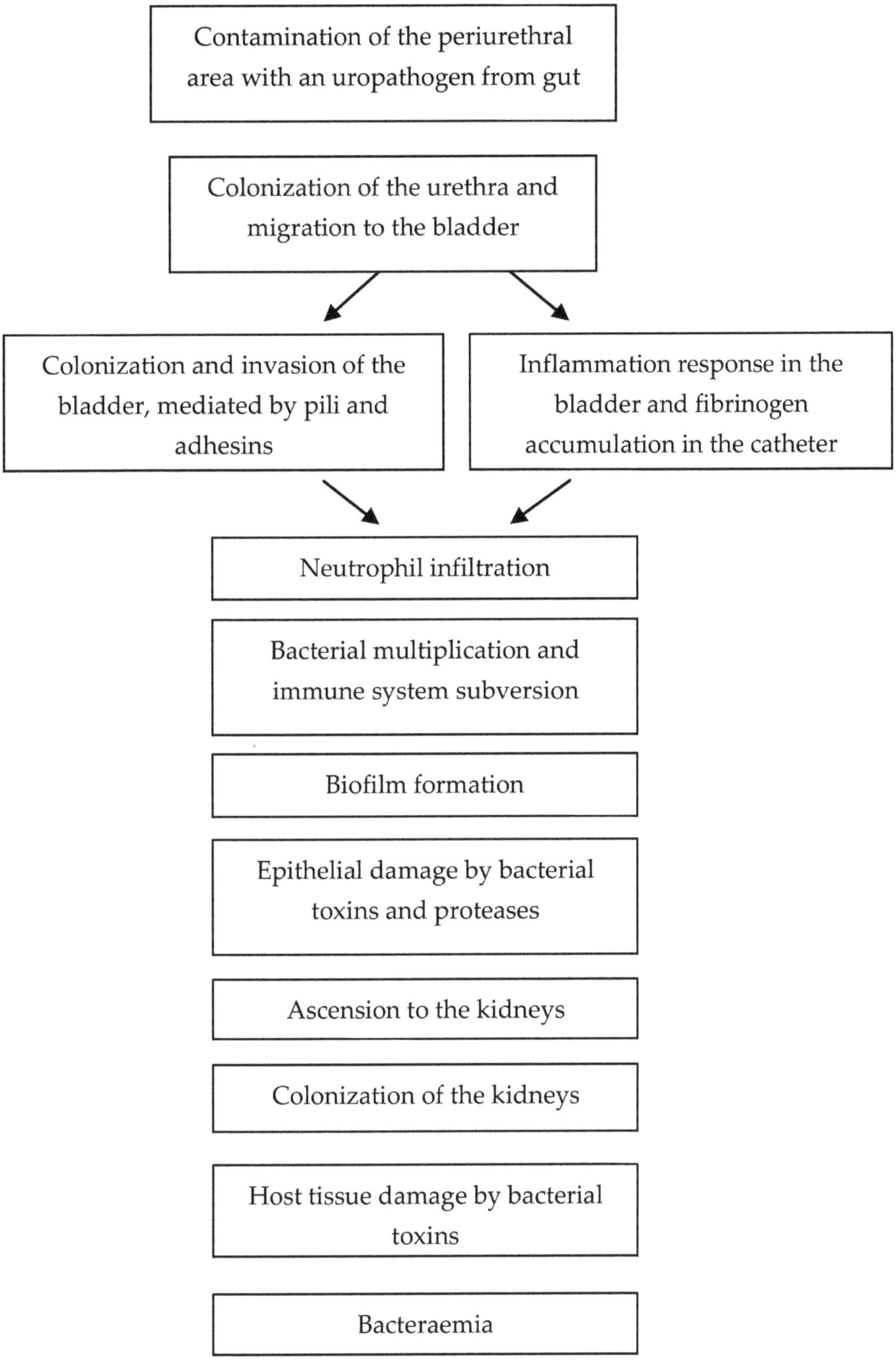

Figure 1. Process involved in pathogenesis of UTI in patients with diabetes.

ascend against the flow of urine, and adhere to the epithelial layer. *E. coli* that successfully invade the urinary tract harbor a specific factor that enables them to survive. These strains of *E. coli* are commonly named uropathogenic *E. coli* (UPEC). Flagellae are thread-like structures which provide *E. coli* with the ability to move. It has been found to bind to TLR5 [19] and is of importance for the immune response to *E. coli* in UTI in mice [20]. A critical step for UPEC is adhesion to avoid being washed out with the urine and the first step in a series of events leading to infection. The type-1 fimbriae are adhesion factors studied in great detail and are critical for adhesion and invasion of UPEC into bladder cells [21, 22]. They are equipped with a protein on the tip called FimH, which is responsible for the interaction with the host cell [23]. It binds to several structures on uroepithelial cells, the most important being uroplakin IA that coats the facet cells of the bladder [24]. They also bind to β-integrin, which triggers cytoskeleton rearrangement leading to bacterial internalization [25]. In renal epithelial cells, complement factor 3, which is secreted by epithelial cells during infection, can link with type 1 fimbriae to form a complex that interacts with CD46 to promote internalization. Other fimbriae like P fimbriae are connected with kidney infection, since they bind to glycosphingolipids on kidney epithelial cells [26].

Flagella provide the bacteria with mobility and may interact with the superficial bladder cell through TLR5. Further adhesion is provided by type 1 fimbriae binding to uroplakin 1A or β1-integrin, which also promote internalization into the cell. Complement secreted upon bacterial infection binds to the bacteria and promotes interaction with the bladder through CD46. In the kidney, P fimbriae of the bacteria bind to glycosphingolipids on the surface of renal epithelial cells. Bacterial invasion is further promoted by TLR4 and TLR5.

5.2. Increased adherence to uroepithelial cells

The uroepithelium is having a very important property of flexibility by which it will allow filling and emptying of the bladder and at the same time impermeable to fluid and able to cope with the varying pH, osmolality, and toxicity, for example, high ammonium concentration. It is composed of different layers of cells with the umbrella or facet cells lining the lumen are multinuclear, large cells with uroplakin facing the urine. Uroplakins are proteins contributing to the impermeability of the epithelium but can also act as a receptor for type 1 fimbriae on the uropathogenic *E. coli* [27].

The important step in the pathogenesis of UTIs is the adherence of uropathogens to the bladder mucosa. Therefore, adhesins (fimbriae) are important virulence factors. Although virulence factors have been distinguished best in *E. coli* (the most common uropathogen), many same principles may be applicable to other Gram-negative uropathogens, for example, Klebsiellae. Type 1 fimbriae mediate the adherence of glycoprotein receptors (uroplakins) on the uroepithelial cells to *E. coli*, whereas P fimbriae bind to glycolipid receptors in the kidney [25].

5.3. Immune dysfunction

It is observed that hyperglycemic environment alters immune function in patients with diabetes. Several aspects of immunity may be affected, including polymorphonuclear leukocyte function and adhesion, phagocytosis, and chemotaxis. This may play a part in the pathogenesis of urinary tract infections in patients with diabetes. Lower urinary concentrations of interleukin-8 and interleukin-6 in women suffering from diabetes have been shown to correlate with a lower urinary WBCs count that may contribute to the increased incidence of UTIs in this patient group [28].

If UPEC comes in contact with the epithelium, within minutes, the antimicrobial peptide cathelicidin is secreted and acts on the bacteria. Within hours, cytokines and chemokines are produced and their signaling will start to fix professional immune cells to the site of infection. The bacteria on the other hand will try to circumvent the immune defense in different ways. One is to enter the cell cytoplasm and form intracellular bacterial communities (IBCs) in order to "hide" from the immune response [29]; another is to down regulate the immune response with different modes of signaling. Depending on the number of bacteria, the host status, and the virulence factors they carry, the bacteria will either survive in the urinary tract or be eliminated and washed out with the urine [29].

If this first line of defense against pathogens entering the urinary tract fails, an inflammatory response is initiated. Attachment to the bladder uroepithelial cells by bacterial fimbriae allows for close contact between host and pathogen. Trans-membrane signaling through TLRs leads to the production of inflammatory mediators such as chemokines with subsequent recruitment of professional immune cells to the infectious focus. Chemokine IL-8 is required for neutrophil recruitment and activation in the urinary tract [30].

When the inflammatory response subsides, bacteria may still be left in the bladder epithelium. Bacteria that form IBCs can escape the different steps in host defense and treatment with antibiotics will be less efficient because of poor antibiotic penetration into the IBCs. From the IBC, bacteria can be expelled from the cells by a TLR4 mediated mechanism or in mature IBCs, and bacteria form filamentous structures and then separate from the cell to colonize adjacent cells. The cells may also be exfoliated, allowing the underlying immature cells to be exposed to further UPEC invasion. Here, they can turn into quiescent intracellular reservoirs (QIRs) for weeks, only to re-emerge to cause recurrent infections. Pyelonephritis may develop if the bacteria ascend further in the urinary tract. In the kidney, bacteria may cause damage of tissue and reach the blood circulation, causing septicemia, commonly called urosepsis. This increases the mortality from 0.3% in pyelonephritis to 7.5–30% in urosepsis [31].

6. Classification of urinary tract infection

UTIs are classified based on laboratory data, clinical symptoms, and microbiological findings. Practically, UTIs have been divided into uncomplicated and complicated UTIs and sepsis. The present guidelines give an outline of a tentative improved system of classification of UTI based on various factors as follows: (Guidelines on Urological Infections by European Association of Urology)

i. Classification based on grade of severity of infections and symptoms

ii. Classification based on underlying risk factors

iii. Classification based on anatomical level of infection

iv. Classification based on microbiological findings

v. Classification based on complications

7. Diagnosis of urinary tract infection in diabetics

Upper and lower UTI can be suspected in diabetic patients with most common symptoms. Symptoms vary in upper and lower UTI. **Table 1** highlights the symptomatic difference between upper and lower UTI.

Diagnosis of urinary tract infection can be done by following methods.

- **Examination of midstream urine specimen:** After the symptomatic identification, a midstream urine sample should be examined for the presence of WBCs, as pyuria is present in almost all cases of UTI.
- **Pyuria detection:** Pyuria can be detected either by microscopic examination (defined as >10 leukocytes/mm^3) or by dipstick leukocyte esterase test (sensitivity of 75–96% and specificity of 94–98%).
- **Colonization:** An absence of pyuria on microscopic assessment can suggest colonization, instead of infection, when there is bacteriuria [32].
- **Microscopic examination:** Allows for visualizing bacteria in urine.
- **Dipstick:** Tests for the presence of urinary nitrite.
  - **Positive test:** Indicates the presence of bacteria in urine.
  - **Negative test:** is the product of low count bacteriuria or bacterial species that lack the ability to reduce nitrate to nitrite (mostly Gram-positive bacteria).
- **Urine culture:** Should be done in all cases of suspected UTI in diabetic patients, prior to initiation of treatment (preferred method of obtaining a urine sample for culture is from voided, clean-catch, and midstream urine) [33].

7.1. Diagnosis of UTI in women patients

All women with recurrent UTI should undergo a physical examination to evaluate urogenital anatomy and vaginal tissues estrogenization. Postvoid residual urine volume also should

Lower UTI	Upper UTI
• Frequency • Urgency • Dysuria • Suprapubic pain	Costovertebral angle pain/tenderness fever and chills, with or without lower urinary tract symptoms

Table 1. Symptomatic difference between upper and lower UTI.

be measured. Diabetes screening is indicated in patients with other risk factors like family history and obesity. Most women do not need extensive urologic investigations. However, women who suffer infection with organisms which is not common causes of UTI, such as *Proteus, Klebsiella, Enterobacter,* and *Pseudomonas,* may have structural abnormalities or renal calculi. They would benefit from imaging studies of the upper urinary tract and cystoscopy. Women who have persistent hematuria after recovery of their infection also require a complete urologic workup. Although empirical therapy based on symptoms is generally accurate and cost-effective, women who are thought to be in the early stages of a problem with recurrent UTI should have documented cultures. Urine culture serves as the gold standard for diagnostic accuracy. The standard definition of a UTI on culture is >100,000 colony forming units per HPF. This value has excellent specificity but a sensitivity of only 50% [34].

8. Complications of urinary tract infection in diabetics

Emphysematous pyelonephritis (EPN) is a severe and necrotizing form of multifocal bacterial nephritis along with gas formation within parenchyma of the kidney. So far, more than 200 cases have been reported in literature. Underlying poorly controlled diabetes mellitus is present in up to 90% of affected patients [28].

The commonest offending organisms are Klebsiella and *Escherichia coli* followed by Proteus. The clinical manifestations are nonspecific and not different from the classic triad of upper UTI (i.e., fever, flank pain and pyuria); due to this, the diagnosis of EPN is often delayed. Disseminated intravascular coagulopathy, acute respiratory distress syndrome, disturbance of consciousness, acute renal failure, and shock can reveal some severe forms. Diabetic ketoacidosis is a very uncommon presentation, and only few cases have been reported so far.

EPN needs a radiological diagnosis. Conventional radiography may indicate gas bubbles overlying the renal fossa. Ultrasonography (US) characteristically shows an enlarged kidney that contains high amplitude echoes within the renal parenchyma. Computed tomography (CT) is the imaging procedure of choice, which confirms the presence and extent of parenchymal gas.

9. Pathogens of UTI in diabetes

A descriptive, cross sectional study was conducted on UTI and antibiotic sensitivity pattern among diabetic patients in National Academy of Medical Sciences (NAMS), Mahabouddha, Kathmandu, Nepal. According to this study, *E. coli* is the most common organism followed by *Klebsiella, Proteus,* and *Pseudomonas*. Most of the urinary isolates were sensitive to Ceftriaxone, Ciprofloxacin, and Cotrimoxazole, whereas resistance was high for ampicillin [35].

A study was conducted to find out the prevalence of UTI in diabetic patients. A total of 1470 diabetic patients (847 women and 623 men) were included in the study, admitted to the Diabetes Clinic of the Emergency Clinical County Hospital Timişoara between January and December 2012. According to this study, 10.7% in overall population had positive urine

Gram-negative microorganisms	Frequency (%)	Gram-positive microorganisms	Frequency (%)
Escherichia coli	56.75	Alpha *Streptococci*	33.33
Klebsiella pneumonia	21.62	*Staphylococcus aureus*	66.66
Pseudomonas aeruginosa	9.54	*S. epidermidis*	0
Enterobacter aerogenes	4.05	–	–
Proteus mirabilis	4.05	–	–
Citrobacter freundii	4.05	–	–

Table 2. Pathogens of UTI in diabetes.

cultures. In this population, almost 78% of patients were having asymptomatic bacteriuria. The most frequent bacteria involved in UTI are *Escherichia coli* (68.9%) [9].

About 10.5% of type 2 and 12.8% of type 1 diabetic patients had UTI. There is no significant difference between type 1 and type 2 diabetes ($p = 0.45$); 4.5% of men and 15.3% of women developed UTI, an extremely significant difference ($p < 0.0001$)

Chiţă et al. concluded that urinary tract infections are more prevalent in diabetic patients. Because of the high proportion of asymptomatic forms among diabetic patients, the urine culture should be done in all hospitalized patients with diabetes.

The pathogens involved in causing urinary tract infection in diabetic patients and their frequency are mentioned in **Table 2**.

10. Management of urinary tract infections in diabetics

Generally, treatment of UTI is similar in both diabetic patients and nondiabetic patients [5]; however, the choice of antibiotics in UTI patients with diabetes is one of the important considerations in the therapeutic management. Possible drug interactions between antimicrobials and antidiabetics or certain antibiotics may lead to impaired glucose homeostasis.

UTI treatment in diabetes patients depends on various factors including [5];

- Presence of symptoms
- Presence of infection in the bladder (lower UTI) or also involves the kidney (upper UTI)
- Presence of urologic abnormalities
- Severity of systemic symptoms
- Occur with metabolic alterations and renal function

Moreover, UTI treatment varies based on patient's age, sex, infecting agent, underlying disease, and whether there is lower or upper urinary tract involvement. Several clinical trials revealed that increasing trends of resistance to many antimicrobials with the increasing trend of antibiotic resistance in *E. coli*, with limited therapeutic options, the management of urinary tract infections is likely to become complicated.

10.1. Treatment recommendations for UTI in diabetes according to Infectious Diseases Society of America (IDSA)

10.1.1. Acute cystitis management in patients with type II diabetes

Acute cystitis treatment should be tailored according to culture results, if obtained. Apart from proper glucose control, one of the following UTI treatments is mandatory for acute cystitis management [36]. **First line treatment management**: Nitrofurantoin 100 mg three times daily for 5 days or fosfomycin trometamol 3 g single dose, or trimethoprim-sulfamethoxazole 960 mg twice daily for 3 days (can be used empirically only if resistance prevalence is known to be less than 20% and medication was not used in previous 3 months). **Second line management**: Quinolones and β-lactams.

10.1.2. Pyelonephritis management in patients with type II diabetes

Hospitalization should be done for the patients with severe symptoms for initial intravenous antibiotic therapy [5, 36]. Empiric antibiotics treatment: broad-spectrum cephalosporins, aminoglycosides, fluoroquinolones, piperacillin-tazobactam, or carbapenems should be started [37]. Severe sepsis presenting patients or those known to harbor-resistant uropathogens or the patients who have received multiple antibiotic courses should receive broad-spectrum coverage, guided by current urinary culture report. Treatment should be tailored when culture reports are available.

11. Antimicrobial agents

There are several types of antimicrobial agents such as antibiotics, antifungals, antivirals, antimalarials, and anthelmintics. Likewise, there are several types of microorganisms such as bacteria, fungi, viruses, and parasites. Microorganisms are responsible for various infectious diseases and sometimes leading to death. Antimicrobial agents play an essential role in decreasing morbidity and mortality associated with infections. Antimicrobial agents increased the life expectancy and quality of life. Different antimicrobial agents and their mechanism of action are mentioned in **Table 3**.

11.1. Benefits of antimicrobial agents

- Prevent and treat infection
- Increased the expected life spans of human being
- Prevent or treat infection after surgery (C section, organ transplants, joint replacements, etc.)
- Prevent or treat infection at the time of chemotherapy treatments
- Antimicrobial drugs decrease the morbidity and mortality caused by food-borne, water-borne, and other poverty-related infections

Antimicrobial agents	Effect on bacteria	Mechanism
Penicillins, cephalosporins, carbapenems, polypeptide antibiotics	Bactericidal	Inhibition of cell wall synthesis
Lincosamides, aminoglycosides, macrolides, tetracyclines, chloramphenicol	Bacteriostatic	Inhibition of protein synthesis
Quinolones, metronidazole	Bactericidal	Inhibits DNA synthesis
Rifamycins	Bactericidal	Inhibitions of RNA transcription
Sulfonamides	Bacteriostatic	Competitive inhibition

Table 3. Different antimicrobial agents and its mechanism of action.

12. Antimicrobial resistance

Resistance to antibiotics and other types of antimicrobial agents is growing and represents the single greatest challenge in the treatment of infectious diseases today. According to WHO, "AMR occurs when microorganisms change when they are exposed to antibiotic and antimicrobial drugs." Due to anti microbial resistance, antimicrobial agents turning ineffective and infections persist in the body, increasing the risk of spread to others. AMR affects the effective prevention, and treatment of infections caused by bacteria, parasites, viruses, and fungi. WHO says that AMR is a growing and alarming threat to global public health that requires lot of action from the government. Moreover, people should get a lot of awareness message regarding antimicrobial resistance. An antimicrobial resistance developing microorganisms are sometimes called as "superbugs" [38].

As per WHO cost analysis data, health care cost of resistant infections is higher than nonresistant infections because of

- Longer duration of illness
- Additional tests
- Use of more expensive drugs

Global WHO statistics says that a total of 480,000 people develop multidrug resistant TB each year, and drug resistance is starting complication in treatment of HIV and malaria as well.

12.1. Emergence of drug-resistant bacteria

Emergence of penicillinase-producing *Staphylococcus aureus* and emergence and spread of multidrug-resistant *S. aureus* in the early 1960s, emergence of MRSA in 1961, emergence of PISP in 1967, emergence of penicillinase-producing *H. influenzae* in 1974, emergence of PRSP in 1977, emergence of BLNAR *H. influenzae* in 1980, emergence of ESBL-producing

Gram-negative bacilli in 1983, emergence of VRE in 1986, increased infections with MRSA, PRSP, BLNAR, etc. and increase of resistant *gonococci* in 1990s, increase of MDRP, and increase of quinolone-resistant *E. coli* in 2000s are the emergence of drug resistance bacteria.

Major reasons for increasing antimicrobial resistance:

- Ineffective infection-control practices
- Noncompliance with infection-control practices
- Using sub-optimal dose of antibiotics for prophylaxis and treatment of infection
- Multiple comorbidities in hospitalized patients
- Prolonged hospitalization
- Increased number and duration of intensive care unit stays
- Colonized patients transfer from hospital to hospital
- Grouping of colonized patients in long-term-care facilities

Major mechanisms for acquired antimicrobial resistance:

- Enzyme that degrades the antimicrobial agent
- Enzyme that alters the antimicrobial agent
- Mutation in the antimicrobial agent's target which reduces the antimicrobial agent binding.
- Posttranslational or posttranscriptional modification of the antimicrobial agent's target, which reduces binding of the antimicrobial agent
- Reduced uptake of the antimicrobial agent
- Active efflux of the antimicrobial agent
- Antimicrobial agent target overproduction

13. Conclusion

Urinary tract infections are more common in the diabetic patients. Diabetic patients are severely affected with urinary tract infection. Treatment of UTI without proper diagnosis may lead to antimicrobial drug resistance. Treatment with antimicrobial agents should be started on the basis of culture reports. Only bacteriuria with symptoms of UTI should be treated with antibiotics to avoid the spread of drug resistant pathogens in the society. This practice can reduce the morbidity and mortality in diabetic patients suffering from urinary tract infection. The multidrug resistant pathogens are a challenge to society.

Author details

Ajay Kumar Prajapati

Address all correspondence to: ajay_prajapati2000@yahoo.co.in

Bharathiar University, Coimbatore, India

References

[1] Kofteridis DP, Papadimitraki E, Mantadakis E, et al. Effect of diabetes mellitus on the clinical and microbiological features of hospitalized elderly patients with acute pyelonephritis. Journal of the American Geriatrics Society. 2009;**57**(11):2125-2128

[2] American Diabetes Association. Diagnosis and classification of diabetes Mellitus. Diabetes Care. 2005;**28**(Suppl 1):537-542

[3] Bastaki S. Review diabetes mellitus and its treatment. International Journal of Diabetes and Metabolism. 2005;**13**:111-134

[4] Ocvirk S, Kistler M, Khan S, Talukder SH, Hauner H. Traditional medicinal plants used for the treatment of diabetes in rural and urban areas of Dhaka: An ethnobotanical survey. Journal of Ethnobiology and Ethnomedicine. 2013;**9**:43-50

[5] Fünfstück R, Nicolle LE, Hanefeld M, Naber KG. Urinary tract infection in patients with diabetes mellitus. Clinical Nephrology. 2012;**77**(1):40-48

[6] Wang MC, Tseng CC, Wu AB, et al. Bacterial characteristics and glycemic control in diabetic patients with *Escherichia coli* urinary tract infection. Journal of Microbiology, Immunology, and Infection. 2013;**46**(1):24-29

[7] Truzzi JC, Almeida FM, Nunes EC, Sadi MV. Residual urinary volume and urinary tract infection: When are they linked? The Journal of Urology. 2008;**180**(1):182-185

[8] Hosking DJ, Bennett T, Hampton JR. Diabetic autonomic neuropathy. Diabetes. 1978; **27**(10):1043-1055

[9] Chita T, Licker M, Sima A, Vlad A, Timar B, Sabo P, et al. Prevalence of urinary tract infections in diabetic patients. Romanian Journal of Diabetes Nutrition and Metabolic Diseases. 2013;**20**:99-105

[10] Saravanan M, Sudha R. Survey on urinary tract infection associated with diabetes mellitus. Journal of Academia and Industrial Research. 2014;**6**:258-262

[11] Sewify M, Nair S, Warsame S, Murad M, Alhubail A, Behbehani K, et al. Prevalence of urinary tract infection and antimicrobial susceptibility among diabetic patients with controlled and uncontrolled Glycemia in Kuwait. Journal Diabetes Research. 2016;**2016**:6573215

[12] Delamaire M, Maugendre D, Moreno M, Le Goff MC, Allannic H, Genetet B. Impaired leucocyte functions in diabetic patients. Diabetic Medicine. 1997;**14**(1):29-34

[13] Valerius NH, Eff C, Hansen NE, et al. Neutrophil and lymphocyte function in patients with diabetes mellitus. Acta Medica Scandinavica. 1982;**211**(6):463-467

[14] Geerlings SE, Brouwer EC, Van, Kessel KC, Gaastra W, Stolk RP, Hoepelman AI. Cytokine secretion is impaired in women with diabetes mellitus. European Journal of Clinical Investigation. 2000;**30**(11):995-1001

[15] Hoepelman AIM, Meiland R, Geerlings SE. Pathogenesis and management of bacterial urinary tract infections in adult patients with diabetes mellitus. International Journal of Antimicrobial Agents. 2003;**22**(Suppl 2):S35-S43

[16] Lye WC, Chan RKT, Lee EJC, et al. Urinary tract infections in patients with diabetes mellitus. The Journal of Infection. 1992;**24**:169-174

[17] Geerlings SE, Brouwer EC, Gaastra W, et al. Effect of glucose and pH on uropathogenic and nonuropathogenic *Escherichia coli*: Studies with urine from diabetic and nondiabetic individuals. Journal of Medical Microbiology. 1999;**48**(6):535-539

[18] Alteri CJ, Smith SN, Mobley HL. Fitness of *Escherichia coli* during urinary tract infection requires gluconeogenesis and the TCA cycle. PLoS Pathogens. 2009;**5**(5):e1000448

[19] Hayashi F, Smith KD, Ozinsky A, et al. The innate immune response to bacterial flagellin is mediated by Toll-like receptor 5. Nature. 2001;**410**(6832):1099-1103

[20] Andersen-Nissen E, Hawn TR, Smith KD, et al. Cutting edge: Tlr5$^{-/-}$ mice are more susceptible to *Escherichia coli* urinary tract infection. Journal of Immunology. 2007;**78**(8): 4717-4720

[21] Connell H, Agace W, Hedlund M, et al. Fimbriae-mediated adherence induces mucosal inflammation and bacterial clearance. Consequences for anti-adhesion therapy. Advances in Experimental Medicine and Biology. 1996;**408**:73-80

[22] Mulvey MA, Lopez-Boado YS, Wilson CL, et al. Induction and evasion of host defenses by type 1-piliated uropathogenic *Escherichia coli*. Science. 1998;**282**(5393):1494-1497

[23] Jones CH, Pinkner JS, Roth R, et al. FimH adhesin of type 1 pili is assembled into a fibrillar tip structure in the Enterobacteriaceae. Proceedings of the National Academy of Sciences of the United States of America. 1995;**92**(6):2081-2085

[24] Zhou G, Mo WJ, Sebbel P, et al. Uroplakin Ia is the urothelial receptor for uropathogenic *Escherichia coli*: Evidence from in vitro FimH binding. Journal of Cell Science. 2001;**114**(22):4095-4103

[25] Eto DS, Jones TA, Sundsbak JL, et al. Integrin-mediated host cell invasion by type 1-piliated uropathogenic *Escherichia coli*. PLoS Pathogens. 2007;**3**(7):e100

[26] Springall T, Sheerin NS, Abe K, et al. Epithelial secretion of C3 promotes colonization of the upper urinary tract by *Escherichia coli*. Nature Medicine. 2001;**7**(7):801-806

[27] Wu XR, Sun TT, Medina JJ. In vitro binding of type 1-fimbriated *Escherichia coli* to uroplakins Ia and Ib: Relation to urinary tract infections. Proceedings of the National Academy of Sciences of the United States of America. 1996;**93**(18):9630-9635

[28] Patterson JE, Andriole VT. Bacterial urinary tract infections in diabetes. Infectious Disease Clinics of North America. 1995;**9**(1):25-51

[29] Hunstad DA, Justice SS. Intracellular lifestyles and immune evasion strategies of uropathogenic *Escherichia coli*. Annual Review of Microbiology. 2010;**64**:203-221

[30] Agace WW, Hedges SR, Ceska M, et al. Interleukin-8 and the neutrophil response to mucosal gram-negative infection. The Journal of Clinical Investigation. 1993;**92**(2):780-785

[31] Mysorekar IU, Hultgren SJ. Mechanisms of uropathogenic *Escherichia coli* persistence and eradication from the urinary tract. Proceedings of the National Academy of Sciences of the United States of America. 2006;**103**(38):14170-14175

[32] Little P, Turner S, Rumsby K, et al. Dipsticks and diagnostic algorithms in urinary tract infection: development and validation, randomised trial, economic analysis, observational cohort and qualitative study. Health Technology Assessment. 2009;**13**(19):iii-iv. ix–xi, 1-73

[33] Bennett JE, Doli R, Blaser, Mandell MJ. Douglas, and Bennetts Principles and Practice of Infectious Diseases. 8th ed. Elsevier Inc; 2015

[34] Guido et al. The diagnosis of urinary tract infection: A systematic review. Deutsches Ärzteblatt International. 2010;**107**(21):361-367

[35] Simkhada R. Urinary tract infection and antibiotic sensitivity pattern among diabetics. Nepal Medical College Journal. 2013;**15**(1):1-4

[36] Gupta K, Hooton TM, Naber KG, et al. Infectious Diseases Society of America; European Society for Microbiology and Infectious Diseases International clinical practice guidelines for the treatment of acute uncomplicated cystitis and pyelonephritis in women: A 2010 update by the Infectious Diseases Society of America and the European Society for Microbiology and Infectious Diseases. Clinical Infectious Diseases. 2011;**52**(5):e103-e120

[37] Nicolle LE. Uncomplicated urinary tract infection in adults including uncomplicated pyelonephritis. The Urologic Clinics of North America. 2008;**35**(1):1-12

[38] Antibiotic Resistance Questions & Answers. Get Smart: Know When Antibiotics Work. Centers for Disease Control and Prevention, USA. June 30, 2009. Retrieved March 20, 2013

2

Virulence Factors and Innovative Strategies for the Treatment and Control of Uropathogenic *Escherichia coli*

Barbara Kot

Abstract

Urinary tract infections (UTIs) are considered to be the most frequent bacterial infections. *Escherichia coli* is the major factor of community-acquired UTI (80–90%) and a large part of nosocomial UTI (30%), including cystitis, pyelonephritis, prostatitis, and asymptomatic bacteriuria. Uropathogenic *E. coli* (UPEC) shows a variety of virulence factors that allow their transition from the intestinal tract to the urinary tract and causing infection. The virulence factors responsible for pathogenesis outside the gastrointestinal tract belong to various functional groups. Antimicrobial resistance among *E. coli* causing UTIs is increasing in many countries around the world. This paper presents key virulence factors of UPEC such as adhesins, toxins, iron acquisition systems, and biofilm formation by UPEC, which are major problems in patients with long-term catheterization. The resistance of UPEC to antibiotics and innovative strategies of treatment and control of UPEC including drug therapy, preventive vaccines, probiotics, cranberry as source of antimicrobial metabolites, bacteriophages, new therapeutic antibiofilm treatment such as engineered phages, nanoparticles, and plant-derived antibacterial agents are also presented.

Keywords: UPEC, UTI, virulence factors, biofilm, antimicrobial resistance, treatment of UPEC, prevention

1. Introduction

Urinary tract infections (UTIs) are considered the most frequent bacterial infections in humans usually caused by *Enterobacteriaceae*. Among them, *Escherichia coli* is a predominant etiological factor of UTI [1]. The pathogenic *E. coli* strains belong to different pathotypes including enteric *E. coli* and extraintestinal *E. coli* (ExPEC). Seven major pathotypes of enteric *E. coli* cause mainly gastroenteritis but sometimes are responsible for diseases outside the intestinal tract [2]. Three pathotypes of the ExPEC are able to exist in the gut but do not cause diseases in this place. Whereas, colonization by the ExPEC strains of other host niches including the central nervous system, blood, and the urinary tract leads to illness in human [3]. Among ExPEC, uropathogenic *E. coli* (UPEC) is the most frequently associated with human diseases. UPEC strains cause 80–90% of community-acquired UTIs and more than 30% of hospital-acquired UTIs [4]. Development of UTIs depends on anatomical factors of host, defense mechanisms, and virulence factors of infecting microorganism. Bacterial infections of the urinary tract are important problem, because about 60% of women in the United States will have at least one UTI during their life. About 8 million physician visits per year are related to these often chronic infections, making UTIs a problem of economic and medical significance [5]. UPEC can colonize the bladder and cause cystitis or may ascend into the kidneys, causing pyelonephritis [3]. *E. coli* may also spread from the urinary tract to the bloodstream causing bacteremia in above 30% of cases and the potential sepsis [6]. The presence of high numbers of *E. coli* in the urine without the clinical symptoms is referred as asymptomatic bacteriuria (ABU) and such infection in healthy, nonpregnant women is generally not treated [7]. Infections of the urinary tract occur when *E. coli* enter through the urethra and effectively colonize the bladder. *E. coli* is the most common pathogen causing cystitis, pyelonephritis with the possibility of causing kidney damage and death. This microorganism can induce acute renal failure and in case of complications after renal transplantation, *E. coli* is the most common clinical isolate [8]. It is considered that human intestinal tract is a primary reservoir of UPEC strains, although in some cases, clonal group of UPEC strains can be transmitted by contaminated food [9]. Host inflammatory responses on the breach of the sterile urinary tract by UPEC consist of the production of cytokines and chemokines, neutrophil influx, the exfoliation of infected bladder epithelial cells, and the generation of reactive nitrogen and oxygen species [5]. Genomic differences among UPEC and other *E. coli* show evolutionary adaptations, which enable UPEC to colonize environmental niches within the urinary tract such as epithelia lining the lumenal walls of the urethra, bladder, renal pelvis, and collecting ducts of the kidneys [10].

UPEC strains have different virulence factors that enable the bacteria to adhere and colonize the uroepithelial cells and to establish the UTIs. UPEC harbor more genes encoding adhesins, iron acquisition systems, and toxins than K12 strains and commensal *E. coli* isolates. These virulence genes are often encoded on mobile genetic elements called pathogenicity islands [11, 12].

This paper describes key virulence factors of UPEC, the role of biofilm formation by UPEC in development of UTIs and in catheter-associated UTIs. The resistance to antibiotics and new therapeutic approaches of treatment and control of UPEC will be also discussed.

2. Virulence factors of UPEC

2.1. Adhesins

Adhesive proteins as the most important determinants of pathogenicity of UPEC strains are arguable [13], but based on many observations of ABU strains, it was found that these strains are nonadherent and nonhemolytic [14]. UPEC adhesins activate host signaling pathways that promote bacterial invasion [15]. Bacterial adherence to urothelium is important in the development of UTI because it allows the bacteria to persist in the urinary tract against flushing by urine flow. Function of type 1 fimbriae as virulence factors in human pathology remains unclear because they are expressed in both commensal and pathogenic *E. coli* strains [16, 17]. The type 1 fimbriae are heteropolymeric surface organelles that consist of several subunits. These fimbriae bind *E. coli* cells to the urothelial mannosylated glycoproteins uroplakin by subunit FimH, which is located at the distal tip of the type 1 fimbriae. UPEC commonly expresses FimH that efficiently bind monomannose- and trimannose-containing glycoprotein receptors. Whereas, commensal *E. coli* strains usually bind to trimannose residues [18]. Binding of FimH to uroplakins that are expressed in the differentiated urothelium of the bladder and urethers causes adhesion and cellular invasion of *E. coli* and promotes formation of intracellular bacterial communities which leads to the acute stage of infection [19, 20]. FimH adhesin enables UPEC to escape before the immune response by internalization within urothelial cells. Inside infected urothelial cells, *E. coli* is harbored within vesicles [21, 22]. Blocking of FimH adhesin with antibodies or inactivity of the *fimH* gene has a negative effect on the ability of UPEC to colonize the bladder epithelium [5]. *fimH* gene is the most commonly identified virulence gene in the isolates causing UTI [17].

About 80% of UPECs express P fimbriae that are frequently associated with acute pyelonephritis [23]. P fimbriae are encoded by *pap*A-K gene operon which can be localized on one or more pathogenic-associated islands [24]. The P-fimbrial–tip adhesins (PapG adhesins) bind to Gal α (1–4) Gal in glycosphingolipids of the membrane of urothelial cells localized in the kidney. The PapG adhesins are encoded by four classes of *papG* genes but only two of them are associated with uropathogenicity. Class II adhesin genes are predominant among the isolates from pyelonephritis and from renal transplant patients, while class III genes are found more frequently among cystitis isolates [25–27]. Attachment of P fimbriae to receptors leads to activation of the immune cell response and to the development of inflammation- and pain-associated with UTIs. P fimbriae improve bacterial colonization of the tubular epithelium that can adversely affect renal filtration leading to total obstruction of the nephron and consequently contributes to the full pathophysiology of pyelonephritis [14].

S fimbriae of *E. coli* bind to sialyl galactosides occurring in the receptors of erythrocytes and renal tubular epithelium cells, and are also involved in UTIs development. S fimbriae show binding to epithelial cells of lower urinary tract and kidney and may facilitate bacterial dissemination within host tissues [15, 28].

E. coli strains harboring operons coding fimbrial Dr and afimbrial Afa adhesins are also associated with UTIs. Dr adhesins bind to decay-accelerating factor (DAF) which is widely distributed along the urinary tract and plays an important role in colonization of urinary tract by Dr adhesin-producing *E. coli* [29]. UPECs with Afa adhesins have a tropism to renal tissue and have the ability to induce chronic or recurrent infection [30]. The research recently conducted by Muenzner et al. [31] showed that uropathogenic *E. coli* strains, which express the Dra/AfaE adhesins, bind to CEACAMs (carcinoembryonic antigen-related cell adhesin molecules) present on epithelial cells. The interaction of CEACAMs with Dra/AfaE adhesins causes increase of integrin activity, promote matrix adhesion, and suppress epithelial exfoliation, which promotes host infection.

Curli are highly adhesive extracellular amyloid fibers produced by UPEC and other *Enterobacteriaceae* [32]. The major subunit of curli is the CsgA [33]. Curli promote adherence to epithelial cells and resistance against the human antimicrobial peptide LL-37, and also cause induction of the proinflammatory cytokine IL-8. They exhibit exclusive role in promoting UPEC biofilms and represent one of the major biofilm components [34]. Curli are produced at limitation of nutrients and salts, at reduced oxygen tension and at temperature below 30°C. However, it is believed that many pathogenic bacteria and commensal strains can also express curli at 37°C during infection in humans [35]. Curli fimbriae interact with serum proteins and this might promote bacterial dissemination in host. UPEC strains-producing curli are more likely to cause urosepticaemia than strains which do not produce curli [36].

2.2. Toxins

Production of toxins by UPEC is an important virulence factor because they may induce an inflammatory response and lead to symptoms of urinary tract infections. The most important virulence factor of UPEC is α-hemolysin (HlyA). This toxin is strongly proinflammatory and leads to secretion of IL-6, IL-8, and chemotaxins that increase clinical severity in UTI patients [27, 37]. HlyA belongs to the family of RTX (repeats in toxin) [38]. HlyA is a lipoprotein of 110 kDa that forms pores in host cells, leading at high concentrations of HlyA to cell lysis, that enable UPEC to defeat mucosal barriers, damage effector immune cells, and gain access to nutrients and iron [39]. At sublytic concentrations, HlyA implicates the inhibition of chemotaxis and bacterial killing by phagocytes and induces apoptosis of neutrophils and renal cells, and also promotes the exfoliation of bladder epithelial cells [40]. Hilbert et al. [41] found that cytotoxicity, cytokine suppression, and HlyA production were tightly linked in clinical strains, and that *E. coli* utilizes HlyA to inhibit epithelial cytokine production *in vitro*. HlyA is responsible for about 50% of UTIs cases which leads to renal complications [27].

Cytotoxic necrotizing factor 1 (CNF1) is produced by approximately one third of UPEC [14]. The toxicity of this protein is linked with its ability to constitutive activation of the Rho GTPases that affect numerous cellular functions such as the formation of actin stress fibers and membrane ruffle formation. The result is the entry of *E. coli* into urothelial cells [42]. CNF1 promote apoptosis of bladder epithelial cells, probably stimulating their exfoliation and increasing bacterial entry to underlying tissue [43]. Besides, CNF1 inhibits activities of neutrophils, reducing phagocytosis and antimicrobial activity [44].

Secreted autotransporter toxin (Sat) is referred to as serine protease autotransporter and is associated with pyelonephritic *E. coli* strains. Sat is considered a virulence factor because it has toxic activity against cell lines of bladder or kidney origin. Sat induces elongation of cells and loosening of cellular junctions in cell lines of kidney. Furthermore, Sat triggers vacuolation within the cytoplasm of both human bladder and kidney cell lines [45]. Another secreted toxin called Vat (vacuolating autotransporter toxin), often expressed by UPEC strains, shows the ability to induce a variety of cytopathic effects in target host cells, including swelling and vacuolation. However, the role of Vat in UTI pathogenesis has not been thoroughly studied [46].

2.3. Iron acquisition systems

Limiting iron availability in the urinary tract is an important host defense against bacterial pathogens. For growth and metabolic activity, bacteria require a cytoplasmic iron concentration of about 10^{-6} M, while free iron concentrations in the mammalian host are extremely low (10^{-25} M in the blood and lower at other sites of organism) [47]. Consequently, pathogenic bacteria have to be equipped with systems for acquisition of iron from the host. Bacteria produce siderophores, low-molecular-weight molecules that bind and transport iron (Fe^{3+}) through the bacterial membrane into cytosol where the iron is released. Iron bound siderophores are transported through (with) specific receptors at the outer membrane that facilitate carrying of siderophore-iron complexes through the bacterial membrane. Common siderophore system is enterobactin and its receptor FebA, which is expressed by both pathogenic and K12 *E. coli* strains, although in the context of infection and also other siderophore systems (salmochelin and IroN, aerobactin and IutA, and yersiniabactin and FyuA) have been observed in UPEC [3]. The occurrence of these systems in UPEC strains difficult to identify certain systems as virulence factors of UPEC [48].

3. Biofilm formation by UPEC

Currently biofilm is defined as a structured bacterial community embedded in a self-produced matrix and attached to an abiotic or living surface [49].

The biofilm matrix is composed with exopolysaccharides, which form a hydrated viscous layer and protects enclosed bacterial cells against dehydration, toxic molecules such as antibiotics, and from immune system of host [50]. Bacteria within the biofilm differ in gene expression resulting in a phenotype different from the planktonic bacteria. The slow growth of pathogens in biofilms is the major factor conferring resistance to antibiotics [51]. The ability of bacteria to form biofilm is associated with pathogenesis of numerous diseases. Biofilm formation results in chronic, persistent infections that are difficult to eradicate with antimicrobial treatment. It is believed that biofilms occur in up to 60% of human infections [52]. UPEC can persist within the bladder tissue in underlying epithelial cells or create biofilm-like pods in the recurrent cystitis [53]. Biofilm of *E. coli* may form on the urothelium and is involved in infections associated with biomaterials such as catheters or prostheses. UPEC strains are frequently isolated from biofilms formed in the lumen of catheters and showing resistance to antibiotic treatment [54]. Catheter-associated urinary tract infection (CAUTI) is the most common nosocomial infection, and approximately 80% of UTIs acquired in the hospital are associated with catheterization [55]. The insertion of indwelling catheter into the bladder increases the susceptibility of patients to UTIs, because these devices are the initiation site of infection by introducing opportunistic organisms into the urinary tract [56]. UPEC strains are capable of colonizing the intestinal and vaginal tracts, and these sites are potential reservoirs of microorganisms for UTIs and CAUTIs [57]. The urinary catheter connects the colonized perineum with the sterile bladder providing a route for bacterial entry along the catheter lumen or the external surface of the catheter [58]. CAUTI is related to the susceptibility of catheter material to microbial colonization. The initial stage of biofilm formation on a urinary catheter includes deposition of conditioning film of host urinary components, such as proteins, electrolytes, and other organic molecules [59]. These molecules on the surface of the urinary catheter may change its surface and neutralize any antiadhesive properties [60]. Planktonic bacteria are attached to the surface of the urinary catheter through hydrophobic and electrostatic interaction [61]. Development of biofilm on surface of the catheter occurs through the division of binding bacterial cells, appending additional planktonic bacteria and secretion of extracellular matrix. Detachment of single cell or group of bacterial cells from the biofilm may result in the passage of pathogens into the urine [51]. For this reason, biofilm formation on the urinary catheters is critical for initiating and maintaining of CAUTIs and is a reservoir of resistant pathogenic bacteria [62]. Several factors contribute to the formation of biofilm by *E. coli*, e.g. fimbriae, curli, and flagella. Type 1 fimbriae involved in biofilm formation may also support the colonization of urinary catheter surface [15]. The risk of CAUTI depends on the duration of catheterization, the quality of catheter care, and host susceptibility. Prolonged catheterization is the most important risk factor associated with CAUTI [62]. Long-term urinary catheter use (more than 30 days) causes permanent bacterial colonization of the urine in 100% cases [63]. Examination of people in a nursing home showed that long-term catheterization was significantly related with bacteriuria, pyelonephritis, and renal inflammation [58]. Forming of biofilm on the urinary catheters is a public health problem for patients who need these medical devices. It is recommended that patients who are chronically catheterized were treated with 5–10 days of targeted antibiotic therapy [64].

4. Antimicrobial resistance of UPEC

Antimicrobial resistance in UPEC is a clinical problem in patients with UTIs, in particular in women with recurrent UTI. The empirical antimicrobial treatment in case of recurrent UTIs exerts significant resistance pressure on the uropathogens and the fecal flora, which serves as resistance reservoirs for potential uropathogens [65–67]. Antimicrobial resistance among *E. coli* causing UTI is increasing in many countries around the world and shows considerable variations during different time periods and in different areas [68, 69].

The level of resistance of UPEC strains from hospitalized patients in Poland and Turkey to ampicillin was 56% [70, 71], while above 85% of UPEC strains from patients in India were resistant to this antibiotic [68]. High percentage (67.3%) of *E. coli* strains resistant to tetracycline was isolated from people with UTI from different parts of India [68].

Sanchez et al. [72] suggested that the increase of resistance of UPEC to ciprofloxacin is a result of widespread use of this antibiotic in the treatment of uncomplicated UTIs in the early 2000s. The most recent published data suggested that the level of resistance to trimethoprim-sulfamethoxazole increased and in different countries was over 21–24.2% [71–73]. This trend has continued for decades and the increasing resistance of *E. coli* to trimethoprim-sulfamethoxazole can be explained by frequent use of this antimicrobial agent because it is recommended as the second-line drug in treating acute uncomplicated cystitis in women. Authors reported low resistance of *E. coli* to nitrofurantoin (0.85–1.6%) and no increase in resistance in the last decade was observed [71, 72].

The extended spectrum of β-lactamases (ESBLs) produced by *Enterobacteriaceae* is responsible for resistance of amino and ureido penicillin, oxyimino cephalosporin, and monobactams, but not to 7-α-substituted β-lactam [74]. The production of ESBLs by UPEC strains complicates treatment because these strains are resistant not only to β-lactam antibiotics but often are also resistant to other classes of antibiotics-like aminoglycosides, quinolones, and cotrimoxazole, such as gentamicin, ciprofloxacin, and trimethoprim-sulfamethoxazole, respectively [75–77]. This reduces the treatment options to a limited number of antibiotics and empirical therapy with cephalosporins and fluoroquinolones often fail in patients with UTI [78]. Hoban et al. [79] found that these resistant microorganisms are more susceptible to the carbapenems, imipenem, and ertapenem, than to other antibiotics. ESBL-producing microorganisms were primarily considered multiresistant organisms originating in hospitals, but in recent years, the number of ESBL producers increased also among outpatients, especially related with UTIs. The authors reported 21 and 21.4% ESBL-producing *E. coli* found in community-acquired UTIs in Turkey [80] and in North India [81], respectively, while in Mexico, 31% of uropathogenic *E. coli* isolated from hospitalized patients [77] and 17.6% *E. coli* from hospitalized European UTI patients [79] were producers of ESBLs. UTIs complicated by ESBL producers tend to lead to uncertain outcomes and prolong hospitalization, especially that these organisms tend to be multidrug resistant [74]. Among ESBLs, the CTX-M enzymes are the most prevalent among isolates of UPE from inpatients and outpatients leading to serious problems for the antimicrobial management of these infections [82, 83]. There is a need for new therapy of UTI caused by multiresistant ESBL-producing UPEC.

5. Treatment and control of UPEC

Currently, the antibiotic therapy is an important part of the therapeutic strategy for UTI. The increased antibiotic resistance in recent years suggests that the choice of antibiotic should be guided by the results of sensitivity assay, although in cases of community-acquired UTI, an empirical therapy is often used [23]. The drugs of first-line choice for empirical treatment of uncomplicated UTI in all European countries are fosfomycin trometamol, pivmecillinam, or nitrofurantoin macrocrystals [84]. Trimethoprim-sulfamethoxazole is also used in countries where resistance to this chemotherapeutic is low. Higher rates of side effects in comparison with other drugs limit the use of quinolones as second-line therapy. Moreover, in many countries in Europe, high resistance rates of *E. coli* strains to nalidixic acid were observed [85], and thus aminoglycosides and carbapenem are the drugs of choice. In patients with recurrent infections of the urinary tract, the antibiotics may be recommended prophylactically. It is believed that two recurrences of UTI within 6 months after therapy or three episodes per year could be considered an indication to establish prophylaxis after treatment. The drugs for this purpose are nitrofurantoin, trimethoprin-sulfamethoxazole, fosfomycin trometamol, and cotrimoxazole at lower doses than therapeutic [86]. However, repeated antibiotic treatment of UTI and prophylactic use of antibiotics frequently results in a rise in resistance to antibiotics and adversely affects microbiota of patients which may lead to secondary infections posttreatment, such as gastrointestinal infection and vaginal yeast infection [87, 88].

For this reason, alternative or additional prophylactic strategies have been investigated. One of them is improving the management of UTI by the development of preventive vaccines. Effective vaccine for UTI will need to generate a strong mucosal immune response in the urinary tract. Designing a UTI vaccine that would be effective against UPEC is difficult due to heterogeneous nature of the UPEC population. UTI vaccine should be designed based on more than one antigen because not all strains express the exact set of virulence genes during infections. A vaccine based on the multiple virulence factors, such as fimbrial adhesins or iron receptors, could be clinically effective against UTI [89]. The vaccine with whole or lysed fractions of inactivated bacteria can be effective to generate protective immunity. Urovac® is one of such vaccines (Solco Basel AG, Birsfelden, Switzerland, and Protein Express, Cincinnati, OH, USA) containing ten heat-killed uropathogens, including six UPEC strains. The UPEC strains in the Urovac® show different virulence factors, such as hemolysin, type 1, P, and S fimbrial adhesins, CNF-1, siderophores, and the *E. coli* CFT073 pathogenicity island marker and many different O and H antigens. Evaluating the efficacy of vaginally administrated Urovac® found that the immunization did not ensure significant long-term protection from UTI or an increase in mean levels of UPEC antibodies in serum, vagina, or urine [90]. However, among the women receiving Urovac, 72% were free from UTIs, while only 30% of women given placebo remained free from UTIs caused by *E. coli*. Moreover, in the Urovac vaccinated group, the number of *E. coli* caused UTIs was significantly lower compared to the control group [91]. Another vaccine which is used in Switzerland since 1988 and sold in other countries worldwide is OM-89/Uro-Vaxom® (OM Pharma, Myerlin, Switzerland). Uro-Vaxom is an oral capsule containing a lyophilized mix of membrane proteins from 18 UPEC strains. The clinical studies showed that Uro-Vaxom was significantly more effective than placebo in preventing recurrent UTI [92].

Other prophylaxis method is use of different *Lactobacillus* species in the form of probiotics which reduced the risk of UTI and vaginal infections. Use of *Lactobacillus* species maintains low pH and produces hydrogen peroxide that inhibits growth of *E. coli* in urinary tract but also activates Toll-like receptor-2 and therefore leads to reduced inflammatory reaction [93]. Beerepoot et al. [94] conducted study in which postmenopausal women with recurrent UTI prophylactically received trimethoprim-sulfamethoxazole or oral capsules containing *L. rhamnosus* GR-1 and *L. reuteri* RC-14. After 12 months of treatment, the reduction in recurrence was more than 50% in both groups. However, in group that received trimethoprim-sulfamethoxazole, the two-fold increase in resistance was observed.

Research on dietary supplementation showed that cranberry juice and its extracts reduced UTI recurrences. The active metabolite of cranberry, proanthocyanidin A prevents bacterial adhesion to the urothelial layer by inhibiting P fimbriae expression [95]. The minimum daily dose of proanthocyanidin A, which is able to reduce significantly the number of urinary *E. coli* to be 36 mg [96]. The study conducted by Wojnicz et al. [97] showed that cranberry extract Żuravit S.O.S.® reduced motility and adhesion to epithelial cells in *E. coli* strains isolated from urine of patients with pyelonephritis and also limited the ability of these strains to form biofilm.

Bacteriophages are highly specific and very effective in lysing bacteria. The use of lytic phages that are able to pass through the extracellular matrix against *E. coli* biofilm causes a reduction of bacteria number in biofilm and also prevents biofilm formation on catheter coated with hydrogel containing bacteriophages [98, 99]. Biofilm-associated UTIs are difficult to treat due to the high level of antimicrobial resistance showed by biofilm structures. Many authors recommend macrolides (erythromycin, clarithromycin, and azithromycin) as the treatment of choice in biofilm-associated infections because these antibiotics inhibit the production of primary component of the matrix, alginate [100, 101]. Ciprofloxacin, norfloxacin, gentamicin, or nitrofurazone are often used as components in coating and impregnating the catheters in the aim to inhibit bacterial attachment and development of biofilm [55, 102]. New therapeutic antibiofilm treatments are studied as alternative to antibiotics in order to inhibit biofilm formation and also to avoid the emergence of resistant bacterial populations. The silver showed antimicrobial activity by interacting with bacterial cell membrane and is used to coat catheters. The study showed a statistically significantly lower frequency of bacterial infection in patients treated with a silver alloy-coated catheter compared to those treated with uncoated catheter. Schaeffer et al. [103] reported that bacteriuria was present in 27% of patients with the silver-coated silicone catheter and in 55% of group with uncoated silicone catheter. It was also demonstrated that silver alloy used in hydrogel-coated urinary catheter reduced of up 45% of CAUTI [104]. However, the study conducted by Desai et al. [105] showed that *E. coli* adherence was not significantly lower on silver-impregnated silicone or latex catheters compared to adherence of *E. coli* on catheters without silver.

The new antibiofilm strategy is phage therapy using engineered bacteriophages that have biofilm-degrading enzymatic activity. It was demonstrated that engineered phages that express biofilm-degrading enzymes are more efficient in removing bacterial biofilms than nonenzymatic phage alone. Lu and Collins [106] generated bacteriophage which expressed biofilm-degrading enzyme (DspB) during infection. The DspB showed simultaneous action against both bacterial cells in the biofilm and the biofilm matrix. The engineered enzymatic phage reduced bacterial biofilm cell in 99.9%. One of the new ways of eliminating biofilm is the use of nanoparticles. Water-based synthesis of yttrium fluoride (YF_3) nanoparticles that showed antibacterial properties against *E. coli* was described. The minimal inhibitory concentration was observed at 0.01 mg/mL. In addition, YF3 nanoparticles-coated catheters were able to significantly reduce bacterial colonization compared to the uncoated surface, which provides the potential to develop the concept of utilizing yttrium fluoride nanoparticles as novel antimicrobial and antibiofilm agents [107].

The alternative strategies to decrease UPEC infection include the use of plant-derived antibacterial agents containing different functional groups in their structure and development of resistance in bacteria to these antimicrobials is less frequent [108]. Borges et al. [109] showed that phenolic acids such as gallic and ferulic acid have prevented biofilm formation and show potential to reduce the mass of biofilms formed by the Gram-negative bacteria including *E. coli*. The antibiofilm effect of trans-cinnamaldehyde (TC) on UPEC was reported by Amalaradjou et al. [110]. These authors showed that TC was effective against UPEC biofilm on polystyrene or latex, and the expression of *E. coli* genes encoding attachment and invasion of bladder cells was significantly decreased by TC [111]. Phytochemicals as alternative antimicrobials in preventing and inactivating *E. coli* biofilm on urinary catheters were also assessed. It was demonstrated that TC at the concentration of 0.5% was highly effective for preventing *E. coli* biofilm formation in the lumen of urinary catheter and after 1 day of completely inhibited biofilm formation. Whereas, completely inactivated biofilm after 1 day was observed at 1.25%

and 1.5% TC solution. *p*-Coumaric and ferulic acids have preventive action on *E. coli* biofilm formation on urinary catheter but complete inactivation of the biofilm formed at presence of these phytochemicals was not observed [112]. Recently showed that two alkaloids, piperine from black pepper and reserpine from Indian snakeroot, decreased swarming and swimming motilities of the uropathogenic *E. coli* CFT073. Additionally, piperine increased penetration of ciprofloxacin and azithromycin in to biofilm of *E. coli* CFT073. Authors suggest that these substances can affect on bacterial colonization by inhibition bacterial motility and also may help in treatment of infection by strengthening the penetration of antibiotic in biofilms [113].

One of the other strategies to prevent colonization, invasion, and biofilm formation by UPEC is inhibition of the assembly of pili by family of bicyclic 2-pyridones, termed pilicides.

The activity of pilicides was evaluated in two different pilus biogenesis systems in UPEC. Hemagglutination mediated by either type 1 or P pili, adherence to bladder cells, and biofilm formation mediated by type 1 pili were all reduced by 90% in laboratory and clinical *E. coli* strains [114]. Pilicide ec240 was found to disrupt type 1 pili, P pili, S pili, and flagellar motility [115]. Other pilicides also inhibit the production of Dr pili that are important in pyelonephritis [116]. Mannosides are FimH receptor analogues and bind to this pilus with high affinity, which results in blocking FimH binding to mannosylated receptors. The use of mannosides is considered a new strategy in treating and preventing UTIs because they prevent bladder colonization and invasion and are effective against multidrug-resistant UPEC and against established UTIs [117].

6. Conclusions

UTIs belong to the most common bacterial infections. *E. coli* is the major factor of community-acquired UTIs and a large part of nosocomial UTIs is also caused by this microorganism. UPECs have a wide range of virulence factors and spread of antimicrobial resistance that threaten effective treatment of UTIs using antibiotics. Intensive research that can identify essential virulence mechanisms of UPEC can lead to the development of UTI treatments and prophylactics. The identification of virulence determinants, especially responsible for initial attachment and adhesion of bacterial cells to receptors can be the basis for the development of targeted therapy that prevents the development of UTI. New strategies of UTIs treatment and prevention include chemical compounds such as pilicides and mannosides that block UPEC adhesion or vaccines against siderophores, pili, and UPEC toxins. However, they are still at the preclinical stage of development. These novel antivirulence therapies for treatment of UTIs still require substantial effort associated with future clinical trials.

Author details

Barbara Kot

Address all correspondence to: barbara.kot@uph.edu.pl

Department of Microbiology, Institute of Biology, Siedlce University of Natural Sciences and Humanities, Siedlce, Poland

References

[1] Kaper JB, Nataro JP, Mobley HL. Pathogenic *Escherichia coli*. Nat Rev Microbiol. 2004;**2**:123-140. DOI:10.1038/nrmicro818

[2] Allocati N, Masulli M, Alexeyev MF, Di Ilio C. *Escherichia coli* in Europe: An overview. Int J Environ Res Public Health. 2013;**10**:6235-6254. DOI:10.3390/ijerph10126235

[3] Wiles TJ, Kulesus RR, Mulvey MA. Origins and virulence mechanisms of uropathogenic *Escherichia coli*. Exp Mol Pathol. 2008;**85**:11-19. DOI:10.1016/j.yexmp.2008.03.007

[4] Samet M, Ghaemi E, Nejad MH, Jamali A. Prevalence of different virulence factors and biofilm production ability of urinary *Escherichia coli* isolates. Int J Biol Med Res. 2014;**5**: 4546-4549.

[5] Bower JM, Eto DS, Mulvey MA. Covert operations of uropathogenic *Escherichia coli* within the urinary tract. Traffic. 2005;**6**:18-31. DOI: 10.1111/j.1600-0854.2004.00251.x

[6] Siegman-Igra Y, Fourer B, Orni-Wasserlauf R, Golan Y, Noy A, Schwartz D, Giladi M. Reappraisal of community-acquired bacteremia: A proposal of a new classification for the spectrum of acquisition of bacteremia. Clin Infect Dis. 2002;**34**:1431-1439. DOI:10.1086/339809

[7] Schneeberger C, Kazemier BM, Geerlings SE. Asymptomatic bacteriuria and urinary tract infections in special patient groups: Women with diabetes mellitus and pregnant women. Curr Opin Infect Dis. 2014;**27**:108-114. DOI: 10.1097/QCO.0000000000000028

[8] Abbott KC, Oliver JD, Hypolite I, Lepler LL, Kirk AD, Ko CW, Hawkes CA, Jones CA, Agodoa LY. Hospitalizations for bacterial septicemia after renal transplantation in the United States. Am J Nephrol. 2001;**21**:120-127. DOI:10.1159/000046234

[9] Manges AR, Johnson JR, Foxman B, O'Bryan TT, Fullerton KE, Riley LW. Widespread distribution of urinary tract infections caused by a multidrug-resistant *Escherichia coli* clonal group. N Engl J Med. 2001;**345**:1007-1013. DOI:10.1056/NEJMoa011265

[10] Welch RA, Burland V, Plunkett G 3rd, Redford P, Roesch P, Rasko D, Buckles EL, Liou SR, Boutin A, Hackett J, Stroud D, Mayhew GF, Rose DJ, Zhou S, Schwartz DC, Perna NT, Mobley HL, Donnenberg MS, Blattner FR. Extensive mosaic structure revealed by the complete genome sequence of uropathogenic *Escherichia coli*. Proc Natl Acad Sci U S A. 2002;**99**:17020-17024. DOI:10.1073/pnas.252529799

[11] Gal-Mor O, Finlay BB. Pathogenicity islands: A molecular toolbox for bacterial virulence. Cell Microbiol. 2006;**8**:1707-1719. DOI:10.1111/j.1462-5822.2006.00794.x

[12] Oelschlaeger TA, Dobrindt U, Hacker J. Pathogenicity islands of uropathogenic *E. coli* and the evolution of virulence. Int J Antimicrob Agents. 2002;**19**:517-521. DOI:10.1016/S0924-8579(02)00092-4

[13] Martinez JJ, Mulvey MA, Schilling JD, Pinkner JS, Hultgren SJ. Type 1 pilus-mediated bacterial invasion of bladder epithelial cells. EMBO J. 2000;**19**:2803-2812. DOI: 10.1093/emboj/19.12.2803

[14] Bien J, Sokolova O, Bozko P. Role of uropathogenic *Escherichia coli* virulence factors in development of urinary tract infection and kidney damage. Int J Nephrol. 2012;**2012**:681473. DOI: 10.1155/2012/681473

[15] Mulvey MA. Adhesion and entry of uropathogenic *Escherichia coli*. Cell Microbiol. 2002; **4**:257-271.

[16] Bergsten G, Wullt B, Schembri MA, Leijonhufvud I, Svanborg C. Do type 1 fimbriae promote inflammation in the human urinary tract? Cell Microbiol. 2007;**9**:1766-1781. DOI: 10.1111/j.1462-5822.2007.00912.x

[17] Yun KW, Kim HY, Park HK, Kim W, Lim IS. Virulence factors of uropathogenic *Escherichia coli* of urinary tract infections and asymptomatic bacteriuria in children. J Microbiol Immunol Infect. 2014;**47**:455-461. DOI:10.1016/j.jmii.2013.07.010

[18] Sokurenko EV, Courtney HS, Maslow J, Siitonen A, Hasty DL. Quantitative differences in adhesiveness of type 1 fimbriated *Escherichia coli* due to structural differences in fimH genes. J Bacteriol. 1995;**177**:3680-3686.

[19] Justice SS, Hung C, Theriot JA, Fletcher DA, Anderson GG, Footer MJ, Hultgren SJ. Differentiation and developmental pathways of uropathogenic *Escherichia coli* in urinary tract pathogenesis. Proc Natl Acad Sci U S A. 2004;**101**:1333-1338. DOI: 10.1128/IAI.73.11.7657-7668.2005

[20] Eto DS, Jones TA, Sundsbak JL, Mulvey MA. Integrin-mediated host cell invasion by type 1-piliated uropathogenic *Escherichia coli*. PLoS Pathog. 2007;**3**:e100. DOI:10.1371/journal.ppat.0030100

[21] Mulvey MA, Schilling JD, Martinez JJ, Hultgren SJ. Bad bugs and beleaguered bladders: Interplay between uropathogenic *Escherichia coli* and innate host defenses. Proc Natl Acad Sci U S A. 2000;**97**:8829-8835.

[22] Bishop BL, Duncan MJ, Song J, Li G, Zaas D, Abraham SN. Cyclic AMP-regulated exocytosis of *Escherichia coli* from infected bladder epithelial cells. Nat Med. 2007;**13**:625-630. DOI: 10.1038/nm1572

[23] Minardi D, d'Anzeo G, Cantoro D, Conti A, Muzzonigro G. Urinary tract infections in women: Etiology and treatment options. Int J Gen Med. 2011;**4**:333-343. DOI:10.2147/IJGM.S11767

[24] Rasko DA, Phillips JA, Li X, Mobley HL. Identification of DNA sequences from a second pathogenicity island of uropathogenic *Escherichia coli* CFT073: Probes specific for uropathogenic populations. J Infect Dis. 2001;**184**:1041-1049. DOI:10.1086/323602

[25] Manning SD, Zhang L, Foxman B, Spindler A, Tallman P, Marrs CF. Prevalence of known P-fimbrial G alleles in *Escherichia coli* and identification of a new adhesin class. Clin Diagn Lab Immunol. 2001;**8**:637-640. DOI: 10.1128/CDLI.8.3.637-640.2001

[26] Marrs CF, Zhang L, Tallman P, Manning SD, Somsel P, Raz P, Colodner R, Jantunen ME, Siitonen A, Saxen H, Foxman B. Variations in 10 putative uropathogen virulence genes

among urinary, faecal and peri-urethral *Escherichia coli*. J Med Microbiol. 2002;**51**:138-142. DOI:10.1099/0022-1317-51-2-138

[27] Marrs CF, Zhang L, Foxman B. *Escherichia coli* mediated urinary tract infections: are there distinct uropathogenic *E. coli* (UPEC) pathotypes? FEMS Microbiol Lett. 2005;**252**:183-190. DOI: 10.1016/j.femsle.2005.08.028

[28] Marre R, Kreft B, Hacker J. Genetically engineered S and F1C fimbriae differ in their contribution to adherence of *Escherichia coli* to cultured renal tubular cells. Infect Immun. 1990;**58**:3434-3437.

[29] Nowicki B, Selvarangan R, Nowicki S. Family of *Escherichia coli* Dr adhesins: decay-accelerating factor receptor recognition and invasiveness. J Infect Dis. 2001;**183**, Suppl 1:S24–S27. DOI:10.1086/318846

[30] Le Bouguénec C. Adhesins and invasins of pathogenic *Escherichia coli*. Int J Med Microbiol. 2005;**295**:471-478.

[31] Muenzner P, Kengmo Tchoupa A, Klauser B, Brunner T, Putze J, Dobrindt U, Hauck CR. Uropathogenic *E. coli* exploit CEA to promote colonization of the urogenital tract mucosa. PLoS Pathog. 2016;**12**:e1005608. DOI:10.1371/journal.ppat.1005608

[32] Cegelski L, Pinkner JS, Hammer ND, Cusumano CK, Hung CS, Chorell E, Åberg V, Walker JN, Seed PC, Almqvist F, Chapman MR, Hultgr SJ. Small-molecule inhibitors target *Escherichia coli* amyloid biogenesis and biofilm formation. Nat Chem Biol. 2009; **5**:913-919. DOI:10.1038/nchembio.242

[33] Barnhart MM, Chapman MR. Curli biogenesis and function. Annu Rev Microbiol. 2006;**60**:131-147. DOI:10.1146/annurev.micro.60.080805.142106

[34] Römling U Characterization of the rdar morphotype, a multicellular behaviour in *Enterobacteriaceae*. Cell Mol Life Sci. 2005;**62**:1234-1246. DOI:10.1007/s00018-005-4557-x

[35] Kai-Larsen Y, Lüthje P, Chromek M, Peters V, Wang X, Holm A, Kádas L, Hedlund KO, Johansson J, Chapman MR, Jacobson SH, Römling U, Agerberth B, Brauner A. Uropathogenic *Escherichia coli* modulates immune responses and its curli fimbriae interact with the antimicrobial peptide LL-37. PLoS Pathog. 2010;**6**:e1001010. DOI: 10.1371/journal.ppat.1001010

[36] Hung C, Marschall J, Burnham CA, Byun AS, Henderson JP. The bacterial amyloid curli is associated with urinary source bloodstream infection. PLoS One. 2014;**9**:e86009. DOI: 10.1371/journal.pone.0086009

[37] Fatima N, Agrawal M, Shukla I, Khan PA. Characterization of uropathogenic *E. coli* in relation to virulence factors. Sci Rep. 2012;1:342. DOI:10.4172/scientificreports.342

[38] Bhakdi S, Mackman N, Nicaud JM, Holland IB. *Escherichia coli* hemolysin may damage target cell membranes by generating transmembrane pores. Infect Immun. 1986;**52**:63-69.

[39] Keane WF, Welch R, Gekker G, Peterson PK. Mechanism of *Escherichia coli* alpha-hemolysin-induced injury to isolated renal tubular cells. Am J Pathol. 1987;**126**:350-357.

[40] Smith YC, Grande KK, Rasmussen SB, O'Brien AD. Novel three-dimensional organoid model for evaluation of the interaction of uropathogenic *Escherichia coli* with terminally differentiated human urothelial cells. Infect Immun. 2006;**74**:750-757. DOI:10.1128/IAI.74.1.750-757.2006

[41] Hilbert DW, Paulish-Miller TE, Tan CK, Carey AJ, Ulett GC, Mordechai E, Adelson ME, Gygax SE, Trama JP. Clinical *Escherichia coli* isolates utilize alpha-hemolysin to inhibit in vitro epithelial cytokine production. Microbes Infect. 2012;**14**:628-638. DOI:10.1016/j.micinf.2012.01.010

[42] Hertting O, Chromek M, Slamova Z, Kadas L, Soderkvist M, Vainumäe I, Tallvik T, Jacobson SH, Brauner A. Cytotoxic necrotizing factor 1 (CNF1) induces an inflammatory response in the urinary tract in vitro but not in vivo. Toxicon. 2008;**51**:1544-1547. DOI: 10.1016/j.toxicon.2008.03.019

[43] Mills M, Meysick KC, O'Brien AD. Cytotoxic necrotizing factor type 1 of uropathogenic *Escherichia coli* kills cultured human uroepithelial 5637 cells by an apoptotic mechanism. Infect Immun. 2000;**68**:5869-5880.

[44] Davis JM, Carvalho HM, Rasmussen SB, O'Brien AD. Cytotoxic necrotizing factor type 1 delivered by outer membrane vesicles of uropathogenic *Escherichia coli* attenuates polymorphonuclear leukocyte antimicrobial activity and chemotaxis. Infect Immun. 2006;**74**:4401-4408. DOI:10.1128/IAI.00637-06

[45] Guyer DM, Radulovic S, Jones FE, Mobley HL. Sat, the secreted autotransporter toxin of uropathogenic *Escherichia coli*, is a vacuolating cytotoxin for bladder and kidney epithelial cells. Infect Immun. 2002;**70**:4539-4546. DOI: 10.1128/IAI.70.8.4539-4546.2002

[46] Ewers C, Li G, Wilking H, Kieβling S, Alt K, Antáo EM, Laturnus C, Diehl I, Glodde S, Homeier T, Böhnke U, Steinrück H, Philipp HC, Wieler LH. Avian pathogenic, uropathogenic, and newborn meningitis-causing *Escherichia coli*: How closely related are they? Int J Med Microbiol. 2007;**297**:163-176. DOI:10.1016/j.ijmm.2007.01.003

[47] Andrews SC, Robinson AK, Rodríguez-Quiñones F. Bacterial iron homeostasis. FEMS Microbiol Rev. 2003;**27**:215-237. DOI: http://dx.doi.org/10.1016/S0168-6445(03)00055-X

[48] Garcia EC, Brumbaugh AR, Mobley HL. Redundancy and specificity of *Escherichia coli* iron acquisition systems during urinary tract infection. Infect Immun. 2011;**79**:1225-1235. DOI:10.1128/IAI.01222-10

[49] Costerton JW, Stewart PS, Greenberg EP. Bacterial biofilms: A common cause of persistent infections. Science. 1999; **284**:1318-1322. DOI: 10.1126/science.284.5418.1318

[50] Soto SM, Marco F, Guiral E, Vila J. Biofilm formation in uropathogenic *Escherichia coli* strains: Relationship with urovirulence factors and antimicrobial resistance. In: Nikibakhsh A, editor. Clinical Management of Complicated Urinary Tract Infection. InTech; 2011. http://www.intechopen.com/books/clinical-management-of-complicated-urinary-tractinfection/biofilm-formation-in-uropathogenic-escherichia-coli-strains-relationship-with-urovirulence-factors-a

[51] Trautner BW, Darouiche RO. Role of biofilm in catheter-associated urinary tract infection. Am J Infect Control. 2004;**32**:177-183. DOI:10.1016/j.ajic.2003.08.005

[52] Ponnusamy P, Natarajan V, Sevanan M. In vitro biofilm formation by uropathogenic *Escherichia coli* and their antimicrobial susceptibility pattern. Asian Pac J Trop Med. 2012;**5**:210-213. DOI:10.1016/S1995-7645(12)60026-1

[53] Anderson GG, Palermo JJ, Schilling JD, Roth R, Heuser J, Hultgren SJ. Intracellular bacterial biofilm-like pods in urinary tract infections. Science. 2003;**301**:105-107. DOI:10.1126/science.1084550

[54] Nicolle LE. Catheter-related urinary tract infections. Drugs Aging. 2005;**22**:627-639.

[55] Ha US, Cho YH. Catheter-associated urinary tract infections: new aspects of novel urinary catheters. Int J Antimicrob Agents. 2006;**28**:485-490. DOI:10.1016/j.ijantimicag.2006.08.020

[56] Jacobsen SM, Stickler DJ, Mobley HL, Shirtliff ME. Complicated catheter-associated urinary tract infections due to *Escherichia coli* and *Proteus mirabilis*. Clin Microbiol Rev. 2008;**21**:26-59. DOI: 10.1128/CMR.00019-07.

[57] Johnson JR. Virulence factors in *Escherichia coli* urinary tract infection. Clin Microbiol Rev. 1991;**4**:80-128.

[58] Warren JW, Muncie HL Jr, Hebel JR, Hall-Craggs M. Long-term urethral catheterization increases risk of chronic pyelonephritis and renal inflammation. J Am Geriatr Soc. 1994;**42**:1286-1290.

[59] Denstedt JD, Wollin TA, Reid G. Biomaterials used in urology: Current issues of biocompatibility, infection, and encrustation. J Endourol. 1998;**12**:493-500. DOI:10.1089/end.1998.12.493

[60] Gristina AG. Biomaterial-centered infection: Microbial adhesion versus tissue integration. Science. 1987;**237**:1588-1595. DOI: 10.1126/science.3629258

[61] Pratt LA, Kolter R. Genetic analysis of *Escherichia coli* biofilm formation: roles of flagella, motility, chemotaxis and type I pili. Mol Microbiol. 1998;**30**:285-293. DOI: 10.1046/j.1365-2958.1998.01061.x

[62] Tambyah PA. Catheter-associated urinary tract infections: diagnosis and prophylaxis. Int J Antimicrob Agents. 2004;**24** Suppl 1:S44–S48. DOI:10.1016/j.ijantimicag.2004.02.008

[63] Djeribi R, Bouchloukh W, Jouenne T, Menaa B. Characterization of bacterial biofilms formed on urinary catheters. Am J Infect Control. 2012;**40**:854-859. DOI:10.1016/j.ajic.2011.10.009

[64] Nicolle LE. The chronic indwelling catheter and urinary infection in long-term-care facility residents. Infect Control Hosp Epidemiol. 2001;**22**:316-321. DOI:10.1086/501908

[65] Raum E, Lietzau S, von Baum H, Marre R, Brenner H. Changes in *Escherichia coli* resistance patterns during and after antibiotic therapy: A longitudinal study among outpatients in Germany. Clin Microbiol Infect. 2008;**14**:41-48. DOI:10.1111/j.1469-0691.2007.01841.x

[66] de Lastours V, Chau F, Tubach F, Pasquet B, Ruppé E, Fantin B. Independent behavior of commensal flora for carriage of fluoroquinolone-resistant bacteria in patients at admission. Antimicrob Agents Chemother. 2010;**54**:5193-5200. DOI:10.1128/IAI.73.9.5301-5310.2005

[67] Lichtenberger P, Hooton TM. Antimicrobial prophylaxis in women with recurrent urinary tract infections. Int J Antimicrob Agents. 2011;**38**:Suppl:36-41. DOI: 10.1016/j.ijantimicag.2011.09.005

[68] Kumar Y, Sood S, Sharma A, Mani KR. Antibiogram and characterization of resistance markers among *Escherichia coli* isolates from urinary tract infections. J Infect Dev Ctries. 2013;**7**:513-519. DOI: 10.3855/jidc.2706

[69] Niranjan V, Malini A. Antimicrobial resistance pattern in *Escherichia coli* causing urinary tract infection among inpatients. Indian J Med Res. 2014;**139**:945-948.

[70] Kot B, Wicha J., Żak-Puławska Z. Susceptibility of *Escherichia coli* strains isolated from persons with urinary tract infections in 2007-2008 to antimicrobial agents. Przegl Epidemiol. 2010;**64**:307-312.

[71] Eryılmaz M, Bozkurt ME, Yildiz MM, Akin A. Antimicrobial resistance of urinary *Escherichia coli* isolates. Trop J Pharm Res. 2010;**9**:205-209.

[72] Sanchez GV, Master RN, Karlowsky JA, Bordon JM. *In vitro* antimicrobial resistance of urinary *Escherichia coli* isolates among U.S. outpatients from 2000 to 2010. Antimicrob Agents Chemother. 2012;**56**:2181-2183. DOI: 10.1128/AAC.06060-11

[73] Ferjani S, Saidani M, Ennigrou S, Hsairi M, Ben Redjeb S. Virulence determinants, phylogenetic groups and fluoroquinolone resistance in *Escherichia coli* isolated from cystitis and pyelonephritis. Pathol Biol. 2012;**60**:270-274. DOI:10.1016/j.patbio.2011.07.006

[74] Calbo E, Romani V, Xercavins M, Gomez L, Vidal CG, Quintana S, Vila J, Garau J. Risk factors for community-onset urinary tract infections due to *Escherichia coli* harbouring extended-spectrum beta-lactamases. J Antimicrob Chemother. 2006;**57**:780-783. DOI:10.1093/jac/dkl035

[75] Machado ETM, Coque R, Canton F, Baquero JC, Peixe L. Dissemination in Portugal of CTX-M-15-, OYA-1-, and TEM-1-producing *Enterobacteriaceae* strains containing the aac(6′)-Ib-cr gene, which encodes an aminoglycoside- and fluoroquinolone-modifying enzyme. Antimicrob Agents Chemother. 2006;**50**:3220-3221. DOI:10.1128/AAC.00473-06

[76] Oteo J, Pérez-Vázquez M, Campos J. Extended-spectrum [beta]-lactamase producing *Escherichia coli*: changing epidemiology and clinical impact. Curr Opin Infect Dis. 2010;**23**:320-326.

[77] Alcántar-Curiel MD, Alpuche-Aranda CM, Varona-Bobadilla HJ, Gayosso-Vázquez C, Jarillo-Quijada MD, Frías-Mendivil M, Sanjuan-Padrón L, Santos-Preciado JI. Risk factors for extended-spectrum β-lactamases-producing *Escherichia coli* urinary tract infections in a tertiary hospital. Salud Publica Mex. 2015;**57**:412-418.

[78] Chaudhary U, Aggarwal R. Extended-spectrum lactamases (ESBL) – An emerging threat to clinical therapeutics. Indian J Med Microbiol. 2004;**22**:75-80.

[79] Hoban DJ, Lascols C, Nicolle LE, Badal R, Bouchillon S, Hackel M, Hawser S. Antimicrobial susceptibility of *Enterobacteriaceae*, including molecular characterization of extended-spectrum beta-lactamase-producing species, in urinary tract isolates from hospitalized patients in North America and Europe: results from the SMART study 2009-2010. Diagn Microbiol Infect Dis. 2012;**74**:62-67. DOI: 10.1016/j.diagmicrobio.2012.05.024

[80] Yumuk Z, Afacan G, Nicolas-Chanoine MH, Sotto A, Lavigne JP. Turkey: A further country concerned by community-acquired *Escherichia coli* clone O25-ST131 producing CTX-M-15. J Antimicrob Chemother. 2008;**62**:284-288. DOI:10.1093/jac/dkn181

[81] Datta P, Gupta V, Sidhu S. Extended spectrum beta lactamase positive uropathogenic *E. coli* – Epidemiological factors and resistance. BJMP 2014;**7**:a718.

[82] Canton R, Coque TM. The CTX-M b-lactamase pandemic. Curr Opin Microbiol. 2006;**9**: 466-475. DOI: 10.1016/j.mib.2006.08.011

[83] Ho PL, Poon WW, Loke SL, Leung MS, Chow KH, Wong RC, Yip KS, Lai EL, Tsang KW; COMBAT study group. Community emergence of CTX-M type extended-spectrum beta-lactamases among urinary *Escherichia coli* from women. J Antimicrob Chemother. 2007;**60**:140-144. DOI:10.1093/jac/dkm144

[84] Schito GC, Gualco L, Naber KG, Botto H, Palou J, Mazzei T, Marchese A. Do different susceptibility breakpoints affect the selection of antimicrobials for treatment of uncomplicated cystitis? J Chemother. 2010;**22**:345-354. DOI:10.1179/joc.2010.22.5.345

[85] Schito GC, Naber KG, Botto H, Palou J, Mazzei T, Gualco L, Marchese A. The ARESC study: An international survey on the antimicrobial resistance of pathogens involved in uncomplicated urinary tract infections. Int J Antimicrob Agents. 2009;**34**:407-413. DOI:10.1016/j.ijantimicag.2009.04.012

[86] Ludwig M, Hoyme U, Weidner W. Recurrent urinary tract infection in women. Long-term antibiotic prophylaxis. Urologe A. 2006;**45**:436-442. DOI:10.1007/s00120-006-1023-9

[87] MacDonald TM, Beardon PH, McGilchrist MM, Duncan ID, McKendrick AD, McDevitt DG. The risks of symptomatic vaginal candidiasis after oral antibiotic therapy. Q J Med. 1993;**86**:419-424. DOI: http://dx.doi.org/419-424

[88] Dethlefsen L, Huse S, Sogin ML, Relman DA. The pervasive effects of an antibiotic on the human gut microbiota, as revealed by deep 16S rRNA sequencing. PLoS Biol. 2008; **6**:e280. DOI: 10.1371/journal.pbio.0060280

[89] Wieser A, Romann E, Magistro G, Hoffmann C, Nörenberg D, Weinert K, Schubert S. A multiepitope subunit vaccine conveys protection against extraintestinal pathogenic *Escherichia coli* in mice. Infect Immun. 2010;**78**:3432-3442. DOI: 10.1128/IAI.00174-10

[90] Uehling DT, Hopkins WJ, Elkahwaji JE, Schmidt DM, Leverson GE. Phase 2 clinical trial of a vaginal mucosal vaccine for urinary tract infections. J Urol. 2003;**170**:867-869. DOI:10.1097/01.ju.0000075094.54767.6e

[91] Hopkins WJ, Elkahwaji J, Beierle LM, Leverson GE, Uehling DT. Vaginal mucosal vaccine for recurrent urinary tract infections in women: Results of a phase 2 clinical trial. J Urol 2007;**177**:1349-1353. DOI:10.1016/j.juro.2006.11.093

[92] Bauer HW, Rahlfs VW, Lauener PA, Blessmann GS. Prevention of recurrent urinary tract infections with immuno-active *E. coli* fractions: A meta-analysis of five placebo-controlled double-blind studies. Int J Antimicrob Agents. 2002;**19**:451-456. DOI:10.1016/S0924-8579(02)00106-1

[93] Amdekar S, Singh V, Singh DD. Probiotic therapy: Immunomodulating approach toward urinary tract infection. Curr Microbiol. 2011;**63**:484-490. DOI:10.1007/s00284-011-0006-2

[94] Beerepoot MAJ, Riet G, Nys S, van der Wal WM, de Borgie CAJM, de Reijke TM, Prins JM, Koeijers J, Verbon A, Stobberingh E, Geerlings SE. Lactobacilli vs antibiotics to prevent urinary tract infections: A randomized, double-blind, noninferiority trial in postmenopausal women. Arch Intern Med. 2012;**172**:704-712. DOI: 10.1001/archinternmed.2012.777

[95] Howell AB. Bioactive compounds in cranberries and their role in prevention of urinary tract infections. Mol Nutr Food Res. 2007;**51**:732-737. DOI:10.1002/mnfr.200700038

[96] Howell AB, Botto H, Combescure C, Blanc-Potard AB, Gausa L, Matsumoto T, Tenke P, Sotto A, Lavigne JP. Dosage effect on uropathogenic *Escherichia coli* anti-adhesion activity in urine following consumption of cranberry powder standardized for proanthocyanidin content: A multicentric randomized double blind study. BMC Infect Dis. 2010;**10**:94. DOI: 10.1186/1471-2334-10-94

[97] Wojnicz D, Sycz Z, Walkowski S, Gabrielska J, Włoch A, Kucharska A, Sokół-Łętowska A, Hendrich AB. Study on the influence of cranberry extract Żuravit S·O·S® on the properties of uropathogenic *Escherichia coli* strains, their ability to form biofilm and its antioxidant properties. Phytomedicine. 2012;**19**:506-514. DOI:10.1016/j.phymed.2011.12.013

[98] Carson L, Gorman SP, Gilmore BF. The use of lytic bacteriophages in the prevention and eradication of biofilms of *Proteus mirabilis* and *Escherichia coli*. FEMS Immunol Med Microbiol. 2010;**59**:447-455. DOI: 10.1111/j.1574-695X.2010.00696.x

[99] Chibeu A, Lingohr EJ, Masson L, Manges A, Harel J, Ackermann HW, Kropinski AM, Boerlin P. Bacteriophages with the ability to degrade uropathogenic *Escherichia coli* biofilms. Viruses. 2012;**4**:471-487. DOI: 10.3390/v4040471

[100] Ichimiya T, Takeoka K, Hiramatsu K, Hirai K, Yamasaki T, Nasu M. The influence of azithromycin on the biofilm formation of *Pseudomonas aeruginosa* in vitro. Chemotherapy. 1996;**42**:186-191.

[101] Soto SM. Importance of biofilms in urinary tract infections: new therapeutic approaches. Adv Biol. 2014; ID 543974, 13 pages. DOI:10.1155/2014/543974

[102] Hamill TM, Gilmore BF, Jones DS, Gorman SP. Strategies for the development of the urinary catheter. Expert Rev Med Devices. 2007;**4**:215-225. DOI:10.1586/17434440.4.2.215

[103] Schaeffer AJ, Story KO, Johnson SM. Effect of silver oxide/trichloroisocyanuric acid antimicrobial urinary drainage system on catheter-associated bacteriuria. J Urol. 1988;**139**: 69-73.

[104] Rupp ME, Fitzgerald T, Marion N, Helget V, Puumala S, Anderson JR, Fey PD. Effect of silver-coated urinary catheters: Efficacy, cost-effectiveness, and antimicrobial resistance. Am J Infect Control. 2004;**32**:445-450. DOI:10.1016/S0196655304004742

[105] Desai DG, Liao KS, Cevallos ME, Trautner BW. Silver or nitrofurazone impregnation of urinary catheters has a minimal effect on uropathogen adherence. J Urol. 2010;**184**:2565-2571. DOI: 10.1016/j.juro.2010.07.036

[106] Lu TK, Collins JJ. Dispersing biofilms with engineered enzymatic bacteriophage. Proc Natl Acad Sci U S A. 2007;**104**:11197-11202. DOI: 10.1073/pnas.0704624104

[107] Lellouche J, Friedman A, Gedanken A, Banin E. Antibacterial and antibiofilm properties of yttrium fluoride nanoparticles. Int J Nanomed. 2012;**7**:5611-5624. DOI: 10.2147/IJN.S37075

[108] Domadia P, Swarup S, Bhunia A, Sivaraman J, Dasgupta D. Inhibition of bacterial cell division protein FtsZ by cinnamaldehyde. Biochem Pharmacol. 2007;**832**:831-840. DOI: 10.1016/j.bcp.2007.06.029

[109] Borges A, Saavedra MJ, Simões M. The activity of ferulic and gallic acids in biofilm prevention and control of pathogenic bacteria. Biofouling 2012;**28**:755-767. DOI: 10.1080/08927014.2012.706751

[110] Amalaradjou MAR, Narayanan A, Baskaran SA, Venkitanarayanan K. Antibiofilm effect of trans-cinnamaldehyde on uropathogenic *Escherichia coli.* J Urol. 2010;**184**:358-363. DOI: 10.1016/j.juro.2010.03.006

[111] Amalaradjou MAR, Narayanan A, Venkitanarayanan K. Trans-cinnamaldehyde decreases attachment and invasion of uropathogenic *Escherichia coli* in urinary tract epithelial cells by modulating virulence gene exptression. J Urol. 2011;**185**:1526-1531. DOI: 10.1016/j.juro.2010.11.078

[112] Kot B, Wicha J, Piechota M, Wolska K, Grużewska A. Antibiofilm activity of trans-cinnamaldehyde, p-coumaric, and ferulic acids on uropathogenic *Escherichia coli.* Turk J Med Sci. 2015;**45**:919-924. DOI:10.3906/sag-1406-112

[113] Dusane DH, Hosseinidoust Z, Asadishad B, Tufenkji N. Alkaloids modulate motility, biofilm formation and antibiotic susceptibility of uropathogenic *Escherichia coli.* PLoS One. 2014;**9**:e112093. DOI: 10.1371/journal.pone.0112093

[114] Pinkner JS, Remaut H, Buelens F, Miller E, Aberg V, Pemberton N, Hedenström M, Larsson A, Seed P, Waksman G, Hultgren SJ, Almqvist F. Rationally designed small compounds inhibit pilus biogenesis in uropathogenic bacteria. Proc Natl Acad Sci U S A. 2006;**103**:17897-17902. DOI: 10.1073/pnas.0606795103

[115] Greene SE, Pinkner JS, Chorell E, Dodson KW, Shaffer CL, Conover MS, Livny J, Hadjifrangiskou M, Almqvist F, Hultgrenet SJ. Pilicide ec240 disrupts virulence circuits in uropathogenic *Escherichia coli.* mBio. 2014;**5**:e02038-14. DOI:10.1128/mBio.02038-14

[116] Piatek R, Zalewska-Piatek B, Dzierzbicka K, Makowiec S, Pilipczuk J, Szemiako K, Cyranka-Czaja A, Wojciechowski M. Pilicides inhibit the FGL chaperone/usher assisted biogenesis of the Dr fimbrial polyadhesin from uropathogenic *Escherichia coli*. BMC Microbiol. 2013 Jun 12;**13**:131. DOI: 10.1186/1471-2180-13-131.

[117] Totsika M, Kostakioti M, Hannan TJ, Upton M, Beatson SA, Janetka JW, Hultgren SJ, Schembri MA. A FimH inhibitor prevents acute bladder infection and treats chronic cystitis caused by multidrug-resistant uropathogenic *Escherichia coli* ST131. J Infect Dis. 2013;**15**; 208: 921-928. DOI: 10.1093/infdis/jit245

3

Resistant Gram-Negative Urinary Tract Bacterial Infections

Nashaat S. Hamza and Abdalla Khalil

Abstract

Urinary tract infection (UTI) is one of the most common infections in both the community as well in hospital settings. It is mostly caused by Gram-negative bacteria (GNBs). Over the past two decades, GNBs have developed complex mechanisms of resistance against most of the potent antibiotics. This has been a global challenge which has been identified by the World Health Organization as "one of the greatest threats to human health." This crisis is mostly attributed to the overuse and misuse of these medications, as well as lack of new drug antimicrobials by the pharmaceutical industry. This resulted in prolonged hospital stay, marked increase in the cost as well as increase in morbidity and mortality. Furthermore, it increases the risks and complications of urological procedures. In this chapter, we review the management of the most common and challenging group of resistant Gram-negative organisms, the extended-spectrum β-lactamases producing organisms (ESBL) and the carbapenem-resistant organisms (CRE/CRP). The latter group includes carbapenem-resistant *Enterobacteriaceae* (CRE), as well as *Pseudomonas aeruginosa* carbapenemases (CRP). When treating these infections, clinicians have few effective antimicrobials options. A critical step in managing these organisms is the early recognition and appropriate empiric therapy. Both showed morbidity and mortality benefits.

Keywords: urinary tract infection (UTI), Gram-negative bacteria (GNBs), complicated urinary tract infections (CUTIs), extended-spectrum β-lactamases producing organisms (ESBL), carbapenem-resistant organisms (CRE/CRP), carbapenems, ceftazidime-avibactam, colistin, fosfomycin, *Enterobacteriaceae*

1. Introduction

Urinary tract infection is the second most common infectious presentation in community as well as in hospital settings. It has been estimated that 150 million people are diagnosed with

UTI each year worldwide [1]. It is mostly caused by GNBs. Over the past two decades, GNBs have developed complex mechanisms of resistance against most of the potent antibiotics. This has been a global challenge which has been identified by the World Health Organization as "one of the greatest threats to human health" [2]. This crisis is mostly man-made as it is attributed to the overuse and misuse of these medications, as well as a lack of new drug development by the pharmaceutical industry seeking better profitable agents.

This resulted in prolonged hospital stay, marked increases in the cost as well as increase in morbidity and mortality [3–6]. Furthermore, bloodstream infections associated with severe complicated urinary tract infections (CUTIs) are associated with high mortality rates of 20–50% among critically ill patients. Many urological procedures are complicated with such infectious manse, frustrating the surgeons and the patients [7].

Multiple mechanisms that enable the organism to become resistant include enzymatic transformation, modification of site of action, active efflux from the cell interior and, the prevention of entry of the molecules into the cell [8].

There are different confusing terminologies in addressing this process. An international panel of experts developed the following definitions: multidrug-resistant (MDROs) means acquiring nonsusceptibility to at least one agent in three or more antimicrobial categories, extensively drug-resistant (XDR) is nonsusceptible to at least one agent in all, but two or fewer antimicrobial categories, and pan-drug-resistant (PDR) isolates are nonsusceptible to any of the available antimicrobial classes [1, 9, 10].

The term "ESKAPE" was one of the former descriptions of pathogens that cause the majority of hospital infections while effectively "escaping" the effects of available therapeutics. Other terms include "SPICE organisms" which include many Gram-negative bacteria that have inducible, chromosomal AmpC β-lactamase genes. The resistance to antibiotics may not be detectable initially, but appears after a period of exposure to β-lactam antibiotics (during therapy or after).

We are focusing in this review on the most common and challenging groups of resistant Gram-negative organisms, the ESBL, and the CRE, as well as CRP. The other highly resistant organism, such as *Acinetobacter baumannii,* less frequently causes urinary tract infection and its therapy is even more complicated [11–13].

When treating these infections, clinicians have a few effective antimicrobials to choose from and many are associated with significant adverse effects. A critical step in managing these organisms is the early recognition and appropriate empiric therapy. Both showed morbidity and mortality benefits. In this chapter we will review the available data on managing UTIs caused by ESBL and the CRE/CRP.

2. Materials and methods

The purpose of this chapter is to review the available data on managing UTIs caused by resistant Gram-negative bacteria. Clinical trials and review articles (in English) were identified from a Medline search (2000–2017), in addition to laboratory data and abstracts from international Conferences.

2.1. Definition: ESBL organisms

The term ESBL was originally applied to plasmid-encoded β-lactamases that are capable of inactivating extended-spectrum cephalosporins and are inhibited by β-lactamase inhibitors, such as clavulanic acid. *Enterobacteriaceae*, primarily *Escherichia coli* and *Klebsiella pneumoniae*, are among the most frequently producing bacteria [9].

ESBLs are plasmid-encoded or chromosomally encoded β-lactamases with broad activity against penicillins and cephalosporins. They are a diverse group of bacterial enzymes that break down and inactivate most β-lactam antibiotics. They are inhibited by the available β-lactamase inhibitors (clavulanic acid, sulbactam, avibactam, and tazobactam) and do not affect cephamycins (e.g., cefoxitin and cefotetan) or carbapenems. β-Lactamases are divided into A, B, C, and D classes according to their amino acid sequence homology (Ambler classification) [14].

These bacteria are usually multi-resistant, as they are frequently capable of resisting other antibiotics, such as the aminoglycosides, tetracyclines, and trimethoprim/sulfamethoxazole though other mechanisms, leaving few treatment options [3]. As these resistant genes are plasmid-mediated, they can be easily disseminated to other bacterial species [15–17]. UTIs caused by these organisms are seen at alarming rates in both hospital infection and in the community settings [15, 18, 19].

Although 95–100% ESBL organisms are still considered sensitive to carbapenems, rapid emergence of carbapenem resistance has been documented globally, and was linked to the over usage of these agents [20].

2.2. Epidemiology

Surveillance in Asia, Latin America, and Europe revealed dramatically increasing resistance to cephalosporins among *E. coli* and *Klebsiella* spp. [21]. In a large study in Turkey (SMART), the rate of ESBL in *E. coli* isolated from urine samples was high (50% hospital isolates and 38% community acquired isolates) [22, 23].

In one study, 21,414 positive urine cultures were collected from a University hospital in the UK. There were 1420 ESBL-positive specimens. There were a 44% increase, from 4.6 to 6.6%, of the ESBL-positive organisms over 2 years.

Multidrug resistance were detected in 75% of ESBL + *Klebsiella* spp. against >6 antibiotic classes [24].

In the CHINET surveillance system data from 2005 to 2014, ESBL production among *E. coli* isolates was between 51.7 and 55.8% [25].

The spreading of such isolates in the community is well documented, so containment of this type of bacterial infection will be real challenging [23]. There were many outbreaks caused by these organisms all over the globe with high morbidity and mortalities [17].

2.3. Risk factors

Many studies have implicated broad-spectrum cephalosporins as the major class associated with ESBL production; others considered fluoroquinolone and β-lactam-β-lactamase inhibitor combinations, as the main risk factors for ESBL infections [26]. Other risk factors include nursing home residence, diabetes, recurrent UTIs, male gender, prolonged hospitalization, intensive care admission, and urinary catheterization [19, 24, 27–29].

Prospective cohort study of 225 healthy German volunteers traveling to 53 different countries (mostly in Asia, Africa, and S. America) evaluated the risk of ESBL colonization. Stool samples were collected before and after traveling. The isolates were examined phenotypically and by PCR amplification sequencing. Among 191 participants that were ESBL-negative before travel, 30% were colonized by ESBL-producing *E. coli* after returning home [29, 30].

The use of antibiotics in farm animals as growth promoters is linked to this global disaster. In a recent study from India, 18 poultry farms were surveyed, 16 of them reported using antimicrobials for growth promotion. There were 1556 *E. coli* isolates, collected and tested. The prevalence of ESBL-positive strains in broiler farms was 87% [31]. Multiple studies have shown the benefit of early identifications of this organism, to offer the appropriate empiric therapy. A simple predicting score for early recognition was recently published. Four risk factors were identified; each was given a score of one. Scores above 2 had a sensitivity of (84%) and a specificity of (92%). These variables include recent antimicrobial use (OR, 15.29), recent invasive procedures (OR, 12.33), nursing home residents (OR, 27.77), and frequent emergency department visits (OR, 9.98) [32].

2.4. Mechanism of resistance

The most common mechanisms include enzymatic inactivation, target modification, reduced permeability, and active efflux. Antibiotic resistance can be intrinsic to specific microorganisms, which can be explained by their inherent characteristics. Point mutations on β-lactamase genes are responsible for emergence of ESBLs. These new genes could be transmitted through small mobile genetic element DNA (plasmid, transposons) to other bacteria from same or other species [5, 8].

A more distinct type of ESBL including CTX-M-type, AmpC, and carbapenemase, can confer phenotypic resistance that widens the resistance abilities against more antibiotics than the classical isolates [33].

2.5. Detection

These organisms are capable of resisting most of the third-generation cephalosporins but they are inhibited by clavulanate. This is the basis of detecting these organisms using routine laboratory tests such as double disk diffusion test or E-test. The size of zone of inhibition around one or more of the β-lactam-containing discs toward the clavulanic acid-containing disc is indicative of some ESBL producers [34, 35].

The detection of specific genes by PCR and sequencing are commonly used for final confirmation of ESBL producers. A commercially available multiplex real-time PCR can detect the predominant class A β-lactamase genes bla_{CTX-M}, bla_{SHV}, bla_{TEM}, and CIT-type AmpCs with high sensitivity and it is much faster than routine cultures [36].

2.6. Carbapenem resistant organisms

The carbapenems are the most potent agents with wide spectra of coverage. They are the most dependent agents in critical infectious syndromes. However, resistance to these agents has increasingly been reported worldwide, rendering them increasingly ineffective. These organisms are also capable of resisting other classes of antibiotics (aminoglycosides, fluoroquinolone, and co-trimoxazole), due to the frequent coexistence of other resistance genes on the same mobile genetic elements, rendering them superbugs. The most recent example is the emergence of colistin resistant genes in isolates which are already resistant to the carbapenems.

K. pneumoniae carbapenemase (KPC-class A) was the first CRE enzyme to be reported in 2001. New Delhi metallo-β-lactamase (NDM-class B) is one of the most recently reported metallo-enzymes. It has spread widely in the Indian sub-continent and now worldwide. The oxacillinase-48 type (OXA-48-class C) has been identified mostly in Mediterranean and southern European countries. Other mechanisms of resistance include efflux pump over activity (pumping the antibiotics out of the bacterial cell), hyper production of AmpC β-lactamase in the already highly resistant ESBL organisms, and changes in porin permeability [8].

Infections with such resistant isolates resulted in high morbidity, prolonged hospital stay, and mortality [37, 38]. In a pooled analysis of the 9 studies (985 patients), the mortality rate was higher among CRE-infected than carbapenem susceptible *Enterobacteriaceae*-infected patients (RR 2.05, 95% CI 1.56–2.69). The authors calculated 26–44% of deaths from 7 studies attributable to carbapenem resistance [39]. The rate was even higher (61%) in patients infected with KPC-expressing *K. pneumoniae* who received initially ineffective therapy [40].

2.7. Epidemiology

A multicenter observational study in 11 hospitals from 7 Latin American countries that included 255 patients with bacteremia was reported. Twenty-three percent of the isolates were CRE/CRP [38].

According to the latest data collected by the European Antimicrobial Resistance Surveillance Network (EARS-Net), the rate of CRE rose from 6.2% in 2012 to 8.1% in 2015 [41].

CRE are more prevalent in Italy and Greece. In an active surveillance study, rectal swabs (and clinical samples) were collected from 15,104 hospitalized patients (over 2 years). *K. pneumoniae* CRE was detected in 496 consecutive non-replicated samples [42].

In a Greek study, 3449 *K. pneumoniae* isolates were recovered over 10 years. Among them, 1668 (48%) were CRE-producing. Sixteen percent of the isolates were resistant to colistin [43].

2.8. Detection

These include antimicrobial susceptibility testing, modified Hodge testing, and inhibitor-based testing. In 2015, the CDC-CRE surveillance definition was revised to one of two criteria: (1) resistance to any carbapenem according to current CLSI breakpoints (MIC ≥ 2 for ertapenem or ≥4 for doripenem, meropenem, or imipenem) or (2) demonstration of carbapenemase production. Several phenotypic assays are available commercially detecting carbapenemase production from bacterial culture within hours. The Carba NP test has high sensitivity and specificity that can differentiate between class A, B, and C CRE. In one study, its specificity and sensitivity were almost 96% [44].

There are many commercially available PCR-based testing for early recognition and confirmation.

2.9. Therapy of urinary tract infections caused by MDROs

2.9.1. ESBL-producing β-lactamases

In general and for serious life threatening infections, the carbapenems are the drugs of choice for infections caused by these organisms [12, 35]. However, the surge in using the carbapenems, resulted in the evolution of CRE/CRP, so there were multiple recent trials evaluating, carbapenem-sparing are regimens, mostly for less severe infections [12, 45–48].

2.9.2. CRE/CRP

In general, there is no clear consensus on managing these organisms. The available data are drawn from expert opinion or from small trials. There are few controlled trials that determined the best therapeutic so far [49, 50].

In the following sections, we will review the available data on different classes of antibiotics that have been used in managing ESBL, and then if applicable, will discuss their roles in treating CRE/CRP.

2.9.2.1. Carbapenems

They have a broad spectrum of antimicrobial activity more than any other classes of antimicrobials, and are potent bactericidal (ertapenem lakes anti-pseudomonas activities) [51–54].

In multiple non-randomized studies that included large number of patients with bacteremia, sepsis, and other serious infections, they showed high cure-improvement rates with great safety profile [54, 55].

Studies of the pharmacokinetic/pharmacodynamics data also showed superiority of this class of antibiotic in achieving the proper concentration above the bacterial minimal inhibitory concentrations (MICs) [56].

In vitro activities against many ESBL isolates are well documented against large collections of ESBL producing *Enterobacteriaceae* and *P. aeruginosa* isolates [57].

For treating CRE/CRP, limited data on combination regimens involving carbapenems (if MICs ≥ 8 mg/L) adding colistin or high-dose tigecycline or aminoglycoside or even triple combinations, seem to confer decent therapeutic advantage over monotherapy. For organisms with higher MIC, a combination of two or even three antibiotics may be needed.

In a recent meta-analysis of 22 studies of using, the most common regimen, carbapenems plus colistin or polymyxin had mortality advantages [38].

On the other hand, a retrospective study of 436 patients were recruited in the INCREMENT study-cohort (26 tertiary hospitals from 10 countries). The main outcome variable was 30 day all-cause mortality in patients with CRE/CRP bloodstream infection. Overall mortality was not different between those receiving combination therapy and monotherapy (35% vs. 41%) [58].

Synergy is another potential benefit arising from the use of antibiotic combinations.

Tigecycline with colistin, colistin with a carbapenem, fosfomycin with a carbapenem, fosfomycin with an aminoglycoside, and a carbapenem with an aminoglycoside have been reported as antibiotic combinations effectively administered to series of patients infected with carbapenemase-producing *Enterobacteriaceae* [4].

Efforts have been exerted to limit the usage of their precious agents by using alternative regimens whenever [46].

2.9.2.2. Piperacillin-tazobactam (PTZ)

PTZ is a broad-spectrum drug combination used in serious infections. However, the extensive usage of this agent accelerated the emergence of resistance [48, 59].

Some ESBL *E. coli* producers' isolates might have high in vitro susceptibility to PTZ; however, its clinical utility in serious UTIs, especially when associated with bacteremia, has been controversial. In a prospective, randomized, open-label comparison of the therapeutic efficacy of (PTZ), cefepime, and ertapenem in nosocomial UTIs with ESBL producers, 66 participants were evenly randomized to the PTZ and ertapenem treatment groups (cefepime arm was eliminated because of high treatment failure rate). The clinical and microbiological responses to both antibiotics were similar around 94% [60].

Similar non-inferiority of PTZ to carbapenems was shown in a retrospective analysis of bloodstream infection by an ESBL-producing organism, if susceptible in vitro [61].

In a post hoc analysis of patients with bloodstream infections due to ESBL producing isolates from 6 published prospective cohorts, the effect of amoxicillin-clavulanic acid, PTZ, and carbapenems were compared. The mortality rates at day 30 were much higher with the first 2 antibiotics than with carbapenems [62].

In a retrospective observational study, 331 patients with ESBL bacteremias were evaluated. Empiric therapy with PTZ was used in 48% while 52% received carbapenems. The adjusted risk of death (14-day mortality) was 1.92 times higher for patients receiving empiric PTZ compared with carbapenem therapy (95% confidence interval, 1.07–3.45) [63].

In an editorial that tried to explain these controversial results, the authors mentioned various variables including the inoculum of the bacteria in the bloodstream, the sources of bacteremia (less fatal if from UTIs than central line infections), selection bias inherent to observational studies, and the presence of different genetic and virulence of the included bacteria [35].

A large recent multicenter randomized controlled open-label non-inferiority trial, MERINO trial, comparing meropenem (standard arm) against PTZ in adult patients with bacteremia caused by *E. coli* or *Klebsiella* spp., is ongoing, and hopefully, it will provide better answer to these conflicting data [61].

2.9.2.3. Cephalosporins

Cephalosporins have been less effective than comparative regimens in treating severe/serious infections with ESBL-producing bacteria. They are rapidly hydrolyzed by many ESBLs stains [60].

In many clinical studies, it was associated with a trend toward clinical and microbiological failure, as well as a trend of increased mortality [64, 65].

Despite their in vitro activities, there are reports of mutations and/or acquiring plasmids encoding AmpC-resistant genes during therapy with these agents. Others concerns about this agent failure include the decreased activity with high bacterial load (inoculum effect) and the failure to meet necessary pharmacodynamics targets due to inadequate dosing and/or interval schedules [50].

The most studied agent in this class is the cefepime. In the above-mentioned recent prospective, randomized, open-label that compared (PTZ), cefepime, and ertapenem in nosocomial UTIs, the microbiological and therapeutic efficacies of cefepime in febrile nosocomial urinary tract infection with ESBL *E. coli* were much less than the other competitors at 33% [60].

Data is more clear in patients with serious infections associated with ESBL-producing organisms' bloodstream infections. In a recent study, the mortality risk was 2.87 times higher for patients receiving cefepime compared with carbapenems (95% confidence interval (0.88–9.41) [66].

Another retrospective study included adult patients with BSI due to ESBL-producing *K. pneumoniae* or *E. coli*. In multivariate analysis, using cefepime as empirical therapy was associated with a trend toward an increased mortality risk, while empirical carbapenem therapy was associated with a trend toward decreased mortality [65].

There is few data from limited studies (with small number of participants) that showed cefepime is effective if used against in vitro susceptible ESBL-producing *Enterobacteriaceae* and as a de-escalation therapy in patients with uncomplicated UTIs [53, 67].

There are less robust data for the efficacy of other cephalosporins, cefmetazole (a cephamycins), in treating patients with extended-spectrum β-lactamase producing [68].

2.9.2.4. Aminoglycosides

Aminoglycosides are very potent antibiotics; however, their use is associated with significant renal and auditory toxicities. They have been successful in treating ESBL-UTIs as a monotherapy or in combinations with other agents. Combinations with other agents were effective in the treatment of CRE/CRP infections if the strain is susceptible to aminoglycosides [69].

Many of the plasmids that carry ESBL-producing genes also carry genes encodes resistant to aminoglycosides, mostly against tobramycin and gentamicin. In contrast, amikacin has retained high susceptibility rates, particularly against *E. coli.*

In a small study of UTI caused by highly resistant ESBL (also resistant to nitrofurantoin, fosfomycin, and quinolones and trimethoprim/sulfamethoxazole), amikacin intramuscular injections for 10 days achieved clinical success in 97.2%. Overall bacteriological success rate was 94.1% on the 7–10 days after treatment [70].

In a review of 20 studies evaluating CRE infections therapy, combination of aminoglycosides and carbapenems displayed the lowest mortality rate (11.1%) [71].

2.9.2.5. Fluoroquinolones

In many parts of the world, *E. coli* fluoroquinolone resistance rates are >20% among patients with community-acquired uncomplicated UTI and 50% among patients with complicated infections. The rate of resistance is even higher against *Klebsiella* spp. up to 70% in one recent international surveillance study [8, 72].

The co-existing of ESBL and fluoroquinolone resistant is extremely high in some areas of the world, in those who uses quinolones prophylaxis and in returned travelers to theses endemic areas [73]. Therefore, they are in general not recommended in the setting of high ESBL isolates [74].

Sitafloxacin is the newest member (fourth generation) of the fluoroquinolone family of antibiotics which has a broad-spectrum activity including many anaerobes [75]. In a recent prospective randomized controlled trial, comparing the clinical and bacteriological efficacy of sitafloxacin and ertapenem for non-bacteremic acute pyelonephritis caused by ESBL-EC was evaluated. Carbapenems were initially given to all patients, and then were randomized to one of the study drugs. The 2 arms were equal in the rates of clinical and microbiological cure [76].

These data suggest that fluoroquinolones may no longer be effective as first-line therapy for Gram-negative UTI in hospitalized patients and definitely in ESBL-producing organisms.

2.9.2.6. Trimethoprim/sulfamethoxazole

Although treatment with trimethoprim/sulfamethoxazole was traditionally effective in treating UTIS, the evolution of resistance is a current major concern. The Infectious Diseases Society of America guideline recommends against using it if local bacterial resistance rate is ≥20% [77]. Genes that encode for ESBLs are usually found on large plasmids accompanied by genetic determinants of resistance against multiple classes of antibiotics, such as aminoglycosides, sulfonamides, and fluoroquinolones. TMP-SMX is not recommended as an empiric treatment option of UTIs caused by resistant strains of *E. coli* or *K. pneumoniae* that reaches 40–66% in some areas in the world [78].

2.9.2.7. Tigecycline

Tigecycline has potent activity against a vast majority of organisms including Gram-negatives, Gram-positives, and anaerobes. It has almost susceptibility rates of 100% against ESBL-producing *E. coli,* however less potency against *K. pneumoniae* isolates producing. However, its use has concerning safety issues [11, 79]. Insufficient urinary excretion of the unchanged drug (15–22% of the dose) has prompted recommendations to avoid tigecycline for UTIs therapy [80, 81].

In a systematic review of the literature, 14 patients received tigecycline for UTIs caused by MDR Gram-negative bacilli. In 12 patients, there were initial microbiological clearance. Eleven patients had evidence of clinical response. However, there were post-therapy growth of tigecycline-resistant organisms in 2 cases [81].

Few studies tried to overcome this obstacle by using higher than the recommended dose for highly resistant organisms (initial dose of 200 mg one time followed by 100 mg every 24 h) [82].

The efficacy of tigecycline is further limited by increasing in vitro resistance in CRE. Serum and urinary levels of tigecycline are low, and most experts discourage the use of tigecycline as monotherapy for bloodstream or urinary tract infections [83].

This agent has no activity against *Pseudomonas, Proteus, Providencia,* and *Morganella.*

2.9.2.8. The polymyxins

The polymyxins are antibacterial agents that are produced from different strains of *Bacillus polymyxa.* Colistin and polymyxin B are available commercially; both have similar chemical structures and antibacterial activity in vitro, however they differ in their pharmacokinetic profiles. They can cause significant nephrotoxicity (reported in 20–60%) and neurotoxicity [69]. However, the spreading of extensively resistant Gram-negative bacteria as well as the paucity of newer effective antimicrobials let to the extensive usage of these agents as a last resort [84]. The vast majority of ESBL-producing *E. coli* and *K. pneumoniae* are susceptible to these drugs.

Currently, they are the backbone of most of the regimens used against the CRE/CRP organisms. Common combination regimens include tigecycline, carbapenem, minocycline, rifampicin, aminoglycosides, ampicillin/sulbactam, and piperacillin-tazobactam. Large clinical trials are underway to clarify the use of polymyxin different combinations [85].

Polymyxin B is administered directly as the active antibiotic, whereas colistin methanesulfonate is converted in vivo to colistin. The optimal dosing of these agents is still controversial.

Higher doses of colistin were proposed for managing serious CRE/CRP associated infections.

A recent systematic review that included 22 studies (observational studies as well as randomized controlled trials) of polymyxin-based combination therapy in adult patients with infections caused by CRE/CRP was published. The primary outcome was a 30-day mortality. Mortality was significantly higher with polymyxin monotherapy compared with combination therapy of polymyxin with tigecycline, aminoglycosides or fosfomycin, of 1.57 (95% CI = 1.06–2.32). However, the authors caution about the low quality of the evidence [86].

The mechanism of colistin resistance can be generally classified intrinsic or acquired by a recently recognized plasmid-mediated resistance gene [87].

In November 2015, plasmid-borne colistin resistance gene mcr-1 was initially identified in animal and clinical samples from China. As of September 2016, the mcr-1 gene was detected in 35 countries worldwide in human sources in 22 countries [88]. This created a real lethal superbug.

2.9.2.9. Fosfomycin (Fosf)

This agent has gained attention, as it has activities against both Gram-positive and Gram-negative MDR and XDR bacteria [89, 90–94]. It exhibits bactericidal activity against many Gram-positive and Gram-negative pathogens including many of the ESBL-producing *E. coli* and *K. pneumoniae* [91]. Fosf achieves very high concentrations within the urine and is therefore an excellent agent for cystitis, but it is not recommended for treating pyelonephritis or bacteremias due to inadequate concentrations in the blood. However, small studies have shown great results in using Fosf in complicated UTIs [95]. It is currently approved by the American Food and Drug Administration for the treatment of uncomplicated cystitis as a one-time dose of 3 g. Several studies have shown clinical efficacy in the treatment of ESBL cystitis when the dosing is extended to 3 g every 48–72 h for 3 doses [96].

A meta-analysis that evaluated the antimicrobial activity, or the clinical effectiveness of Fosf, reviewed 17 studies. Out of a total of 5057 clinical isolates of *Enterobacteriaceae*, 4448 were ESBL producers. Almost 90% of the isolates were susceptible to Fosf. Eighty percent of 748 *K. pneumoniae* isolates produced ESBL and were susceptible to Fosf [94].

In a prospective study of 47 patients with UTI caused by *E. coli*-ESBL-producing organisms, the outcome was evaluated. Fosfomycin was used in 27 patients and 20 patients received meropenem. The clinical and microbiological success was similar in 2 groups; however, the costs were significantly lower in the Fosf group ($p < 0.001$). Fosfomycin was used orally 3 g sachet every other night total of 3 doses, while meropenem was used as a dose for 14 days [95].

In a retrospective study, 60 patients were treated for MDR UTI. There were cases infected with *Enterobacteriaceae*, *P. aeruginosa*, and *VRE*. The clinical response rate was 55%. Chronic kidney disease was associated clinical failure ($p = 0.04$) [92].

For the carbapenem-producing organisms, a very few clinical data on using this agent are available.

In Europe, an intravenous Fosf formulation is available. In a small (in 11 ICU patients) European study, intravenous Fosf (2–4 g q6 h) in combination with other antibiotics was associated with good bacteriological and clinical outcomes in all patients with carbapenem-resistant *K. pneumoniae* infections [96].

In an in vitro study, 365 isolates out of 2229 urine samples were evaluated. ESBL producers were detected in 65% were, 16% were carbapenem-resistant *Enterobacteriaceae*, almost 95% of the total isolates were susceptible to Fosf [97].

A recent, albeit pessimistic, data came from China. A study collected 233 clinical isolates CRE/CRP *Carbapenem Resistant Enterobacteriaceae/Carbapenem Resistant Pseudomonas* at four different hospitals. Forty-five percent of the strains (105/233) were resistant to Fosf. Plasmid-mediated fosfomycin-modifying enzymes fosA, fosA2, fosA3, and fosA5 genes were identified [98].

2.9.2.10. Nitrofurantoin

Another oral antimicrobial agent that can be considered for the treatment of ESB cystitis is nitrofurantoin. One study showed clinical cure rates of 69% in patients with ESBL cystitis in which all isolates were also resistant to SMX/TMP and ciprofloxacin [99].

Nitrofurantoin should only be used for lower UTI and should be avoided in patients with a creatinine clearance less than 60 (few studies accepted GFR more than 40) mL/min as reduced renal function results in decreased active drug within the urine [100]. It is contraindicated in pregnancy.

2.9.2.11. Cefoperazone-sulbactam

In a larger in vitro study, against the GNBs, a total of 18,386 organisms including 13,224 *Enterobacteriaceae* and 3536 *Pseudomonas* were collected (2013–2014) as part of the SENTRY Antimicrobial Surveillance Program. Cefoperazone/sulbactam inhibited 94% of *Enterobacteriaceae* [101]. There are limited clinical data on the usefulness of this agent against ESBL or CRE/CRP organisms in the urinary tract.

2.9.2.12. Ceftazidime-avibactam (Cef-Avb)

Ceftazidime, a third-generation cephalosporin, when combined with avibactam has potent activities against β-lactamase-producing Gram-negative pathogens including ESBL, AmpC β-lactamases, and *CRE*. Currently, Cef-Avb is approved for complicated UTIs (limited to patients without other treatment options in the empiric and documented treatment of MDROs).

In an in vitro study, it was tested against collection of international urinary isolates (1797 isolates were collected from 159 medical centers). All ESBL isolates as well as meropenem-non-susceptible *E. coli* and *K. pneumoniae* isolates were susceptible to Cef-Avb [102].

In another study, 34,062 isolates of *Enterobacteriaceae* from patients (with mostly UTIs) were collected (International Network for Optimal Resistance Monitoring, surveillance from 39 countries). Overall, 99.5% of isolates were susceptible to Cef-Avb. It was also active (99.9%) against molecularly confirmed ESBL-producing, plasmid-mediated AmpC-producing (100%), and ESBL- and AmpC-producing (100%). It lacks activity against the metallo-β-lactamase producers (NDM-1 enzyme) [103].

The REPRISE, an international, randomized, open-label trial, recruited 333 patients from 16 countries worldwide. The study recruited patients mostly with complicated UTIs caused by ceftazidime-resistant *Enterobacteriaceae* or *P. aeruginosa*. They were randomly assigned, 165 to Cef-Avb and 168 to best available therapy. The overall proportions of patients with a clinical cure were similar in the 2 arms [104].

In another clinical study, Cef-Avb was compared to imipenem-cilastatin in hospitalized adults with serious complicated UTI due to Gram-negative pathogens. Patients were allowed to switch to oral ciprofloxacin after at least 4 days on the study drug. Patients in the Cef-Avb group had a better microbiological response (70% vs. 71%) [105].

The RECAPTURE study recruited 033 patients, who were randomized in 2 arms, 393 received Cef-Avb and 417 received doripenem, with possible oral antibiotic switch (total duration was 10–14 days). Combined symptomatic resolution/microbiological were similar in the 2 arms (70.2% vs. 66.2%, respectively) [106].

In a recent study, the outcome of therapy with ceftazidime-avibactam (38 patients) was compared to the outcome of therapy with colistin (99 patients) with CRE infections. Most patients received additional anti-CRE agents as part of their treatment. All-cause hospital mortality at 30 days and after were 9% vs. 32%, respectively [107].

Salvage therapy: in a case series of 36 patients, mostly with life-threatening infections received Cef-Avb as a salvage therapy. The causative organisms were CRE (2 were CRP). In 65.8% of patients, other concurrent antibiotics were used. More than 70% of the patients experienced clinical and/or microbiological cure [108].

Resistance: in less than 2 years since its approval, resistant strains have been isolated. Cef-Avb-resistant *K. pneumoniae* emerged in 3 patients after using Cef-Avb for 10–19 days [109].

2.9.2.13. Ceftolozane-tazobactam (Cef-Taz)

This agent was approved in 2015 for the treatment of complicated urinary tract infections (adults with limited or no other therapeutic options) [110]. There are many in vitro studies that demonstrated activity against Gram-negative and Gram-positive microorganisms, including *E. cloacae, E. coli, K. oxytoca, K. pneumoniae, Proteus mirabilis, P. aeruginosa* as well as coverage of most ESBL-producing organisms and some anaerobes [110, 111].

Cef-Taz was tested in vitro against 3851 *P. aeruginosa* isolates collected from 32 U.S. hospitals. It was active against 97.0% of the isolates, which was better than 7 other broad spectra antibiotics. A total of 363 isolates were classified as extensively drug resistant; Cef-Taz was active against 76.9% of these isolates [112].

The ASPECT is a randomized, double-blind, double-dummy, non-inferiority trial over 25 countries. 1083 patients enrolled, of whom 82% had pyelonephritis. Patients were randomly assigned to receive Cef-Taz or intravenous high-dose levofloxacin for 7 days. Overall, the composite cure rates were higher in the Cef-Taz group than in the levofloxacin. In a subgroup analysis, clinical cure was seen in 90% compared with 73% in patients with ESBL-producing uropathogens [113].

2.9.2.14. Ceftaroline/avibactam

Ceftaroline is a cephalosporin with broad-spectrum activity against Gram-positive and Gram-negative organisms. When Ceftaroline combined with avibactam, it gains activities against many ESBL-producing organisms in vitro. It was tested in one study against 272 ESBL *Enterobacteriaceae* strains. All isolates were inhibited by ceftaroline-avibactam at ≤4 μg/mL; however, it exhibited limited activity against *Acinetobacter* spp. and *P. aeruginosa* [114].

There are no clinical studies that tested the activity of this agent on UTIs caused by any MDROs.

2.9.2.15. Ceftriaxone + sulbactam + disodium edetate (Elores)

It is a novel molecule, which combines β-lactam plus β-lactamase inhibitor. It has shown activities against many resistant Gram-negative bacterial infections. There is a limited data on its spectrum, usage (mostly in India), and its role in urinary tract infections in specific.

In one study, Elores activity was compared to other comparators (including carbapenems) in treating various infectious syndromes. There were 2500 patients enrolled in the study, in which 24% of the patients had UTIs (no specifics on severity or the causative organisms). The clinical cure/improvement was achieved in 98%. There was no clear description on the types or the incidence of resistant organisms in the study [115].

2.10. ESBL and CRE urinary tract infections with pregnancy

Few studies have been conducted regarding the prevalence of ESBL-producing organisms in pregnant women. In Ireland, a low figure of 1.63% of pregnant patients was colonized with ESBL organisms (perianal). Similar rates were seen in a Norwegian study (2.9%) [116].

Higher rates have been reported in other countries: 5.4% in Argentina and 15% in India [117]. In India, 47% in *E. coli*-related UTIs in pregnant patients were ESBL-producing *E. coli* [117–119].

Peripartum maternal transmission of ESBL organism to newborn infants was documented [120].

Recently, first outbreak of a CTX-M ESBL-producing *E. coli* in an Irish neonatal intensive care unit was reported. This outbreak was mediated by mother to neonate transmission [121].

Carbapenem are the drugs of choice for treating complicated UTIs and pyelonephritis due to ESBL pathogens in pregnancy [122]. In small studies, orally administered fosfomycin have been used to treat cystitis with ESBL pathogens with good success.

A case control study compared outcomes in pregnant women with ESBL-UTIs. Suboptimal treatment was noted in the majority of cases involving ESBL-UTIs (89%, n = 40), which was far more likely than what was observed for non-ESBL infections. Data support the importance of more aggressive treatment and follow-up of pregnant women with ESBL-UTIs to prevent secondary clinical pyelonephritis [123].

There are very limited data on CRE/CRP UTI in pregnancy. A case report of community-acquired pyelonephritis caused by KPC-producing isolate was reported in Australia [124].

Authors were refrained from using colistin, because of its toxicity in pregnancy (category C). Tigecycline was not considered either (category D). Rather, they added cefepime, which is regarded as safe in pregnancy (category B) and offers potential synergistic activity with fosfomycin, which is also an inhibitor of cell wall synthesis. In that study, the isolate was resistant to cefepime in vitro. By using 6 g/day as a continuous infusion, they estimated that levels in plasma of 20–30 μg/mL were maintained; moreover, cefepime achieved a very high concentration in the urine. Therefore, it has been reasoned that concentrations of cefepime sufficient to inhibit the growth of *K. pneumoniae* (MIC >32 μg/mL) would be maintained in the urine and genitourinary tract. This approach was successful, as proven by sterile urine cultures (obtained weekly while the patient was on cefepime and 6 weeks after the end of therapy) and the absence of symptoms.

For these challenging cases, a new drug (see above), ceftazidime-avibactam, has shown great activities against most of the ESBL and many of the CRE/CRP organisms. This novel agent is safe during pregnancy. However, there are no randomized trials to show this activity, and it should be considered as a salvage therapy [125].

2.11. Duration of therapy

The optimal length of treatment UTI with highly resistant organisms has not been extensively studied. As there are many different causes of underlying abnormality, a simple recommendation cannot be made. 10 to 14 days of antibiotics are usually recommended for patients with bacteremia, hypotension, and other signs of severe sepsis. Recent clinical trials included complicated urinary tract infections with resistant organisms that have used the study drugs for 10–14 days [93, 105, 106].

2.12. Infection-control

A successful infection program should be able to recognize, screen, and isolate both colonized and infected patients. Standard and transmission-based precautions are strictly applied at all times. Other basic measures including hand hygiene, use of personal protective barriers, and aggressive environmental cleaning are very beneficial. Implementation of simple items-bundles (multiple-drug resistant bundles MDROs) have shown to be very effective in controlling outbreaks.

Hospital-wide vs. high risk areas (ICU, dialysis centers) (routine vs. on outbreaks based) and clinical and bacteriological surveillance have been useful in early identifications and isolation of index cases. The use of molecular technologies including polymerase chain reaction (PCR) optimized the surveillance process [14].

A strict protocol including the above-mentioned interventions showed a great success in reducing the nosocomial spreading of the highly resistant organisms. During the intervention, nosocomial CRE acquisition in acute care declined from a monthly high of 55.5 to an annual low of 4.8 cases per 100,000 patient-days ($p < 0.001$) [126].

2.13. Antimicrobial stewardship

Multidisciplinary program including physicians, pharmacists, and microbiologists that aims to control the usage of antimicrobial is mandatory. In one study, carbapenem use was strictly restricted through antimicrobial stewardship in an effort to control MDROs spreading in an ICU setting. The study protocol also included strict environmental cleaning and disinfection in addition to basic infection control measures. The rate of hospital acquired MDRO *Acinetobacter* decreased from 22.82 cases per 1000 patient-days to 2.68 cases per 1000 patient-days after the protocol implementation ($p < 0.001$) [127].

2.14. Summary of recommended therapy

2.14.1. ESBL producing organisms

In general, carbapenems are the most reliable treatment for infections caused by ESBL-producing bacteria. As shown above, the over usage of these agents resulted in the emergence of the CRE. Multiple trials have shown other effective-carbapenem sparing regimens.

We proposed the following:

A. Uncomplicated cystitis caused by ESBL producing *E. coli* and without any indwelling catheters or obstruent: fosfomycin would be effective (and approved) therapy. In cystitis caused by other ESBL producing organism, fosfomycin alone was associated with significant clinical and microbiological failures.

On the other hand, our (and others) clinical exercise with monotherapy and single dose of fosfomycin was also associated with high rates of relapse. We also have great concerns about the rapid progression of fosfomycin resistance. This will require further research.

Meanwhile, we are proposing fosfomycin 3 g oral sachets twice a week for 3–4 doses with nitrofurantoin 100 mg twice a day for 10 days (if susceptible).

B. For complicated UTIs: monotherapy with carbapenems, piperacillin-tazobactam, aminoglycosides or ceftazidime-avibactam would be effective.

2.14.2. CRE/CRP producing organisms

Treatment of carbapenem-resistant organisms is a real challenge because of limited choices for effective reliable regimens. There are no randomized controlled trials evaluating different antibiotic options for carbapenemase producers. There are many observational studies; combination therapy appears to be superior to single-drug therapy. Combinations of a polymyxin, tigecycline, and meropenem have met with the greatest success. Meropenem has been used in these combinations despite a lack of in vitro susceptibility. Recently ceftazidime-avibactam is showing promising results. It has good activity against (nearly) all class A and class C β-lactamases as well as OXA-48 carbapenemases. However, it lacks activity against the metallo enzymes.

If we can summarize the data above:

2.15. For complicated UTIs/critically ill patients

1. Aminoglycosides (amikacin or gentamicin) or colistin.

   Plus: a carbapenem or

2. Ceftazidime-avibactam (single agent).
3. Tigecycline plus colistin or aminoglycosides: have been tried in few trials.
4. Triple combinations including aminoglycoside, carbapenem, colistin, rifampicin, tigecycline, and fosfomycin have demonstrated synergistic or bactericidal effects in few small studies.

Even with the above-mentioned regimens, failure of therapy is very common, as tigecycline and polymyxin do not have good clearance in the urine.

3. Conclusion

The rapid and global spread of antimicrobial-resistant organisms in recent years is a global challenge. The overuse of antimicrobial use in humans and animals coupled with increased global connectivity facilitated the transmission of Gram-negative infections harboring extended-spectrum β-lactamases. When treating these infections, clinicians have a few effective antimicrobials to choose from and many are associated with significant adverse effects. Definitive therapy should always be guided by susceptibility testing. Expert consultation with an infectious disease specialist is recommended.

Declaration of interest

The authors report no conflicts of interest.

Author details

Nashaat S. Hamza* and Abdalla Khalil

*Address all correspondence to: nashaat11@hotmail.com

The International Medical Center, Jeddah, KSA

References

[1] Flores-Mireles AL, Walker JN, Caparon M. Urinary tract infections: Epidemiology, mechanisms of infection and treatment options. Nature Reviews. Microbiology. 2015;**13**:269-284. DOI: 10.1038/nrmicro3432

[2] Thaden JT, Pogue JM, Kaye KS. Role of newer and re-emerging older agents in the treatment of infections caused by carbapenem-resistant Enterobacteriaceae. Virulence. 2016;**7**:1-14. DOI: 10.1080/21505594.2016.1207834

[3] de Kraker ME, Wolkewitz M, Davey PG. Burden of antimicrobial resistance in European hospitals: Excess mortality and length of hospital stay associated with bloodstream infections due to *Escherichia coli* resistant to third-generation cephalosporins. The Journal of Antimicrobial Chemotherapy. 2011;**66**:398-407. DOI: 10.1093/jac/dkq412

[4] Falagas ME, Lourida P, Poulikakos P. Antibiotic treatment of infections due to carbapenem-resistant Enterobacteriaceae: Systematic evaluation of the available evidence. Antimicrobial Agents and Chemotherapy. 2014;**58**:654-663. DOI: 10.1128/AAC.01222-13

[5] Majeed A, Alarfaj S, Darouiche R. An update on emerging therapies for urinary tract infections. Expert Opinion on Emerging Drugs. 2017;**22**:53-62. DOI: 10.1080/14728214.2017.1293650

[6] Tumbarello M, Viale P, Viscoli C. Predictors of mortality in bloodstream infections caused by *Klebsiella pneumoniae* carbapenemase-producing *K. pneumoniae*: Importance of combination therapy. Clinical Infectious Diseases. 2012;**55**:943-950. DOI: 10.1093/cid/cis588

[7] Zowawi HM, Harris PN, Roberts MJ. The emerging threat of multidrug-resistant Gram-negative bacteria in urology. Nature Reviews Urology. 2015;**12**:570-584. DOI: 10.1038/nrurol.2015.199

[8] Ruppe E, Woerther PL, Barbier F. Mechanisms of antimicrobial resistance in Gram-negative bacilli. Annals of Intensive Care. 2015;**5**:61. DOI: 10.1186/s13613-015-0061-0

[9] Magiorakos AP, Srinivasan A, Carey RB. Multidrug-resistant, extensively drug-resistant and pandrug-resistant bacteria: An international expert proposal for interim standard definitions for acquired resistance. Clinical Microbiology and Infection. 2012;**18**:268-281. DOI: 10.1111/j.1469-0691.2011.03570.x

[10] Kallen AJ, Srinivasan A. Current epidemiology of multidrug-resistant gram-negative bacilli in the United States. Infection Control and Hospital Epidemiology. 2010;**31**(Suppl 1):S51-S54. DOI: 10.1086/655996

[11] Pallett A, Hand K. Complicated urinary tract infections: Practical solutions for the treatment of multiresistant Gram-negative bacteria. Journal of Antimicrobial Chemotherapy. 2010;**65**(Suppl 3):iii25-iii33. DOI: 10.1093/jac/dkq298

[12] Bader MS, Loeb M, Brooks AA. An update on the management of urinary tract infections in the era of antimicrobial resistance. Postgraduate Medicine. 2017;**129**:242-258. DOI: 10.1080/00325481.2017.1246055

[13] Ena J, Arjona F, Martinez-Peinado C. Epidemiology of urinary tract infections caused by extended-spectrum beta-lactamase-producing *Escherichia coli*. Urology. 2006;**68**:1169-1174. DOI: 10.1016/j.urology.2006.08.1075

[14] van Duin D, Doi Y. The global epidemiology of carbapenemase-producing Enterobacteriaceae. Virulence. 2017;**8**:460-469. DOI: 10.1080/21505594.2016.1222343

[15] Padmini N, Ajilda AA, Sivakumar N. Extended spectrum beta-lactamase producing *Escherichia coli* and *Klebsiella pneumoniae*: Critical tools for antibiotic resistance pattern. Journal of Basic Microbiology. 2017;**57**. DOI: 10.1002/jobm.201700008

[16] Bradford PA. Extended-spectrum beta-lactamases in the 21st century: Characterization, epidemiology, and detection of this important resistance threat. Clinical Microbiology Reviews. 2001;**14**:933-951, table of contents. DOI: 10.1128/CMR.14.4.933-951.2001

[17] Rupp ME, Fey PD. Extended spectrum beta-lactamase (ESBL)-producing Enterobacteriaceae: Considerations for diagnosis, prevention and drug treatment. Drugs. 2003;**63**:353-365

[18] Peirano G, Costello M, Pitout JD. Molecular characteristics of extended-spectrum beta-lactamase-producing *Escherichia coli* from the Chicago area: High prevalence of ST131 producing CTX-M-15 in community hospitals. International Journal of Antimicrobial Agents. 2010;**36**:19-23. DOI: 10.1016/j.ijantimicag.2010.02.016

[19] Briongos-Figuero LS, Gomez-Traveso T, Bachiller-Luque P. Epidemiology, risk factors and comorbidity for urinary tract infections caused by extended-spectrum beta-lactamase (ESBL)-producing enterobacteria. International Journal of Clinical Practice. 2012;**66**:891-896. DOI: 10.1111/j.1742-1241.2012.02991.x

[20] Fernando MM, Luke WA, Miththinda JK. Extended spectrum beta lactamase producing organisms causing urinary tract infections in Sri Lanka and their antibiotic susceptibility pattern—A hospital based cross sectional study. BMC Infectious Diseases. 2017;**17**:138. DOI: 10.1186/s12879-017-2250-y

[21] Zhang J, Zhou K, Zheng B. High prevalence of ESBL-producing *Klebsiella pneumoniae* causing community-onset infections in China. Frontiers in Microbiology. 2016;**7**:1830. DOI: 10.3389/fmicb.2016.01830

[22] Koksal I, Yilmaz G, Unal S. Epidemiology and susceptibility of pathogens from SMART 2011-12 Turkey: Evaluation of hospital-acquired versus community-acquired urinary tract infections and ICU- versus non-ICU-associated intra-abdominal infections. The Journal of Antimicrobial Chemotherapy. 2017;**72**:1364-1372. DOI: 10.1093/jac/dkw574

[23] Castillo-Tokumori F, Irey-Salgado C, Malaga G. Worrisome high frequency of extended-spectrum beta-lactamase-producing *Escherichia coli* in community-acquired urinary tract infections: A case-control study. International Journal of Infectious Diseases. 2017;**55**:16-19. DOI: 10.1016/j.ijid.2016.12.007

[24] Toner L, Papa N, Aliyu SH. Extended-spectrum beta-lactamase-producing Enterobacteriaceae in hospital urinary tract infections: Incidence and antibiotic susceptibility profile over 9 years. World Journal of Urology. 2016;**34**(7):1031. DOI: 10.1007/s00345-015-1718-x

[25] Hu FP, Guo Y, Zhu DM. Resistance trends among clinical isolates in China reported from CHINET surveillance of bacterial resistance, 2005-2014. Clinical Microbiology and Infection. 2016;**22**(Suppl 1):S9-14. DOI: 10.1016/j.cmi.2016.01.001

[26] Wener KM, Schechner V, Gold HS. Treatment with fluoroquinolones or with beta-lactam-beta-lactamase inhibitor combinations is a risk factor for isolation of extended-spectrum-beta-lactamase-producing Klebsiella species in hospitalized patients. Antimicrobial Agents and Chemotherapy. 2010;**54**:2010-2016. DOI: 10.1128/AAC.01131-09

[27] Azap OK, Arslan H, Serefhanoglu K. Risk factors for extended-spectrum beta-lactamase positivity in uropathogenic *Escherichia coli* isolated from community-acquired urinary tract infections. Clinical Microbiology and Infection. 2010;**16**:147-151. DOI: 10.1111/j.1469-0691.2009.02941.x

[28] Suarez CJ, Lolans K, Villegas MV. Mechanisms of resistance to beta-lactams in some common Gram-negative bacteria causing nosocomial infections. Expert Review of Anti-infective Therapy. 2005;**3**:915-922. DOI: 10.1586/14787210.3.6.915

[29] Soraas A, Sundsfjord A, Sandven I. Risk factors for community-acquired urinary tract infections caused by ESBL-producing enterobacteriaceae—A case-control study in a low prevalence country. PLoS One. 2013;**8**:e69581. DOI: 10.1371/journal.pone.0069581

[30] Lubbert C, Straube L, Stein C. Colonization with extended-spectrum beta-lactamase-producing and carbapenemase-producing Enterobacteriaceae in international travelers returning to Germany. International Journal of Medical Microbiology. 2015;**305**:148-156. DOI: 10.1016/j.ijmm.2014.12.001

[31] Brower CH, Mandal S, Hayer S. The prevalence of extended-spectrum beta-lactamase-producing multidrug-resistant *Escherichia coli* in poultry chickens and variation according to farming practices in Punjab, India. Environmental Health Perspectives. 2017;**125**:077015. DOI: 10.1289/EHP292

[32] Dickstein Y, Geffen Y, Andreassen S. Predicting antibiotic resistance in urinary tract infection patients with prior urine cultures. Antimicrobial Agents and Chemotherapy. 2016;**60**:4717-4721. DOI: 10.1128/AAC.00202-16

[33] Zowawi HM, Balkhy HH, Walsh TR. Beta-lactamase production in key gram-negative pathogen isolates from the Arabian peninsula. Clinical Microbiology Reviews. 2013;**26**: 361-380. DOI: 10.1128/CMR.00096-12

[34] Singh RM, Singh HL. Comparative evaluation of six phenotypic methods for detecting extended-spectrum beta-lactamase-producing Enterobacteriaceae. Journal of Infection in Developing Countries. 2014;**8**:408-415. DOI: 10.3855/jidc.4052

[35] Perez F, Bonomo RA. Editorial commentary: Bloodstream infection caused by extended-spectrum beta-lactamase-producing Gram-negative bacteria: How to define the best treatment regimen? Clinical Infectious Diseases. 2015;**60**:1326-1329. DOI: 10.1093/cid/civ007

[36] Chavda KD, Satlin MJ, Chen L. Evaluation of a multiplex PCR assay to rapidly detect Enterobacteriaceae with a broad range of beta-lactamases directly from perianal swabs. Antimicrobial Agents and Chemotherapy. 2016;**60**:6957-6961. DOI: 10.1128/AAC.01458-16

[37] Ben-David D, Kordevani R, Keller N. Outcome of carbapenem resistant *Klebsiella pneumoniae* bloodstream infections. Clinical Microbiology and Infection. 2012;**18**:54-60. DOI: 10.1111/j.1469-0691.2011.03478.x

[38] Villegas MV, Pallares CJ, Escandon-Vargas K. Characterization and clinical impact of bloodstream infection caused by Carbapenemase-producing Enterobacteriaceae in seven Latin American countries. PLoS One. 2016;**11**:e0154092. DOI: 10.1371/journal.pone.0154092

[39] Falagas ME, Tansarli GS, Karageorgopoulos DE. Deaths attributable to carbapenem-resistant Enterobacteriaceae infections. Emerging Infectious Diseases. 2014;**20**:1170-1175. DOI: 10.3201/eid2007.121004

[40] Tumbarello M, Sanguinetti M, Montuori E. Predictors of mortality in patients with bloodstream infections caused by extended-spectrum-beta-lactamase-producing Enterobacteriaceae: Importance of inadequate initial antimicrobial treatment. Antimicrobial Agents and Chemotherapy. 2007;**51**:1987-1994. DOI: 10.1128/AAC.01509-06

[41] Weist K, Hogberg LD. ECDC publishes 2015 surveillance data on antimicrobial resistance and antimicrobial consumption in Europe. Euro Surveillance. 2016;**21**. DOI: 10.2807/1560-7917.ES.2016.21.46.30399

[42] Parisi SG, Bartolini A, Santacatterina E. Prevalence of *Klebsiella pneumoniae* strains producing carbapenemases and increase of resistance to colistin in an Italian teaching hospital from January 2012 to December 2014. BMC Infectious Diseases. 2015;**15**:244. DOI: 10.1186/s12879-015-0996-7

[43] Spyropoulou A, Papadimitriou-Olivgeris M, Bartzavali C. A ten-year surveillance study of carbapenemase-producing *Klebsiella pneumoniae* in a tertiary care Greek university hospital: Predominance of KPC- over VIM- or NDM-producing isolates. Journal of Medical Microbiology. 2016;**65**:240-246. DOI: 10.1099/jmm.0.000217

[44] Poirel L, Nordmann P. Rapidec Carba NP test for rapid detection of Carbapenemase producers. Journal of Clinical Microbiology. 2015;**53**:3003-3008. DOI: 10.1128/JCM.00977-15

[45] Yoon YK, Kim JH, Sohn JW. Role of piperacillin/tazobactam as a carbapenem-sparing antibiotic for treatment of acute pyelonephritis due to extended-spectrum beta-lactamase-producing *Escherichia coli*. International Journal of Antimicrobial Agents. 2017;**49**:410-415. DOI: 10.1016/j.ijantimicag.2016.12.017

[46] Gibble AM, Gross AE, Huang AM. Examining the clinical effectiveness of non-carbapenem beta-lactams for the treatment of extended-Spectrum beta-lactamase-producing Enterobacteriaceae. Antibiotics (Basel). 2015;**4**:653-666. DOI: 10.3390/antibiotics4040653

[47] Pilmis B, Parize P, Zahar JR. Alternatives to carbapenems for infections caused by ESBL-producing Enterobacteriaceae. European Journal of Clinical Microbiology & Infectious Diseases. 2014;**33**:1263-1265. DOI: 10.1007/s10096-014-2094-y

[48] D'Angelo RG, Johnson JK, Bork JT. Treatment options for extended-spectrum beta-lactamase (ESBL) and AmpC-producing bacteria. Expert Opinion on Pharmacotherapy. 2016;**17**:953-967. DOI: 10.1517/14656566.2016.1154538

[49] Lee CH, Chu FY, Hsieh CC. A simple scoring algorithm predicting extended-spectrum beta-lactamase producers in adults with community-onset monomicrobial Enterobacteriaceae bacteremia: Matters of frequent emergency department users. Medicine (Baltimore). 2017;**96**:e6648. DOI: 10.1097/MD.0000000000006648

[50] Tamma PD, Rodriguez-Bano J. The use of Noncarbapenem beta-lactams for the treatment of extended-spectrum beta-lactamase infections. Clinical Infectious Diseases. 2017;**64**:972-980. DOI: 10.1093/cid/cix034

[51] Breilh D, Texier-Maugein J, Allaouchiche B. Carbapenems. Journal of Chemotherapy. 2013;**25**:1-17. DOI: 10.1179/1973947812Y.0000000032

[52] Carbapenems for Multi-Drug Resistant Infections: A Review of Guidelines. CADTH Rapid Response Reports. Ottawa (ON): Canadian Agency for Drugs and Technologies in Health; 2016

[53] Golan Y. Empiric therapy for hospital-acquired, Gram-negative complicated intra-abdominal infection and complicated urinary tract infections: A systematic literature review of current and emerging treatment options. BMC Infectious Diseases. 2015;**15**:313. DOI: 10.1186/s12879-015-1054-1

[54] Kaniga K, Flamm R, Tong SY. Worldwide experience with the use of doripenem against extended-spectrum-beta-lactamase-producing and ciprofloxacin-resistant Enterobacteriaceae: Analysis of six phase 3 clinical studies. Antimicrobial Agents and Chemotherapy. 2010;**54**:2119-2124. DOI: 10.1128/AAC.01450-09

[55] Gutierrez-Gutierrez B, Bonomo RA, Carmeli Y. Ertapenem for the treatment of bloodstream infections due to ESBL-producing Enterobacteriaceae: A multinational pre-registered cohort study. The Journal of Antimicrobial Chemotherapy. 2016;**71**:1672-1680. DOI: 10.1093/jac/dkv502

[56] Watanabe A, Fujimura S, Kikuchi T. Evaluation of dosing designs of carbapenems for severe respiratory infection using Monte Carlo simulation. Journal of Infection and Chemotherapy. 2007;**13**:332-340. DOI: 10.1007/s10156-007-0562-3

[57] Betriu C, Gomez M, Lopez-Fabal F. Activity of doripenem against extended-spectrum beta-lactamase-producing Enterobacteriaceae and *Pseudomonas aeruginosa* isolates. European Journal of Clinical Microbiology & Infectious Diseases. 2010;**29**:1179-1181. DOI: 10.1007/s10096-010-0974-3

[58] Gutierrez-Gutierrez B, Salamanca E, de Cueto M. Effect of appropriate combination therapy on mortality of patients with bloodstream infections due to carbapenemase-producing Enterobacteriaceae (INCREMENT): A retrospective cohort study. The Lancet Infectious Diseases. 2017;**17**:726-734. DOI: 10.1016/S1473-3099(17)30228-1

[59] Drawz SM, Bonomo RA. Three decades of beta-lactamase inhibitors. Clinical Microbiology Reviews. 2010;**23**:160-201. DOI: 10.1128/CMR.00037-09

[60] Seo YB, Lee J, Kim YK. Randomized controlled trial of piperacillin-tazobactam, cefepime and ertapenem for the treatment of urinary tract infection caused by extended-spectrum beta-lactamase-producing *Escherichia coli*. BMC Infectious Diseases. 2017;**17**:404. DOI: 10.1186/s12879-017-2502-x

[61] Harris PN, Peleg AY, Iredell J. Meropenem versus piperacillin-tazobactam for definitive treatment of bloodstream infections due to ceftriaxone non-susceptible *Escherichia coli* and Klebsiella spp (the MERINO trial): Study protocol for a randomised controlled trial. Trials. 2015;**16**:24. DOI: 10.1186/s13063-014-0541-9

[62] Rodriguez-Bano J, Navarro MD, Retamar P. Beta-lactam/beta-lactam inhibitor combinations for the treatment of bacteremia due to extended-spectrum beta-lactamase-producing *Escherichia coli*: A post hoc analysis of prospective cohorts. Clinical Infectious Diseases. 2012;**54**:167-174. DOI: 10.1093/cid/cir790

[63] Tamma PD, Han JH, Rock C. Carbapenem therapy is associated with improved survival compared with piperacillin-tazobactam for patients with extended-spectrum beta-lactamase bacteremia. Clinical Infectious Diseases. 2015;**60**:1319-1325. DOI: 10.1093/cid/civ003

[64] Dewar S, Reed LC, Koerner RJ. Emerging clinical role of pivmecillinam in the treatment of urinary tract infection in the context of multidrug-resistant bacteria. The Journal of Antimicrobial Chemotherapy. 2014;**69**:303-308. DOI: 10.1093/jac/dkt368

[65] Chopra T, Marchaim D, Veltman J. Impact of cefepime therapy on mortality among patients with bloodstream infections caused by extended-spectrum-beta-lactamase-producing *Klebsiella pneumoniae* and *Escherichia coli*. Antimicrobial Agents and Chemotherapy. 2012;**56**:3936-3942. DOI: 10.1128/AAC.05419-11

[66] Lee NY, Lee CC, Huang WH. Cefepime therapy for monomicrobial bacteremia caused by cefepime-susceptible extended-spectrum beta-lactamase-producing Enterobacteriaceae: MIC matters. Clinical Infectious Diseases. 2013;**56**:488-495. DOI: 10.1093/cid/cis916

[67] Guet-Revillet H, Emirian A, Groh M. Pharmacological study of cefoxitin as an alternative antibiotic therapy to carbapenems in treatment of urinary tract infections due to extended-spectrum-beta-lactamase-producing *Escherichia coli*. Antimicrobial Agents and Chemotherapy. 2014;**58**:4899-4901. DOI: 10.1128/AAC.02509-14

[68] Matsumura Y, Yamamoto M, Nagao M. Multicenter retrospective study of cefmetazole and flomoxef for treatment of extended-spectrum-beta-lactamase-producing *Escherichia coli* bacteremia. Antimicrobial Agents and Chemotherapy. 2015;**59**:5107-5113. DOI: 10.1128/AAC.00701-15

[69] Kaye KS, Gales AC, Dubourg G. Old antibiotics for multidrug-resistant pathogens: From in vitro activity to clinical outcomes. International Journal of Antimicrobial Agents. 2017;**49**:542-548. DOI: 10.1016/j.ijantimicag.2016.11.020

[70] Ipekci T, Seyman D, Berk H. Clinical and bacteriological efficacy of amikacin in the treatment of lower urinary tract infection caused by extended-spectrum beta-lactamase-producing *Escherichia coli* or *Klebsiella pneumoniae*. Journal of Infection and Chemotherapy. 2014;**20**:762-767. DOI: 10.1016/j.jiac.2014.08.007

[71] Tzouvelekis LS, Markogiannakis A, Piperaki E. Treating infections caused by carbapenemase-producing Enterobacteriaceae. Clinical Microbiology and Infection. 2014;**20**:862-872. DOI: 10.1111/1469-0691.12697

[72] Talan DA, Takhar SS, Krishnadasan A. Fluoroquinolone-resistant and extended-spectrum beta-lactamase-producing *Escherichia coli* infections in patients with pyelonephritis, United States (1). Emerging Infectious Diseases. 2016;**22**:1594-1603. DOI: 10.3201/eid2209.160148

[73] Kantele A, Mero S, Kirveskari J. Fluoroquinolone antibiotic users select fluoroquinolone-resistant ESBL-producing Enterobacteriaceae (ESBL-PE)—Data of a prospective traveller study. Travel Medicine and Infectious Disease. 2017;**16**:23-30. DOI: 10.1016/j.tmaid.2017.01.003

[74] Someshwaran R, Prakash KG, Deshpande SA. Adherence to hospital antibiotic policy for treatment of *Escherichia coli* ESBL in urine. Journal of Clinical and Diagnostic Research. 2016;**10**:DC01-4. DOI: 10.7860/JCDR/2016/16084.7382

[75] Tiengrim S, Phiboonbanakit D, Thunyaharn S. Comparative in vitro activity of sitafloxacin against bacteria isolated from Thai patients with urinary tract infections and lower respiratory tract infections. Journal of the Medical Association of Thailand. 2012;**95**(Suppl 2):S6-17

[76] Malaisri C, Phuphuakrat A, Wibulpolprasert A. A randomized controlled trial of sitafloxacin vs. ertapenem as a switch therapy after treatment for acute pyelonephritis caused by extended-spectrum beta-lactamase-producing *Escherichia coli*: A pilot study. Journal of Infection and Chemotherapy. 2017;**23**. DOI: 10.1016/j.jiac.2017.05.005

[77] Gupta K, Hooton TM, Naber KG. International clinical practice guidelines for the treatment of acute uncomplicated cystitis and pyelonephritis in women: A 2010 update by the Infectious Diseases Society of America and the European Society for Microbiology and Infectious Diseases. Clinical Infectious Diseases. 2011;**52**:e103-e120. DOI: 10.1093/cid/ciq257

[78] Karlowsky JA, Denisuik AJ, Lagace-Wiens PR. In vitro activity of fosfomycin against *Escherichia coli* isolated from patients with urinary tract infections in Canada as part of the CANWARD surveillance study. Antimicrobial Agents and Chemotherapy. 2014;**58**:1252-1256. DOI: 10.1128/AAC.02399-13

[79] Kaewpoowat Q, Ostrosky-Zeichner L. Tigecycline: A critical safety review. Expert Opinion on Drug Safety. 2015;**14**:335-342. DOI: 10.1517/14740338.2015.997206

[80] Drekonja DM, Johnson JR. Tigecycline treatment for urinary tract infections: Case report and literature review. Journal of Chemotherapy. 2011;**23**:168-170. DOI: 10.1179/joc.2011.23.3.168

[81] Brust K, Evans A, Plemmons R. Tigecycline in treatment of multidrug-resistant Gram-negative bacillus urinary tract infections: A systematic review. The Journal of Antimicrobial Chemotherapy. 2014;**69**(10):2606. DOI: 10.1093/jac/dku189

[82] Cunha BA. Pharmacokinetic considerations regarding tigecycline for multidrug-resistant (MDR) *Klebsiella pneumoniae* or MDR *Acinetobacter baumannii* urosepsis. Journal of Clinical Microbiology. 2009;**47**:1613. DOI: 10.1128/JCM.00404-09

[83] van Duin D, Cober ED, Richter SS. Tigecycline therapy for carbapenem-resistant *Klebsiella pneumoniae* (CRKP) bacteriuria leads to tigecycline resistance. Clinical Microbiology and Infection. 2014;**20**:O1117-O1120. DOI: 10.1111/1469-0691.12714

[84] Zavascki AP, Nation RL. Nephrotoxicity of Polymyxins: Is there any difference between Colistimethate and Polymyxin B? Antimicrobial Agents and Chemotherapy. 2017;**61**: e02319-16. DOI: 10.1128/AAC.02319-16

[85] Lenhard JR, Nation RL, Tsuji BT. Synergistic combinations of polymyxins. International Journal of Antimicrobial Agents. 2016;**48**:607-613. DOI: 10.1016/j.ijantimicag.2016.09.014

[86] Zusman O, Altunin S, Koppel F. Polymyxin monotherapy or in combination against carbapenem-resistant bacteria: Systematic review and meta-analysis. The Journal of Antimicrobial Chemotherapy. 2017;**72**:29-39. DOI: 10.1093/jac/dkw377

[87] Liu YY, Wang Y, Walsh TR. Emergence of plasmid-mediated colistin resistance mechanism MCR-1 in animals and human beings in China: A microbiological and molecular biological study. The Lancet Infectious Diseases. 2016;**16**:161-168. DOI: 10.1016/S1473-3099(15)00424-7

[88] Giamarellou H. Epidemiology of infections caused by polymyxin-resistant pathogens. International Journal of Antimicrobial Agents. 2016;**48**:614-621. DOI: 10.1016/j.ijantimicag.2016.09.025

[89] Falagas ME, Vouloumanou EK, Samonis G. Fosfomycin. Clinical Microbiology Reviews. 2016;**29**:321-347. DOI: 10.1128/CMR.00068-15

[90] Jacobson S, Junco Noa L, Ahmed S. Efficacy and safety of oral fosfomycin for urinary tract infections in hospitalized patients. Antimicrobial Agents and Chemotherapy. 2016;**60**:1952. DOI: 10.1128/AAC.02971-15

[91] Sastry S, Doi Y. Fosfomycin: Resurgence of an old companion. Journal of Infection and Chemotherapy. 2016;**22**:273-280. DOI: 10.1016/j.jiac.2016.01.010

[92] Seroy JT, Grim SA, Reid GE. Treatment of MDR urinary tract infections with oral fosfomycin: A retrospective analysis. The Journal of Antimicrobial Chemotherapy. 2016;**71**:2563-2568. DOI: 10.1093/jac/dkw178

[93] Linsenmeyer K, Strymish J, Weir S. Activity of Fosfomycin against extended-spectrum-beta-lactamase-producing uropathogens in patients in the community and hospitalized patients. Antimicrobial Agents and Chemotherapy. 2016;**60**:1134-1136. DOI: 10.1128/AAC.02614-15

[94] Falagas ME, Kastoris AC, Kapaskelis AM. Fosfomycin for the treatment of multidrug-resistant, including extended-spectrum beta-lactamase producing, Enterobacteriaceae infections: A systematic review. The Lancet Infectious Diseases. 2010;**10**:43-50. DOI: 10.1016/S1473-3099(09)70325-1

[95] Senol S, Tasbakan M, Pullukcu H. Carbapenem versus fosfomycin tromethanol in the treatment of extended-spectrum beta-lactamase-producing *Escherichia coli*-related complicated lower urinary tract infection. Journal of Chemotherapy. 2010;**22**:355-357. DOI: 10.1179/joc.2010.22.5.355

[96] Michalopoulos A, Virtzili S, Rafailidis P. Intravenous fosfomycin for the treatment of nosocomial infections caused by carbapenem-resistant *Klebsiella pneumoniae* in critically ill patients: A prospective evaluation. Clinical Microbiology and Infection. 2010;**16**:184-186. DOI: 10.1111/j.1469-0691.2009.02921.x

[97] Banerjee S, Sengupta M, Sarker TK. Fosfomycin susceptibility among multidrug-resistant, extended-spectrum beta-lactamase-producing, carbapenem-resistant uropathogens. Indian Journal of Urology. 2017;**33**:149-154. DOI: 10.4103/iju.IJU_285_16

[98] Huang L, Hu YY, Zhang R. Prevalence of fosfomycin resistance and plasmid-mediated fosfomycin-modifying enzymes among carbapenem-resistant Enterobacteriaceae in Zhejiang, China. Journal of Medical Microbiology. 2017;**66**:1332-1334. DOI: 10.1099/jmm.0.000578

[99] Tasbakan MI, Pullukcu H, Sipahi OR. Nitrofurantoin in the treatment of extended-spectrum beta-lactamase-producing *Escherichia coli*-related lower urinary tract infection. International Journal of Antimicrobial Agents. 2012;**40**(6):554. DOI: 10.1016/j.ijantimicag.2012.08.003

[100] Oplinger M, Andrews CO. Nitrofurantoin contraindication in patients with a creatinine clearance below 60 mL/min: Looking for the evidence. The Annals of Pharmacotherapy. 2013;**47**:106-111. DOI: 10.1345/aph.1R352

[101] Pfaller MA, Flamm RK, Duncan LR. Antimicrobial activity of tigecycline and cefoperazone/sulbactam tested against 18,386 Gram-negative organisms from Europe and the Asia-Pacific region (2013-2014). Diagnostic Microbiology and Infectious Disease. 2017;**88**:177-183. DOI: 10.1016/j.diagmicrobio.2017.02.020

[102] Flamm RK, Sader HS, Farrell DJ. Ceftazidime-avibactam and comparator agents tested against urinary tract isolates from a global surveillance program (2011). Diagnostic Microbiology and Infectious Disease. 2014;**80**:233-238. DOI: 10.1016/j.diagmicrobio.2014.07.005

[103] Karlowsky JA, Biedenbach DJ, Kazmierczak KM. Activity of ceftazidime-avibactam against extended-spectrum- and AmpC beta-lactamase-producing Enterobacteriaceae collected in the INFORM global surveillance study from 2012 to 2014. Antimicrobial Agents and Chemotherapy. 2016;**60**:2849-2857. DOI: 10.1128/AAC.02286-15

[104] Carmeli Y, Armstrong J, Laud PJ. Ceftazidime-avibactam or best available therapy in patients with ceftazidime-resistant Enterobacteriaceae and *Pseudomonas aeruginosa* complicated urinary tract infections or complicated intra-abdominal infections (REPRISE): A randomised, pathogen-directed, phase 3 study. The Lancet Infectious Diseases. 2016;**16**:661-673. DOI: 10.1016/S1473-3099(16)30004-4

[105] Vazquez JA, Gonzalez Patzan LD, Stricklin D. Efficacy and safety of ceftazidime-avibactam versus imipenem-cilastatin in the treatment of complicated urinary tract infections, including acute pyelonephritis, in hospitalized adults: Results of a prospective, investigator-blinded, randomized study. Current Medical Research and Opinion. 2012;**28**:1921-1931. DOI: 10.1185/03007995.2012.748653

[106] Roberts MJ, Bennett HY, Harris PN. Prostate biopsy-related infection: A systematic review of risk factors, prevention strategies, and management approaches. Urology. 2017;**104**:11-21. DOI: 10.1016/j.urology.2016.12.011

[107] van Duin D, Lok JJ, Earley M. Colistin vs. Ceftazidime-avibactam in the treatment of infections due to Carbapenem-resistant Enterobacteriaceae. Clinical Infectious Diseases. 2017;**65**. DOI: 10.1093/cid/cix783

[108] Temkin E, Torre-Cisneros J, Beovic B. Ceftazidime-Avibactam as salvage therapy for infections caused by Carbapenem-resistant organisms. Antimicrobial Agents and Chemotherapy. 2017;**61**:e01964-16. DOI: 10.1128/AAC.01964-16

[109] Shields RK, Chen L, Cheng S. Emergence of Ceftazidime-Avibactam resistance due to plasmid-borne blaKPC-3 mutations during treatment of Carbapenem-resistant *Klebsiella pneumoniae* infections. Antimicrobial Agents and Chemotherapy. 2017;**61**:e02097-16 DOI: 10.1128/AAC.02097-16

[110] Pfaller MA, Bassetti M, Duncan LR. Ceftolozane/tazobactam activity against drug-resistant Enterobacteriaceae and *Pseudomonas aeruginosa* causing urinary tract and intraabdominal infections in Europe: Report from an antimicrobial surveillance programme (2012-15). The Journal of Antimicrobial Chemotherapy. 2017;**72**:1386-1395. DOI: 10.1093/jac/dkx009

[111] Scott LJ. Ceftolozane/tazobactam: A review in complicated intra-abdominal and urinary tract infections. Drugs. 2016;**76**:231-242. DOI: 10.1007/s40265-015-0524-5

[112] Shortridge D, Castanheira M, Pfaller MA. Ceftolozane-tazobactam activity against *Pseudomonas aeruginosa* clinical isolates from U.S. Hospitals: Report from the PACTS Antimicrobial Surveillance Program, 2012 to 2015. Antimicrobial Agents and Chemotherapy. 2017;**61**:e0465-17. DOI: 10.1128/AAC.00465-17

[113] Wagenlehner FM, Umeh O, Steenbergen J. Ceftolozane-tazobactam compared with levofloxacin in the treatment of complicated urinary-tract infections, including pyelonephritis: A randomised, double-blind, phase 3 trial (ASPECT-cUTI). Lancet. 2015;**385**:1949-1956. DOI: 10.1016/S0140-6736(14)62220-0

[114] Castanheira M, Sader HS, Farrell DJ. Activity of ceftaroline-avibactam tested against Gram-negative organism populations, including strains expressing one or more beta-lactamases and methicillin-resistant *Staphylococcus aureus* carrying various staphylococcal cassette chromosome mec types. Antimicrobial Agents and Chemotherapy. 2012;**56**:4779-4785. DOI: 10.1128/AAC.00817-12

[115] Chaudhary M, Mir MA, Ayub SG. Safety and efficacy of a novel drug elores (ceftriaxone+sulbactam+disodium edetate) in the management of multi-drug resistant bacterial infections in tertiary care centers: A post-marketing surveillance study. The Brazilian Journal of Infectious Diseases. 2017;**21**:408-417. DOI: 10.1016/j.bjid.2017.02.007

[116] Rettedal S, Lohr IH, Bernhoff E. Extended-spectrum beta-lactamase-producing Enterobacteriaceae among pregnant women in Norway: Prevalence and maternal-neonatal transmission. Journal of Perinatology. 2015;**35**:907-912. DOI: 10.1038/jp.2015.82

[117] Pathak A, Chandran SP, Mahadik K. Frequency and factors associated with carriage of multi-drug resistant commensal Escherichia Coli among women attending antenatal clinics in central India. BMC Infectious Diseases. 2013;**13**:199. DOI: 10.1186/1471-2334-13-199

[118] Villar HE, Aubert V, Baserni MN. Maternal carriage of extended-spectrum beta-lactamase-producing *Escherichia coli* isolates in Argentina. Journal of Chemotherapy. 2013;**25**:324-327. DOI: 10.1179/1973947813Y.0000000081

[119] Rizvi M, Khan F, Shukla I. Rising prevalence of antimicrobial resistance in urinary tract infections during pregnancy: Necessity for exploring newer treatment options. Journal of Laboratory Physicians. 2011;**3**:98-103. DOI: 10.4103/0974-2727.86842

[120] Peretz A, Skuratovsky A, Khabra E. Peripartum maternal transmission of extended-spectrum beta-lactamase organism to newborn infants. Diagnostic Microbiology and Infectious Disease. 2017;**87**:168-171. DOI: 10.1016/j.diagmicrobio.2016.11.004

[121] O'Connor C, Philip RK, Kelleher J. The first occurrence of a CTX-M ESBL-producing *Escherichia coli* outbreak mediated by mother to neonate transmission in an Irish neonatal intensive care unit. BMC Infectious Diseases. 2017;**17**:16. DOI: 10.1186/s12879-016-2142-6

[122] Hutley EJ, Chand MA, Hounsome G. Fosfomycin: An oral agent for urinary infection caused by extended spectrum beta-lactamase producing organisms. The Journal of Infection. 2010;**60**:308-309. DOI: 10.1016/j.jinf.2010.01.006

[123] Eppes CS, Clark SL. Extended-spectrum beta-lactamase infections during pregnancy: A growing threat. American Journal of Obstetrics and Gynecology. 2015;**213**:650-652. DOI: 10.1016/j.ajog.2015.03.020

[124] Khatri A, Naeger Murphy N, Wiest P. Community-acquired pyelonephritis in pregnancy caused by KPC-producing *Klebsiella pneumoniae*. Antimicrobial Agents and Chemotherapy. 2015;**59**(8):4375. DOI: 10.1128/AAC.00553-15

[125] van Duin D, Bonomo RA. Ceftazidime/Avibactam and Ceftolozane/Tazobactam: Second-generation beta-lactam/beta-lactamase inhibitor combinations. Clinical Infectious Diseases. 2016;**63**:234-241. DOI: 10.1093/cid/ciw243

[126] Schwaber MJ, Carmeli Y. An ongoing national intervention to contain the spread of carbapenem-resistant enterobacteriaceae. Clinical Infectious Diseases. 2014;**58**:697-703. DOI: 10.1093/cid/cit795

[127] Cheon S, Kim MJ, Yun SJ. Controlling endemic multidrug-resistant *Acinetobacter baumannii* in intensive care units using antimicrobial stewardship and infection control. The Korean Journal of Internal Medicine. 2016;**31**:367-374. DOI: 10.3904/kjim.2015.178

4

The Pathogenesis of *Escherichia Coli* Urinary Tract Infection

Timothy Kudinha

Abstract

Urinary tract infections (UTIs) are the commonest human bacterial infections and are responsible for substantial morbidity and mortality, resulting in increased healthcare costs. Most UTIs are caused by specialized *Escherichia coli* (*E. coli*) strains referred to as uropathogenic *E. coli* (UPEC). UPEC possess a variety of virulence factors (VFs), which the organism uses to attach, invade, and injure the host. These VFs include adhesins, toxins, iron acquisition factors, lipopolysacharide capsules, and other invasins. Most studies on UTI pathogenesis have targeted VFs. The source of UPEC is the host's fecal flora. According to the pathogenicity theory, UPEC strains with special VFs move from the host's fecal flora to the urogenital tract and cause UTI. However, another theory states that the numerically abundant strain is responsible for UTI. Effective UTI management is hampered by the recent rise in antibiotic resistance, specifically, the recent emergence of multidrug-resistant *E. coli* sequence type 131. The distribution of VFs and other bacterial characteristics among different patient groups and UTI syndromes, is crucial understanding UTI pathogenesis, which would guide clinical decision making. For ST131 clonal group, further epidemiological studies are needed to clarify transmission pathways, risk factors for spread, and reservoirs, so that effective control measures can be devised.

Keywords: *Escherichia coli*, urinary tract infections, virulence factors, multidrug resistance

1. Introduction

Urinary tract infections (UTIs) are an important medical problem, being the second most com mon bacterial infection of humans after respiratory tract infection. They are often recurrent, frequently difficult to treat, and can cause parenchymal damage to the kidney, leading to renal insufficiency and further complications [1–3]. UTIs impose a substantial burden on society and the health care system in relation to diagnosis, management, lost productivity, morbidity, and sometimes death [4–6]. Furthermore, increasing resistance to therapeutically important antimicrobial agents and the recent emergence of the virulent and multidrug-resistant ST131 clonal group have made UTI management progressively more costly and challenging [7, 8]. Several studies suggest that a greater array of VFs is generally needed to cause more invasive UTIs, although the extent appears to differ according to age and gender. Thus, further studies targeting VFs, which have been proposed as the best target for vaccine development, are needed. A better understanding of UTI pathogenesis, especially for the most common cause of UTI, namely *Escherichia coli,* is crucial for treatment and prevention of UTIs.

2. Etiology of UTI

UTIs are mainly caused by bacteria, although fungi and some viruses have also been implicated. Among bacteria, Gram-negative bacteria of the *Enterobacteriaceae* family, including *E. coli, Klebsiella, Enterobacter, Proteus* species, *etc.*, are mostly involved. However, some Gram-positive organisms, principally *Staphylococcus aureus, Staphylococcus saprophyticus* and *Streptococcus agalactiae,* also play a role especially among young women. *E. coli* is the dominant causative agent in all patient groups, causing 80–90% of all UTIs [5]. Consequently, *E. coli* serves as a model pathogen for studying UTI pathogenesis.

Escherichia coli is a normal constituent of the intestinal microbiota of humans and animals [9, 10]. The distinctive *E. coli* strains that cause most UTIs have been designated uropathogenic *E. coli* (UPEC). They possess diverse virulence-associated factors (VFs) that assist them in attaching to, invading, and injuring the host, and include adhesins, toxins, siderophores, protective polysaccharide coatings, invasins, and serum resistance-associated proteins. The presence and numbers of such VFs predicts *in vivo* virulence [11].

3. Epidemiology and risk factors for *E. coli* UTI

Overall, UTI is more prevalent among females than males, attributable to the close proximity of the urogenital tract to the anus in females, the greater length of the male urethra, and the antibacterial activity of prostatic fluid in men [12, 13]. Functional, hormonal, and anatomical changes that occur during pregnancy predispose pregnant women to UTI [14]. UTI during pregnancy can result in devastating maternal and neonatal complications, including maternal sepsis, preterm labor, and premature delivery [14]. Thirty percent of patients with untreated asymptomatic bacteriuria (ASB) develop symptomatic cystitis and up to 50% develop pyelonephritis [13]. ASB is also associated with intrauterine growth retardation and low-birth-weight infants [13]. Up to 27% of preterm births have been associated with UTI in pregnancy [14].

Among bacterial infections in children, UTI ranks highly, even outnumbering bacterial meningitis, pneumonia, and bacteremia [15]. About 1% of infants < 3 months old develop UTI, with more males affected than females. Proper and urgent UTI management is crucial in children as an estimated 10–15% of children with UTI will develop permanent kidney damage, leading to other chronic diseases such as hypertension and renal insufficiency [16, 17].

The propensity of UTIs to recur, often within a few weeks or months after an initial acute infection, is a problem in UTI management. Approximately 20–30% of women will have a recurrent bladder infection within 6 months after an initial episode, and an additional 3% will experience a third infection [18, 19].

4. *E. coli* UTI pathogenesis

UTI pathogenesis is a complex process that is influenced by various host biological and behavioral factors, and by properties of the infecting pathogen, including VFs. This presents a challenge in epidemiological studies regarding the role of specific VFs in UTI pathogenesis because of the confounding effect of host factors.

In most noncompromised individuals, the urinary tract is normally sterile, and the entry of exogenous microorganisms is prevented by urine flow, secreted and tissue-associated antibacterial factors, and the bactericidal activities of effector immune cells. In most cases, the host fecal flora is the source of the infecting *E. coli* strain, and spreads via the perineal, vaginal, and periurethral areas to the lower urinary tract (i.e., urethra and bladder) where they may establish colonization [20]. Two hypotheses have been proposed to explain the movement of the organism from the fecal flora to the urinary tract. The prevalence hypothesis holds that the numerically most prevalent *E. coli* clones in the feces will be involved, whilst the pathogenicity theory holds that *E. coli* strains with enhanced virulence potential will be selected [20]. These two mechanisms may not be mutually exclusive, but instead may jointly contribute to UTI pathogenesis [21].

Although the host's fecal flora is the major source of the *E. coli* infecting strain, other proximal external reservoirs of the organism have been described. Community outbreaks of UTI have been reported [22–24], but without any evidence of person-to-person transmission. Foods and water have been proposed as possible vehicles of such outbreaks [22–24]. Specifically, extensive molecular similarities between *E. coli* from retail meat products and healthy or infected humans have been described [22]. Within-household spread of *E. coli* among co-habitating humans and their pets, including between sexual partners, have been confirmed [4, 10, 11]. The VFs of the invading bacteria and the host's defense mechanisms determine the outcome of the infection [25]. A variety of host factors, such as age, gender, pregnancy, or immunological status, may predispose to UTI and allow less virulent pathogens to cause the disease [20]. If the infection is confined to the lower urinary tract, with symptoms such as dysuria and frequency of urination, the infection is referred to as acute cystitis. If the infection spreads to the upper urinary tract with symptoms such as flank pain, fever, and malaise, the infection is defined as an acute pyelonephritis.

5. Uropathogenic *E. coli* (UPEC) and virulence factors (VFs)

Virulence refers to the ability of an organism to cause disease, and is a function of the presence of distinct accessory traits, referred to as virulence factors (VFs). VFs are specific properties that enable organisms to overcome host defenses and cause disease [26]. However, although several VFs have been identified in UPEC, experimental and epidemiological data have shown that none uniquely defines these pathogens.

UPEC VFs are grouped by functional categories as adhesins, toxins, iron acquisition systems, and protectins. VFs are encoded by genes located on chromosomes or plasmids, with some being exclusively chromosomal (e.g., *pap* and *hly*), others exclusively or principally plasmid-associated, e.g., *iss* and *traT*, and some either chromosomal or plasmid-associated (*afa*). Consequently, VFs may be vertically or horizontally transmitted, further contributing to the complexity of understanding the role played by specific VF genes in UTI pathogenesis.

6. Structure of adhesins

Adhesins, which appear as hair-like fibers called fimbriae (or pili), facilitate the colonization with *E. coli* in the urinary tract by attaching to host epithelial cells. This attachment promotes the persistence of the organism in the bladder, and serves as a reservoir for ascending infection in the urinary tract [27].

Various adhesins have been identified and are classified mainly according to receptor specificity, with some being mannose resistant and others sensitive. P fimbriae (or pili), the best-described group of mannose-resistant adhesins of UPEC, are so named because they specifically bind to the Gal(α1–4) Gal disaccharide galabiose, which is an antigen within the human P blood group system [26]. Different components of the P fimbriae have been described, including four different units that are at the tip of the fibrillum, including PapG, PapE, PapF, and PapK [28–30]. These fimbrial proteins and other accessory proteins are encoded by a chromosomal multicistronic gene cluster termed *pap* (pilus associated with pyelonephritis), which can be carried on large chromosomal insertions called pathogenicity associated islands (PAIs) [31].

Actual attachment of the organism to host epithelial cells is effected through PapG by recognition of glycolipid receptors expressed on host kidney cells and red blood cells [32]. Three variants of PapG, encoded by distinct alleles of the corresponding gene, *pap*, have been identified, namely PapGI, PapGII, and PapGIII [32–34]. Most studies indicate that allele II is the main PapG variant in *E. coli* bacteremia (regardless of primary source), acute pyelonephritis, and acute prostatitis, whilst allele III predominates in acute cystitis [33, 9]. Other studies found statistically significant associations between allele III and several compromising host conditions, such as urinary anatomical abnormalities, diabetes [33, 35].

Type 1 fimbriae are the commonest adhesive organelles of *E. coli*. They mediate adhesion of the organism to secreted and cell-bound mannosylated glycoproteins and exhibit mannose sensitive hemagglutination of guinea pig erythrocytes [36]. The ubiquitous distribution of these fimbriae in *E. coli* makes it difficult to show an association with UTI outside an experimental setting. However, type 1 fimbriae exhibit several different phenotypes due to allelic variation of the gene for the lectin subunit, fimH, and these phenotypes have been shown to be distributed differentially among fecal and UTI isolates [37–39]. Type 1 fimbriae are encoded by a chromosomal fim gene cluster that contains genes for a structural subunit, an adhesin, several accessory proteins, and regulatory proteins (fimACDFGH) [30, 39].

Phase variation controls the expression of type 1 fimbriae by site specific recombination. A 314-bp phase-variable invertible element, that contains the promoter, controls the transcription of the fimbrial genes fimACDFGH. The promoter drives the expression of type 1 fimbriae when the switch is in the ON orientation but not when it is in the OFF orientation [40]. It has been shown that the expression of type 1 fimbriae coordinately affects the expression of P fimbriae in an inverse manner, providing evidence of a direct communication between genes related to pathogenesis [41, 42].

Although most studies have confirmed that type 1 fimbriae are particularly important in bladder colonization [43, 44], the proportions of UPEC strains from urine and feces expressing type 1 fimbriae appear to be similar [26], ranging from a high of 71% among isolates from cystitis patients to a low of 58% among those from patients with ASB, with fecal strains in the mid-range at 60% [26]. However, in contrast, the level of expression of type 1 fimbriae among UPEC blood isolates (81%) is significantly different from that of fecal strains [45, 46].

Another adhesin family is the Afa/Dr family, which consists of adhesins that include the uropathogen-associated fimbrial adhesin Dr, along with other nonfimbrial adhesins, including Afa-1, Afa-2, Afa-3, Afa 4, NFu1, and Dr-11. These adhesins have a different structure from other *E. coli* fimbrial adhesins in that they appear as fine mesh, a coil-like structure or as a filamentous capsule coating on the cell surface [45, 47, 48]. Epidemiological studies show that *E. coli* strains that express adhesins of the Afa/Dr family are involved in 25–50% of cases of cystitis in children, and 30% of cases of pyelonephritis in pregnant women [49]. Moreover, *E. coli* strains expressing Dr adhesins have been associated with a two-fold increase in the risk of a second UTI. It has also been shown that UPEC encoding the Dr adhesin could survive for more than 1 year within renal tissue [49, 50]. These findings suggest a possible role for Dr/Afa adhesins in recurrent or chronic UTI.

Finally, the closely-related S fimbriae and F1C (fimbriae of serotype 1C), so named because of their binding specificity for terminal sialyl-galactoside residues, mediate X-type mannose resistant hemagglutination of human erythrocytes [51–53]. They agglutinate human and bovine red cells [54, 55]. S fimbriae have a similar, but less well defined, structure to both type 1 and P fimbriae. Just like type 1 and P fimbriae, expression of S fimbriae exhibits phase variation [51]. Binding sites for S fimbriae are located on epithelial cells of the proximal and distal tubules, collecting ducts and glomerulus [55]. In humans, S-fimbriated *E. coli* strains are more closely associated with meningitis and bacteremia than with UTI [56]. They could therefore be important in the movement of the organism from the urinary tract to the blood stream. Few studies have been carried out on the role played by these two types of fimbriae in UTI pathogenesis. FIC fimbriae are expressed by about 14% of UPEC and 7% of *E. coli* fecal isolates [53].

7. Iron acquisition systems for UPEC

Bacteria and the host compete for available iron, which is needed for oxygen transport and storage, DNA synthesis, electron transport, and metabolism of peroxides [57, 58]. Pathogenic bacteria, including UPEC, have devised ways of accessing iron by producing siderophore-mediated iron transport systems. UPEC exhibit multiple mechanisms for extracting iron from the host, mainly siderophore-siderophore receptor systems, but also heme uptake [59–62]. Siderophores, which are secreted low molecular weight molecules, have a high affinity for ferric (Fe^{3+}) iron, which is insoluble as a free cation. UPEC retrieve iron-bound siderophores through receptors that facilitate the transportation of siderophore-iron complexes through the bacterial membrane and into the cytosol where the iron is concentrated and utilized. While all *E. coli* can produce the siderophore enterobactin, production of alternative siderophores has been shown to increase virulence of strains causing bacteremia [10].

Several enterobacteria contain a gene cluster called the high pathogenicity island (HPI), which encodes proteins for biosynthesis of the yersiniabactin siderophore and its uptake system [63, 64]. The HPI is widespread among members of the *Enterobacteriaceae* family, and is essential for virulence in *Yersinia* and certain pathotypes of *E. coli* [63]. One of the important genes residing on the HPI is *fyuA* encoding the 71 kDa outer membrane protein *FyuA* (ferric siderophore uptake), which act as a receptor for Fe-yersiniabactin uptake [65]. FyuA, which was first described in *Yersinia species*, is associated with virulence in many members of the *Enterobacteriaceae* family [65]. Studies by Hancock and Klemm have confirmed that the ferric yersiniabactin receptor (FyuA) is required by UPEC for efficient biofilm formation [66].

Aerobactin is another important hydroxamate siderophore synthesized from the condensation of two lysine and one citrate molecules. In UPEC, the aerobactin system is encoded by a five-gene operon with four genes encoding the enzymes needed for aerobactin synthesis and a fifth encoding the outer membrane receptor protein [67, 68]. The synthesis genes are designated *iuc*, for iron uptake and chelation and the receptor gene is *iut*, for iron uptake and transport [69]. Successive steps in the biosynthesis of aerobactin are catalyzed by the iuc genes and involve hydroxylation of lysine and acetylation of the hydroxyl group to form hydroxamic acid molecules which react with citrate to form aerobactin [69].

Previous studies have shown that the aerobactin system and P fimbriae are commonly found together in UPEC isolates from patients with UTI and urosepsis [70, 71]. However, among urosepsis patient isolates, this association is only true for chromosomally encoded aerobactin [71]. An association of chromosomally encoded aerobactin with hemolysin among urosepsis or UTI patient isolates has also been confirmed [71]. These observations suggest that the association of aerobactin with other VFs differs between plasmid and chromosomal aerobactin. Plasmids carrying the aerobactin region sometimes also carry antimicrobial resistance genes [71–73]. The aerobactin system is found more commonly among UPEC strains from patients with pyelonephritis (73%), cystitis (49%), or bacteremia (58%) than among ASB patient isolates (38%) or fecal strains (41%), which suggest that aerobactin contributes to virulence both within and outside of the urinary tract. The association of aerobactin with more serious forms of UTI is seen specifically in infants, girls, and women [26, 9].

Finally, UPEC produce salmochelins in order to access iron during invasion of the host. The salmochelin siderophore system, so named because it was first shown to be characteristic of *Salmonella* strains [74], is also present in UPEC. This siderophore system is encoded by *iroA* gene cluster, which is made up of five genes, *iroB, iroC, iroD, iroE,* and *iroN*. *iroN* gene encodes an outer membrane siderophore receptor which transports different catechol siderophores, including N-(2,3-dihydroxybenzoy)-L-serine and enterochelin. *iroB* encodes a glucosyltransferase that glucosylates enterobactin, *iroC* encodes an ABC transporter required for transport of salmochelins, whilst *iroD* and *iroE* encode a cytoplasmic esterase, and a periplasmic hydrolase, respectively [75]. The salmochelin receptor iroN may play a dual role as an iron uptake receptor as well as an internalization factor [10]. Using a neonatal rat model, it was shown that *iroN* plays a major role during the bacteremic step of the disease [76]. These findings suggest that *iroN* is associated with increased virulence. Studies by Bauer et al. showed that *iroN* occurred 2.1–4 times more frequently in UTI isolates than in rectal isolates [77].

8. Toxins produced by UPEC

Most hemolytic UPEC strains secrete a heat-labile cytolytic protein toxin known as alpha hemolysin [78], which is encoded by a polycistronic operon, consisting of four genes arranged in the order of hly-CADB [79]. The product of hlyC is important in the activation of the hemolytic toxin, which is the product of the *hlyA* gene. The gene products of *hlyB* and *hlyD* together with TolC are involved in secretion of the hemolysin through the bacterial cell wall [80]. The hemolysin determinants are located on the bacterial chromosome in human isolates of *E. coli*, in contrast to the plasmid location among animal strains [32].

Alpha hemolysin lyses red cells of all mammals and even of fish [81], and is toxic to host cells resulting in inflammation, tissue injury, and impaired host defenses. Hemolysin stimulates super-oxide anion and hydrogen peroxide release from and oxygen consumption by renal tubular cells, including histamine release from mast cells and basophils [82, 83]. Hemolytic uropathogenic strains almost always also express P fimbriae [84]. Hemolysin production is found most commonly in UPEC strains from patients with pyelonephritis (49%), followed by cystitis isolates and ASB [85]. These data demonstrate an association of hemolysin production with invasive uropathogenic strains. UPEC strains that produce increased amounts of alpha hemolysin are also more resistant to the complement action of human serum when compared to strains that are nonhemolytic or produce reduced amounts of hemolysin [81].

UPEC also produce a toxin referred to as cytotoxic necrotising factor type 1 (CNF-1). CNF-1 is a chromosomally encoded UPEC toxin that catalyzes the glutamine deamination of the small GTPases RhoA, Rac, and Cdc 42 [86], leading to the disturbance of numerous eukaryotic cellular functions including formation of actin stress fibers, lamellipodia, filopodia, and modulation of inflammatory signaling pathways [87, 88].

Yamamoto et al. showed that 61% of UTI isolates and 38% of bacteremia isolates produced CNF-1 as opposed to only 10% of commensal fecal isolates [89]. Of these isolates, approximately 98% that produced CNF-1 also produced hemolysin. Studies by Mitsumori et al. showed a

CNF-1 prevalence of 64% among UPEC isolates from prostatitis and 36% from pyelonephritis. These results suggest that CNF-1 is associated with increased virulence in UTI pathogenesis. CNF-1 production may also increase the inflammatory response of the host [90]. Specifically, Elliott et al. reported that CNF-1 evokes edema and necrosis and is associated with inflammation in the intestines of rabbits in a diarrhea model of infection [90]. Human neutrophils have been observed to be less effective at killing CNF-1 positive, than CNF-1 negative bacteria.

9. Protectins

UPEC also express outer membrane proteins, such as traT and Iss, which may enhance serum resistance through avoidance of complement killing [26]. Bacteria are killed by normal human serum through the lytic activity of the complement system [91]. The alternative pathway is activated by bacteria in the absence of specific antibody and plays a more important role in serum killing than the classic pathway [92]. Resistance of *E. coli* to killing by serum results from the individual or combined effects of capsular polysaccharide, O-polysaccharide side chains, and surface proteins [93].

Although the K1 capsule is important in certain strains, other mechanisms appear to be more significant determinants of serum resistance in some populations of *E. coli* isolates. On the whole, smooth strains are more serum resistant than rough strains [94] and the degree of serum resistance is proportional to the amount of lipopolysaccharide (O antigen) the strain contains [95]. Serum-resistant strains are usually more nephropathogenic than comparable serum-sensitive strains in a variety of models of UTI [96, 97] even though these resistant strains may not be associated with increased lethality [96].

9.1. Outer membrane protease T

Outer membrane protease T (OmpT) of *E. coli* is a surface membrane serine protease and is the prototypical member of the omptin family of Gram-negative bacteria [98]. OmpT is an enzyme that catalyzes the activation of plasminogen to plasmin [99, 100], a function that is physiologically relevant for the virulence of *Yersinia pestis* and for clinical *E. coli* isolates [101, 102]. OmpT also plays a role in virulence by cleavage of protamine and other cation peptides with antibiotic activity [103, 104]. Studies by Hui et al. indicated that OmpT promotes *E. coli* persistence in the urinary tract by interfering with the antimicrobial activity of urinary cationic peptides [100].

9.2. Uropathogenic specific protein

Uropathogenic specific protein (Usp) in *E. coli*, which was discovered by chance, is encoded by *usp* located on PAIs [105]. Usp, which is homologous to the *Vibrio cholerae* zonula occludens toxin gene [106], is significantly more prevalent among UPEC isolates than fecal *E. coli* isolates from healthy individuals. Several studies have shown various roles for Usp in UTI pathogenesis in different UTI syndromes and patient groups. Studies by Rijavec et al. showed a strong association between Usp and bacteremia of urinary tract origin, suggesting that Usp is important in the migration of UPEC from the urogenital tract to the blood stream [107]. Other studies have shown comparable prevalences of Usp in cystitis, pyelonephritis, and prostatitis isolates [108]. Furthermore, Usp has (frequently) been associated with all common serotypes of UPEC [109].

10. Biofilm production by UPEC

Biofilm production by *E. coli* is an important VF which may also protect bacteria from antibiotic action and so contribute to resistance [110–113]. Recent studies have shown that biofilm production in *E. coli,* mediated by co-expression of curli and cellulose, supports long-term survival of UPEC in the urinary tract by surrounding the organism with an inert, hydrophobic extracellular matrix [110, 113, 114]. Most studies of biofilm formation in UTI have addressed its role in recurrences.

Curli belong to a class of fibers known as amyloids and are involved in adhesion to surfaces, cell aggregation and, finally, biofilm development. Curli fibers are encoded in the curling subunit gene (*csg*) gene cluster, made up of two differently transcribed operons. One operon codes for *csgB, csgA,* and *csgC,* and the other one for *csgD, csgE,* and *csgG* [115]. Expression of both curli operons is important for curli fiber assembly. Curli fibers are also essential for internalization of bacteria during an infection [30].

Co-expression of curli and cellulose tends to decrease in prevalence from more severe to less severe UTI, then to commensal isolates, suggesting that biofilm may facilitate progression from the lower to upper urinary tract [110]. Furthermore, co-expression of both biofilm components is associated with a high prevalence of individual VF genes, high VF scores, and phylogenetic group B2, consistent with heightened urovirulence of such strains. Notably, there may be an interaction between classic VFs and biofilm formation. For example, in one study, all isolates that co-expressed both biofilm components also harbored fyuA, implying that iron uptake via the yersiniabactin system may play a significant role in biofilm growth [64]. Additionally, recent studies have shown that the biofilm components, curli fimbriae and cellulose, also play important roles in adhesion, invasion, and long-term survival of UPEC within the host urinary tract [110, 111].

11. Phylogenetic group and VF distribution among patient groups and clinical syndromes

E. coli is commonly classified into four main phylogenetic groups namely A, B1, B2, and D [116] as defined by multilocus enzyme electrophoresis and multilocus sequence typing [117]. Several studies have shown that *E. coli* pathogenic strains from extraintestinal infections mostly derive from group B2, and to a less extent group D [21, 118, 119]. Most studies quote prevalence rates around 63–65% for group B2 in pathogenic strains, and 10–15% for group D [21]. Commensal

E. coli are mainly associated with phylogenetic groups A or B1, and are mainly devoid of virulence determinants [118, 120, 121]. The overlapping associations of VFs and phylogeny with clinical virulence makes it difficult to understand which directly determines virulence. However, some studies in children showed that pyelonephritis isolates more often belonged to group B2, contained on average higher prevalences of individual VF genes, and consequently had higher VF scores than did cystitis or fecal isolates, suggesting that both VF repertoire and phylogenetic background play important roles in UTI pathogenesis.

UTI syndrome-specific differences among *E. coli* clinical and fecal isolates from men are consistent with findings from women, which have shown a gradient of virulence from *E. coli* strains causing more invasive UTI syndromes, such as pyelonephritis and febrile UTI, through those causing cystitis, to fecal strains [9, 122]. However, men are less likely than women or girls, to develop cystitis due to low-virulence strains, which is consistent with a previous observation that isolates from men with febrile UTI appeared relatively virulent, even in the presence of host compromise [122].

In most patient groups, pyelonephritis isolates tend to exhibit the highest prevalences of many individual VFs, have the highest VF scores, and are the most likely to belong to phylogenetic group B2, ST131, and a UTI-associated O type. The reported higher prevalence of pap operon genes (encoding P fimbriae) in pyelonephritis than cystitis isolates correlates with increased tropism for the kidney of P fimbriated strains [121, 123]. papGII has been shown, experimentally, to contribute to pathogenesis of pyelonephritis [124, 125], and OmpT is strongly associated with febrile UTI in men [122, 126]. However, it is not clear whether these VFs act individually or in concert with other known or unknown VFs in causing pyelonephritis.

In men and women, although cystitis and pyelonephritis isolates differ in inferred molecular virulence, phylogenetic group distribution is similar between the two clinical syndromes. However, within each phylogenetic group, VF scores exhibit a gradient across source groups (fecal < cystitis < pyelonephritis), suggesting the presence of different virulence strata within each phylogenetic group, with more virulent strains selectively causing pyelonephritis and less virulent strains being associated with cystitis and fecal isolates in that order. This suggests that VF repertoire is as, or more, important than phylogenetic background for predicting pathogenic behavior in UPEC [122, 127].

Although cystitis and pyelonephritis isolates differ significantly in inferred virulence in various patient groups, no single VF profile is unique to any clinical syndrome or patient group, implying that UTI pathogenesis is multiply determined, as suggested by several previous studies [122, 128]. Thus, intervention strategies based on VF genes might have to involve multiple targets, which would offer the extra advantage of protection against a wide range of UTI syndromes.

12. Transmission of VFs

The genes encoding specific UPEC VFs can be exclusively chromosomal (e.g., *pap* and *hly*); exclusively or principally plasmid-associated (e.g., *iss* and *traT*); or can occur in either location (e.g., the aerobactin operon and afa/drab). Plasmid-borne VFs have an obvious vehicle for horizontal transmission among *E. coli* lineages. Such VFs tend to be distributed more broadly but more sporadically within the species than are chromosomal VFs [129]. Studies have demonstrated that certain VFs commonly occur together, in a way that suggests co-selection or direct genetic linkage [130, 131]. Direct genetic linkage of VFs has been shown on PAIs and plasmids [132–134].

13. Antimicrobial drugs and uropathogenic *Escherichia coli*

Managing UTI caused by UPEC has become challenging over the years due to increasing resistance to the commonly used antibiotics [135–139], which poses a great threat to future capacity to treat UTI caused by UPEC. Although TMP-SMX has traditionally been used as a first-line treatment for UTI [140], there are reports of increased resistance to this antibiotic, which in some countries is in the range 15–20% [137]. Many UPEC strains resistant to TMP-SMZ are also resistant to amoxicillin and cephalexin. Nitrofurantoin remains highly effective against UPEC, but is mainly used for cystitis treatment due to its inability to attain sufficient serum levels to treat invasive or systemic infections [137], and all have excellent bioavailability and achieve high urinary concentrations. However, increased FQ use has resulted in a rise in the prevalence of resistance, and FQ-resistant *E. coli* has become a major problem in several countries [141].

14. Relationship between antibiotic resistance and virulence or phylogenetic background in UPEC

Previous studies show that in *E. coli* isolates from patients with urosepsis, resistance to antimicrobial agents such as ampicillin, sulfonamides, tetracycline, chloramphenicol, and streptomycin is negatively associated with virulence and a phylogenetic group B2, but positively associated with host compromise (immune deficiency, diabetes, and other urinary anatomical abnormalities) [26]. There is a similar negative association between FQ resistance and VFs and group B2 [142–144]. This suggests that, resistance may provide a greater fitness advantage to *E. coli* than traditional VFs or a group B2 background, allowing them to cause infections in compromised hosts with weakened defenses who are frequently exposed to antibiotics.

15. *E. coli* sequence type 131 (ST131)

Determining the clonal types of UPEC is crucial for understanding the role of clonal spread to emerging antimicrobial resistance, which is important for defining and interrupting transmission pathways. Multidrug-resistant *E. coli* sequence type 131 (ST131) has emerged over the past decade as a globally disseminated cause of extraintestinal infections in humans and animals [145–147]. The recent emergence of this clone has coincided with an increase in antibiotic resistance among *E. coli* generally, suggesting a contributing role for ST131 in resistance.

In contrast to traditional antimicrobial resistant *E. coli,* which mostly derive from low virulence phylogenetic groups A and B1, ST131 derives exclusively from phylogenetic group B2, which is traditionally known to be enriched for VF genes. This, plus limited experimental evidence of virulence and several case reports of unusually severe or fatal extraintestinal infections due to ST131, suggests that the emergence of ST131 may be due to a high virulence potential (in addition to antibiotic resistance) compared with other *E. coli* types. However, despite this, some studies have reported absence of traits commonly associated with B2 phylogeny, particularly adhesins (e.g., P, S, and FIC fimbriae) and toxins (e.g., hemolysin and cnf1).

Most ST131 clinical isolates are FQ resistant, and many are also co-resistant to aminoglycosides and/or trimethoprim-sulfamethoxazole (TMP-SMZ). A minority produces extended-spectrum beta-lactamases (ESBLs) that confer resistance to extended-spectrum cephalosporins. *E. coli* clonal group ST131 may be associated with other beta-lactamases but some isolates are cephalosporin susceptible [148, 149].

Despite limited epidemiological evidence of increased virulence of ST131, a recent study revealed that ST131 exhibits a marked prevalence gradient across source groups, from pyelonephritis to cystitis isolates, and finally to fecal isolates [126]. This is consistent with increased urovirulence, and provides epidemiological evidence of increased virulence for ST131, which has been presumed but without evidence from experimental animal models [8, 150]. The antibiotic resistance advantage, in combination with the possible presence of enhanced virulence, could explain the recent worldwide emergence of ST131. The increasing prevalence of ESBL-producing *E. coli* has been associated with the emergence of CTX-M-ST131 pandemic clonal group [151]. Available evidence supports that ST131 is an important contributor to the spread of ESBLs among reproductive-age women in some regions, albeit limited research in many parts worldwide [141, 152].

Four VF genes (*iutA, ompT, usp,* and *traT*) are associated with ST131 isolates, and so could represent potential targets for vaccines or other interventions, particularly if a functional role in virulence or dissemination can be demonstrated for them. Most of the ST131 isolates (85%) are of the O25b variant, and the remainder are type O16 [153, 154].

Resistance of ST131 to extended-spectrum cephalosporins is often due to production of ESBLs. The initial descriptions of ST131 emphasized its association with CTX-M-15, but subsequent studies have shown that it is more commonly ESBL-negative but FQ-resistant [154–156]. Previous studies in Australia and Japan showed that ST131-O25b, ST131-O16, and group D-ST405 clonal groups contribute to the spread of ESBL-producing *E. coli* [151, 152]. The dominant ESBL, in *E. coli,* globally and in Australia [157] is CTX-M-15, which is frequently encoded on plasmids carried by the ST131 pandemic clonal group.

16. Conclusions

A wide range of UPEC VFs have been established epidemiologically or experimentally (*in vivo*) as being important in UTI pathogenesis. No single VF profile has been proven to be important in causing any particular UTI syndrome. Indeed, studies have suggested that

UTI pathogenesis is multiply determined. Thus, intervention strategies based on VF genes might have to involve multiple targets, which would offer the extra advantage of protection against a wide range of UTI syndromes. This observation, which is in agreement with previous studies, provides evidence that VF repertoire is as, or more, important than phylogenetic background for predicting pathogenic behavior in UPEC.

The prevalence of antibiotic resistance among human urine *E. coli* isolates has risen substantially in recent years, especially to first line agents such as fluoroquinolones and trimethoprim-sulphamethoxazole. Furthermore, multidrug-resistant *E. coli* ST131 has shown rapid global dissemination among humans and animals, which has coincided with the general increase in resistance among *E. coli* clinical isolates. A better understanding of the microbiological basis for the emergence of UPEC antibiotic resistance is necessary for guiding efforts aimed at interrupting this process. Further studies on ST131 are clearly needed to explain its impressive emergence so that control measures can be devised and implemented.

Author details

Timothy Kudinha

Address all correspondence to: tkudinha@yahoo.com

Charles Sturt University, Orange, NSW, Australia

References

[1] Draghijeva E. Virulence factors in *Escherichia coli* from children with pyelonephritis. Clinical Microbiology and Infection. 1999;**6**:328-333

[2] Leroy S, Chalumeau T, Ulinski T, et al. Impressive renal damage after acute pyelonephritis in a child. Pediatric Nephrology. 2010;**25**:1365-1368

[3] Prakash Kalra OM, Raizada A. Approach to a patient with urosepsis. Journal of Global Infectious Diseases. 2009;**1**:57-63

[4] Foxman B, Barlow R, D'Arcy H, Gillespie B, Solbel J. Urinary tract infection: Self-reported incidence and associated costs. Annals of Epidemiology. 2000;**10**:509-515

[5] Foxman B, Brown P. Epidemiology of urinary tract infections: Transmission and risk factors, incidence, and costs. Infectious Disease Clinics of North America. 2003;**17**:227-241

[6] Griebling TL. Urologic diseases in America project: Trends in resource use for urinary tract infections in men. Journal of Urology. 2005;**173**:1288-1294

[7] Ikram R, Rebecca Psutka R, Carter A, Priest P. An outbreak of multi-drug resistant *Escherichia coli* urinary tract infection in an elderly population: A case-control study of risk factors. BMC Infectious Diseases. 2015;**15**:224

[8] Johnson JR, Porter SB, Zhanel G, Kuskowski MA, Denamur E. Virulence of *Escherichia coli* clinical isolates in a murine sepsis model in relation to sequence type ST131 status, fluoroquinolone resistance, and virulence genotype. Infection and Immunity. 2012;**80**:1554-1562

[9] Ruiz J, Simon K, Horcajada JP, Velasco M, Barranco M, Roig G, Moreno-Martinez A, Martinez JA, Jimenez de Anta T, Mensa J, Vila J. Differences in virulence factors among clinical isolates of *Escherichia coli* causing cystitis and pyelonephritis in women and prostatitis in men. Journal of Clinical Microbiology. 2002;**40**:4445-4449

[10] Zhang L, Foxman B. Molecular epidemiology of *Escherichia coli* mediated urinary tract infections. Frontiers in Bioscience. 2003;**8**:e235–e244

[11] Johnson JR, Kuskowski MA, O'Bryan TT, Colodner R, Raz R. Virulence genotype and phylogenetic origin in relation to antibiotic resistance profile among *Escherichia coli* urine sample isolates from Israeli women with acute uncomplicated cystitis. Antimicrobial Agents and Chemotherapy. 2005;**49**:26-31

[12] Lipsky BA. Urinary tract infections in men. Epidemiology, pathophysiology, diagnosis, and treatment. Annals of Internal Medicine. 1989;**110**:138-150

[13] Gupta K, Stamm WE. Urinary tract infections. In: Dale DC, Federman DD, editors. ACP Medicine. New York: WebMD; 2005. Section 7, chap. 23

[14] Ovalle A, Levancini M. Urinary tract infections in pregnancy. Current Opinion in Urology. 2001;**11**:55-59

[15] Wald E. Urinary tract infections in infants and children: A comprehensive overview. Current Opinion in Pediatrics. 2004;**16**:85-88

[16] Schlager TA. Urinary tract infections in children younger than 5 years of age: Epidemiology, diagnosis, treatment, outcomes and prevention. Paediatrics Drugs. 2001;**3**: 219-227

[17] Chen M, Jahnukainen T, Bao W, Dare E, Ceccatelli S, Celsi G. Uropathogenic *Escherichia coli* toxins induce caspase-independent apoptosis in renal proximal tubules via ERK signaling. American Journal of Nephrology. 2003;**23**:140-151

[18] Scholes D, Hooton TM, Roberts PL, Stapleton AE, Gupta K, Stamm WE. Risk factors for recurrent urinary tract infection in young women. The Journal of Infectious Diseases. 2000;**182**:1177-1182

[19] Eto DS, Jones TA, Sundsbak JL, Mulvey MA. Integrin-mediated host cell invasion by type-1piliated uropathogenic *E. coli*. PLos Pathogens. 2007;**3**:e100, 0949-0960

[20] Moreno E, Andreu A, Perez T, Sabate M, Johnson JR, Prats G. Relationship between *Escherichia coli* strains causing urinary tract infection in women and the dominant faecal flora of the same hosts. Epidemiology and Infection. 2006;**134**:1015-1023

[21] Moreno E, Andreu A, Pigrau C, Kuskowski MA, Johnson JR, Prats G. Relationship between *Escherichia coli* strains causing acute cystitis in women and the fecal *E. coli* population of the host. Journal of Clinical Microbiology. 2008;**46**:2529-2534

[22] Manges AR, Johnson JR, Foxman B, O'Bryan TT, Fullerton KE, Riley LW. Widespread distribution of urinary tract infections caused by a multidrug-resistant *Escherichia coli* clonal group. The New England Journal of Medicine. 2001;**345**:1007-1013

[23] Manges AR, Tabar H, Tellis P, Vincent C, Tellier PP. Endemic and epidemic lineages of *Escherichia coli* that cause urinary tract infections. Emerging Infectious Diseases. 2008;**14**:1575-1583

[24] Pitout JD, Gregson DB, Church DL, Elsayed S, Lampland KB. Community-wide outbreaks of clonally related CTX-M-14 beta-lactamase-producing *Escherichia coli* strains in the Calgary health region. Journal of Clinical Microbiology. 2005;**43**:2844-2849

[25] Svanborg C, Bergsten G, Fischer H, et al. Uropathogenic *Escherichia coli* as a model of host-parasite interaction. Current Opinion in Microbiology. 2005;**9**:33-39

[26] Johnson JR. Virulence factors in *Escherichia coli* urinary tract infection. Clinical Microbiology Reviews. 1991;**4**:80-128

[27] Mobley HL, Island MD, Massad G. Virulence determinants of uropathogenic *Escherichia coli* and *Proteus mirabilis*. Kidney International Supplements. 1994;**47**:S129-S136

[28] Kuehn MJ, Heuser J, Normark S, Hultgren SJ. P pili in uropathogenic *E. coli* are composite fibres with distinct fibrillar adhesive tips. Nature. 1992;**356**:252-255

[29] Xiang-Qi Mu, Bullitt E. PNAS. Structure and assembly of P-pili: A protruding hinge region used for assembly of a bacterial adhesion filament. 2006;**26**:9861-9866. DOI: 10.1073_pnas.0509620103

[30] Antao E, Wieler LH, Ewers C. Adhesive threads of extraintestinal pathogenic *Escherichia coli*. A review. Gut Pathogens. 2009;**1**:22

[31] Lane MC, Mobley HL. Role of P-fimbrial-mediated adherence in pyelonephritis and persistence of uropathogenic *Escherichia coli* (UPEC) in the mammalian kidney. Kidney International. 2007;**72**:19-25

[32] Johnson JR. *papG* alleles among *Escherichia coli* strains causing urosepsis: Associations with other bacterial characteristics and host compromise. Infection and Immunity. 1998;**66**:4568-4571

[33] Johnson JR, Brown JJ, Maslow JN. Clonal distribution of the three alleles of the Gal (α1-4) Gal-specific adhesin gene *papG* among *Escherichia coli* strains from patients with bacteremia. The Journal of Infectious Diseases. 1998;**177**:651-661

[34] Manning SD, Zhang L, Foxman B, Spindler A, Tallman P, Marrs CF. Prevalence of known P-fimbrial G alleles in *Escherichia coli* and identification of a new adhesin class. Clinical and Diagnostic Laboratory Immunology. 2001;**8**:637-640

[35] Flores-Mireles AL, Walker JN, Caparon M, and Hultgren SJ. Urinary tract infections: Epidemiology, mechanisms of infection and treatment options. Nature Reviews Microbiology. 2015;**13**:269-284

[36] O'Hanley P, Low D, Romero I, Lark D, Vosti K, Falkow S, et al. Gal-Gal binding and haemolysin phenotypes and genotypes associated with uropathogenic *Escherichia coli*. The New England Journal of Medicine. 1985;**313**:414-420

[37] Sokurenko EV, Chesnokova V, Doyle RJ, Hasty DL. Diversity of the *Escherichia coli* type 1 fibrial lectin. Journal of Biological Chemistry. 1997;**272**:17880-17886

[38] Sokurenko EV, Chesnokova V, Dykhuizen DE, Ofek I, Wu XR, Krogfelt KA, Struve C, Schembri MA, Hasty DL. Pathogenic adaptation of *Escherichia coli* by natural variation of the FimH adhesion. Proceedings of the National Academy of Sciences of the United States of America. 1998;**95**:8922-8926

[39] Schembri MA, Klemm P. Coordinate gene regulation by fimbriae induced signal transduction. EMBO Journal. 2001;**20**:3074-3081

[40] Simms AN, Mobley HLT. Multiple genes repress motility in uropathogenic *Escherichia coli* constitutively expressing type 1 fimbriae. Journal of Bacteriology. 2008;**190**:3747-3756

[41] Snyder JA, Hagen BJ, Lockatell CV, Maroncle N, Hagan EC, Johnson DE, Welch RA, Mobley HLT. Coordinate expression of fimbriae in uropathogenic *E. coli*. Infection and Immunity. 2005;**73**:7588-7596

[42] Schwan WR, Lee JL, Lenard FA, Matthews BT, Beck MT. Osmolarity and pH growth conditions regulate fim gene transcription and type 1 pilus expression in uropathogenic *Escherichia coli*. Infection and Immunity. 2002;**70**:1391-1402

[43] Hull RA, Donovan WH, Del Terzo M, Stewart C, Rogers M, and Darouiche RO. Role of Type 1 fimbria- and P fimbria-specific adherence in colonization of the neurogenic human bladder by *Escherichia coli*. Infection and Immunity. 2002;**70**:6481-6484

[44] Staerk K, Khandige S, Kolmos HJ, Moeller-Jensen J, Anderson TE. Uropathogenic *Escherichia coli* express type 1 fimbriae only in surface adherent populations under physiological growth conditions. The Journal of Infectious Diseases. 2016;**213**:386-394

[45] Opal SM, Gemski AS, Lyhte LW. Aerobactin and alpha-hemolysin as virulence determinants in *Escherichia coli* isolated from human blood, urine and stool. The Journal of Infectious Diseases. 1990;**161**:794-796

[46] Johnson JR, Roberts PL, Stamm WE. P fimbriae and other virulence factors in *Escherichia coli* urosepsis: Association with patients' characteristics. The Journal of Infectious Diseases. 1987;**156**:225-229

[47] Arthur M, Johnson CE, Rubin RH, Arbeit RD, Campanelli C, Kim C, Steinbach S, Agarwal M, Wilkinson R, Goldstein R. Molecular epidemiology of adhesin and hemolysin virulence factors among uropathogenic *Escherichia coli*. Infection and Immunity. 1989;**57**:303-313

[48] Orskov I, Orskov F. Serologic classification of fimbriae. Current Topics in Microbiology and Immunology. 1990;**151**:71-90

[49] Nowicki B, Selavarangan R, Nowicki S. Family of *Escherichia coli* Dr adhesins: Decay-accelerating factor recognition and invasiveness. The Journal of Infectious Diseases. 2001;**183**:524-527

[50] Servin, AL. Pathogenesis of Afa/Dr diffusely adhering *Escherichia coli*. Clinical Microbiology Reviews. 2005;**18**:264-292

[51] Mulvey MA. Adhesion and entry of uropathogenic *Escherichia coli*. A mini review. Cell Microbiology. 2002;**4**:257-271

[52] Mitsumori K, Terai A, Yamamoto S, Yoshid O. Identification of S, F1C and three PapG fimbrial adhesins in uropathogenic *Escherichia coli* by polymerase chain reaction. FEMS Immunology and Medical Microbiology. 1998;**21**:261-268

[53] Khan SA, Kniep B, Oelschlaeger TA, Van Die I, Korhonen T, Hacker J. Receptor structure for F1C fimbriae of uropathogemic *Escherichia coli*. Infection and Immunity. 2000; **68**:3541-3547

[54] Virkola R, Parkkinen J, Hacker J, Korhonen TK. Sialyloligosaccharide chains of laminin as an extracellular matrix target for S fimbriae of *Escherichia coli*. Infection and Immunity. 1993;**61**:4480-4484

[55] Korhonen TK, Virkola R, Holthofer H. Localization of binding sites for purified *Escherichia coli* P fimbriae in the human kidney. Infection and Immunity. 1986;**54**:328-332

[56] Ott M, Hacker J, Schmoll T, Jarchau T, Korhonen TK, Goebel W. Analysis of the genetic determinants coding for the S-fimbrial adhesion (*sfa*) in different *Escherichia coli* strains causing meningitis or urinary tract infections. Infection and Immunity. 1986;**54**:646-653

[57] Andrews SC, Robinson AK, Rodríguez-Quiñones F. Bacterial iron homeostasis. FEMS Microbiology Reviews. 2003;**27**:215-237

[58] Bagg A, Neilands JB. Ferric uptake regulation protein acts as a repressor, employing iron (II) as a cofactor to bind the operator of an iron transport operon in *Escherichia coli*. Biochemistry. 1987;**26**:5471-5477

[59] Russo TA, Carlino UB, Johnson JR. Identification of *ireA*, a novel iron regulated virulence gene in an extraintestinal pathogenic isolate of *Escherichia coli*. Infection and Immunity. 2001;**69**:6209-6216

[60] Torres AG, Redford P, Welch RA, Payne SM. TonB-dependent systems of uropathogenic *Escherichia coli*: Aerobactin and heme transport and TonB are required for virulence in the mouse. Infection and Immunity. 2001;**69**:6179-6185

[61] Watts RE, Totsika M, Challinor VL, Mabbett AN, Ulett GC, De Voss JJ, Schembri MA. Contribution of siderophore systems to growth and urinary tract colonization of asymptomatic bacteriuria *Escherichia coli*. Infection and Immunity. 2011;**80**:333-3434

[62] Garcia EC, Brumbaugh AR, Mobley HLT. Redundancy and specificity of *Escherichia coli* iron acquisition systems during urinary tract infection. Infection and Immunity. 2011;**79**:1225-1235

[63] Schubert S, Rakin A, Heesenman J. The Yersinia high-pathogenicity island (HPI). Evolutionary and functional aspects. International Journal of Medical Microbiology. 2004;**274**:883-894

[64] Hancock V, Ferrieres L, Klemm P. The ferric yersiniabactin uptake receptor *fyuA* is required for efficient biofilm formation by urinary tract infections *Escherichia coli* in human urine. Microbiology. 2008;**154**:167-175

[65] Schubert S, Picard B, Gouriou AS, Heesemann J, Denamur E. Yersinia high-pathogenicity island contributes to virulence in *Escherichia coli* causing extraintestinal infections. Infection and Immunity. 2002;**70**:5335-5337

[66] Hancock V, Klemm P. Global gene expression profiling of asymptomatic bacteriuria *Escherichia coli* during biofilm growth in human urine. Infection and Immunity. 2007;**75**:966-976

[67] Carbonetti NH, Boonchai S, Parry SH, Väisänen-Rhen V, Korhonen TK, Williams PH. Aerobactin-mediated iron uptake by *Escherichia coli* isolates from human extraintestinal infections. Infection and Immunity. 1986;**51**:966-968

[68] Crosa JH. Genetics and molecular biology of siderophore-mediated iron transport in bacteria. Microbiological Reviews. 1989;**53**:517-530

[69] De Lorenzo V, Bindereif A, Paw BH, Neilands JB. Aerobactin biosynthesis and transport genes of plasmid Co1V-K30 in *Escherichia coli* K-1. Journal of Bacteriology. 1986;**165**:570-578

[70] Jacobson SH, Hammarlind M, Lidefeldt KJ, Osterberg E, Tullus K, Brauner A. Incidence of aerobactin-positive *Escherichia coli* strains in patients with symptomatic urinary tract infection. European Journal of Clinical Microbiology and Infectious Diseases. 1988;**7**:630-634

[71] Colonna B, Nicoletti M, Visca P, Casalino M, Valenti P, Maimone F. Composite IS1 elements encoding hydroxamate-mediated iron uptake in FIme plasmids from epidemic *Salmonella* spp. Journal of Bacteriology. 1985;**162**:307-316

[72] Bennett PM. Plasmid encoded antibiotic resistance: Acquisition and transfer of antibiotic resistance genes in bacteria. British Journal of Pharmacology. 2008;**153**:S347-S357

[73] Phillips I, Eykyn S, King A, Gransden WR, Rowe B, Frost JA, Gross RJ. Epidemic multiresistant *Escherichia coli* infection in West Lambeth Health District. Lancet. 1988;**7**:1038-1041

[74] Hantke K, Nicholson G, Rabsch W, Winkelmann G. Salmochelins, siderophores of *Salmonella enterica* and uropathogenic *Escherichia coli* strains, are recognized by the outer membrane receptor *iroN*. Proceedings of the National Academy of Sciences of the United States of America. 2002;**100**:3677-3682

[75] Caza M, Lepine F, Milot S, Dozois CM. Specific roles of the *iroBCDEN* genes in virulence of an avian pathogenic *Escherichia coli* O78 strain and in production of salmochelins. Infection and Immunity. 2008;**76**:3539-3549

[76] Negre VL, Bonacorsi S, Schubert S, Bidet P, Nassif X, Bingen E. The siderophore receptor iroN but not the high-pathogenicity island or the hemin receptor chuA contributes to the bacteremic step of *Escherichia coli* neonatal meningitis. Infection and Immunity. 2004;**72**:1216-1220

[77] Bauer R, Zhang L, Foxman B, Siitonen A, Jantunen M, Saxen H, Marrs C. Molecular epidemiology of 3 putative virulence genes for *Escherichia coli* urinary tract infection-*usp, iha, and* $iroN_{(E.\ coli)}$. Journal of Infectious Diseases. 2002;**185**:1521-1524

[78] Kucheria R, Dasgupta P, Sacks SH, Khan MS, Sheerin NS. Urinary tract infections: New insights into a common problem. Postgraduate Medical Journal. 2005;**81**:83-86

[79] Burgos Y, Benton L. Common origin of plasmid encoded alpha-hemolysin genes in *Escherichia coli*. BMC Microbiology. 2010;**193**:1-13

[80] Holland IB, Schimdt L, Young J. Type I protein secretion in bacteria, the ABC-transport dependent pathway (review). Molecular Membrane Biology. 2005;**22**:29-39

[81] Birosova E, Siegfried L, Kmetova M, et al. Detection and virulence factors in alpha-haemolytic *Escherichia coli* strains isolated from various clinical materials. CMI. 2004;**10**:569-573

[82] König B, König W, Scheffer J, Hacker J, Goebel W. Role of *Escherichia coli* alpha-hemolysin and bacterial adherence in infection: Requirement for release of inflammatory mediators from granulocytes and mast cells. Infection and Immunity. 1986;**54**:886-892

[83] Scheffer J, König W, Hacker J, Goebel W. Bacterial adherence and hemolysin production from *Escherichia coli* induces histamine and leukotriene release from various cells. Infection and Immunity. 1985;**50**:271-278

[84] Czirók E, Milch H, Csiszár K, Csik M. Virulence factors of *Escherichia coli*. Correlation with *Escherichia coli* pathogenicity of haemolysin production, haemagglutinating capacity, antigens K1, K5, and colicinogenicity. Acta Microbiologica Hungarica. 1986;**33**:69-83

[85] Marrs C, Zhang L, Foxman B. *Escherichia coli* mediated urinary tract infections: Are there distinct uropathogenic *E.coli* (UPEC) pathotypes? FEMS Microbiology Letters. 2005;**252**:183-190

[86] Lemonnier M, Landraud L, Lemichez E. Rho GTPase-activating bacterial toxins: From bacterial virulence regulation to eukaryotic cell biology. FEMS Microbiology Review. 2007;**31**:515-534

[87] Etienne-Manneville S, Hall A. Rho GTPases in cell biology. Nature. 2002;**420**:629-635

[88] Bower JM, Eto DS, Mulvey MA. Covert operations of uropathogenic *Escherichia coli* within the urinary tract. Traffic. 2005;**6**:18-31

[89] Yamamoto S, Terai A, Yuri K, Kurazono H, Takeda Y, Yoshida O. Detection of urovirulence factors in *Escherichia coli* by multiplex polymerase chain reaction. FEMS Immunology & Medical Microbiology. 1995;**12**:85-90

[90] Rippere-Lampe KE, O'Brien AD, Conrau R, Lockman HA. Mutation of the gene encoding cytotoxic necrotizing factor type 1 (cnf1) attenuates the virulence of uropathogenic *Escherichia coli*. Infection and Immunity. 2001;**69**:3954-3964

[91] Elliott SJ, Srinivas S, Albert MJ, et al. Characterization of the roles of hemolysin and other toxins in enteropathy caused by alpha-hemolytic *Escherichia coli* linked to human diarrhea. Infection and Immunity. 1998;**66**:2040-2051

[92] Taylor PW. Bactericidal and bacteriolytic activity of serum against gram-negative bacteria. Microbiological Reviews. 1983;**47**:46-83

[93] Montenegro MA, Bitter-Suermann D, Timmis JK, et al. *traT* gene sequences, serum resistance and pathogenicity-related factors in clinical isolates of *Escherichia coli* and other gram-negative bacteria. The Journal of General and Applied Microbiology. 1985;**131**:1511-1521

[94] Timmis KN, Boulnois GJ, Bitter-Suermann D, Cabello FC. Surface components of *Escherichia coli* that mediate resistance to the bactericidal activities of serum and phagocytes. Current Topics in Microbiology and Immunology. 1985;**118**:197-218

[95] Goldman RC, Joiner K, Leive L. Serum-resistant mutants of *Escherichia coli* O111 contain increased lipopolysaccharide, lack an O antigen-containing capsule, and cover more of their lipid A core with O antigen. Journal of Bacteriology. 1984;**159**:877-882

[96] Domingue GJ, Laucirica R, Baliga P, Covington S, Robledo JA, Li SC. Virulence of wild-type *E. coli* uroisolates in experimental pyelonephritis. Kidney International. 1998;**34**:761-765

[97] Iwahi T, Abe Y, Tsuchiya K. Virulence of *Escherichia coli* in ascending urinary-tract infection in mice. Journal of Medical Microbiology. 1982;**15**:303-316

[98] Mangel W, Toledo DL, Brown MT, Worzalla K, Lee M, Dunn JJ. Omptin: An *Escherichia coli* outer membrane proteinase that activates plasminogen. Methods in Enzymology. 1994;**244**:384-399

[99] Leytus SP, Bowles LK, Konisky K, Mangel WF. Activation of plasminogen to plasmin by a protease associated with outer membrane of *Escherichia coli*. Proceedings of the National Academy of Sciences of the United States America. 1981;**78**:1485-1489

[100] Hui CY, Guo Y, He QS, et al. *Escherichia coli* outer membrane protease OmpT confers resistance to urinary cationic peptides. Microbiology and Immunology. 2010;**54**:452-459

[101] Lundrigan MD, Webb RM. Prevalence of *ompT* among *Escherichia coli* isolates of human origin. FEMS Microbiology Letters. 1992;**76**:51-56

[102] McCarter JD, Stephens D, Shoemaker K, Rosenberg S, Kirsch JF, Georgiou G. Substrate specificity of *Escherichia coli* outer membrane protease ompT. Journal of Bacteriology. 2004;**186**:5919-5925

[103] Guina T, Yi EC, Wang H, Hackett M, Miller SI. A PhoP-regulated outer membrane protease of *Salmonella enterica* serovar Typhimurium promotes resistance to alpha-helical antimicrobial peptides. Journal of Bacteriology. 2000;**182**:4077-4086

[104] Stumpe S, Schmid R, Stephens DL, Georgiou G, Bakker E. Identification of OmpT as the protease that hydrolyzes the antimicrobial peptide protamine before it enters growing cells of *Escherichia coli*. Journal of Bacteriology. 1998;**180**:4002-4006

[105] Kanamura S, Kurazono H, Ishitoya S, et al. Distribution and genetic association of putative uropathogenic virulence factors *iroN, iha, kpsMT, ompT* and *usp* in *Escherichia coli* isolated from urinary tract infections in Japan. Journal of Urology. 2003;**170**:2490-2493

[106] Nakano M, Yamamoto S, Terai A, Ogawa O, Makino S, Hayashi H, Nair GB, Kurazono H. Structural and sequence diversity of the pathogenicity island of uropathogenic *Escherichia coli* which encodes the USP protein. FEMS. 2001;**205**:71-76

[107] Rijavec M, Muller-Premru M, Zakotnik B, Zgur-Bertok D. Virulence factors and biofilm production among *E. coli* strains causing bacteremia of urinary tract origin. Journal of Medical Microbiology. 2008;**57**:1329-1334

[108] Kanamaru S, Kurazono H, Nakano M, Terai A, Ogawa O, Yamamoto S. Subtyping of uropathogenic *Escherichia coli* according to the pathogenicity island encoding uropathogenic-specific protein: Comparison with phylogenetic groups. International Journal of Urology. 2006;**13**:754-760

[109] Yamamoto S. Molecular epidemiology of uropathogenic *Escherichia coli*. Journal of Infection and Chemotherapy. 2007;**13**:68-73

[110] Kai-Larsen Y, Luthje P, Chromek M, et al. Uropathogenic *Escherichia coli* modulates immune responses and its curli fimbriae interact with the antimicrobial peptide LL-37. PLoS Pathogens. 2010;**6**:e1001010

[111] Luthje P, Brauner A. Ag43 promotes persistence of uropathogenic *Escherichia coli* isolates in the urinary tract. Journal of Clinical Microbiology. 2010;**48**:2316-2317

[112] Schroeder M, Brooks BD and Brooks AE. The complex relationship between virulence and antibiotic resistance. Genes (Basel). 2017;**8**:39

[113] Kostakioti M, Hadjifrangiskou M, Hultgren SL. Bacterial biofilms: Development, dispersal, and therapeutic strategies in the dawn of the post-antibiotic era. Cold Spring Harbor Perspectives in Medicine. 2013;**3**:a010306

[114] De la Fuente-Núñez C, Reffuveille F, Fernández L, Hancock RE. Bacterial biofilm development as a multicellular adaptation: Antibiotic resistance and new therapeutic strategies. Current Opinion in Microbiology. 2013;**16**:580-589

[115] Gophna U, Barlev M, Sejffers R, Oelschlager TA, Hacker J, Ron EZ. Curli fibers mediate internalization of *Escherichia coli* by eukaryotic cells. Infection and Immunity. 2001;**69**:2659-2665

[116] Bailey JK, Pinyon JL, Ananthan S, Hall RM. Distribution of human commensal *Escherichia coli* phylogenetic groups. Journal of Clinical Microbiology. 2010;**48**:3455-3456

[117] Johnson JR, Russo TA. Extraintestinal pathogenic *Escherichia coli*: "The other bad *E. coli*." Journal of Clinical Medicine. 2002;**139**:155-162

[118] Kuntaman K, Lestari ES, Severin JA, Kershof, et al. Fluoroquinolone resistant *Escherichia coli*, Indonesia. Emerging Infectious Diseases. 2005;**11**:1363-1369

[119] Takahashi A, Kanamaru S, Kurazono H, Kunishima Y, Tsukamoto T, Ogawa O, Yamamoto S. *Escherichia coli* isolates associated with uncomplicated and complicated cystitis and asymptomatic bacteriuria possess similar phylogenies, virulence genes, and O-serogroup profiles. Journal of Clinical Medicine. 2006;**44**:4589-4592

[120] Picard B, Garcia JS, Gouriou S, et al. The link between phylogeny and virulence in *Escherichia coli* extra-intestinal infection. Infection and Immunity. 1999;**67**:546-553

[121] Johnson JR, Russo TA. Molecular epidemiology of extra-intestinal pathogenic (uropathogenic) *Escherichia coli*. A review. The Indian Journal of Medical Microbiology. 2005;**295**:383-404

[122] Johnson JR, Kuskowski MA, Gajewski A, et al. Extended virulence genotypes and phylogenetic background of *Escherichia coli* isolates from patients with cystitis, pyelonephritis, or prostatitis. The Journal of Infectious Diseases. 2005;**191**:46-50

[123] Johnson JR. Microbial virulence determinants and the pathogenesis of urinary tract infection. Infectious Disease Clinics of North America. 2003;**17**:261-278

[124] Goluszko P, Moseley SL, Truong LD, et al. Development of experimental model of chronic pyelonephritis with *Escherichia coli* O75:K5:H-bearing Dr fimbriae: Mutation in the *dra* region prevented tubulo-interstitial nephritis. Journal of Clinical Investigation. 1997;**99**:1662-1672

[125] Roberts JA, Marklund B, I Ilver D, et al. The Gal alpha (1-4) Gal-specific tip adhesin of *Escherichia coli* P-fimbriae is needed for pyelonephritis to occur in the normal urinary tract. Proceedings of the National Academy of Sciences of the United States of America. 1994;**91**:11889-11893

[126] Kudinha T, Johnson JR, Andrew SD, Kong F, Anderson P, Gilbert GL. Distribution of phylogenetic groups, sequence type ST131, and virulence associated traits among *Escherichia coli* isolates from men with pyelonephritis or cystitis and healthy controls. Clinical Microbiology and Infection. 2013;**19**:E173-E180

[127] Piatti G, Mannini A, Balistreri M, Schito AM. Virulence factors in urinary *Escherichia coli* strains: Phylogenetic background and quinolone and fluoroquinolone resistance. Journal of Clinical Microbiology. 2008;**46**:480-487

[128] Kudinha T, Johnson JR, Andrew SD, Kong F, Anderson P, Gilbert GL. Genotypic and phenotypic characterization of *Escherichia coli* isolates from children with urinary tract infection and from healthy carriers. The Pediatric Infectious Disease Journal. 2013;**32**:543-548

[129] Johnson JR, Delavari P, Kuskowski MA, Stell AL. Phylogenetic distribution of extra-intestinal virulence-associated traits in *Escherichia coli*. The Journal of Infectious Diseases. 2001;**183**:78-88

[130] Johnson JR, Stell AL. Extended virulence genotypes of *Escherichia coli* strains from patients with urosepsis in relation to phylogeny and host compromise. The Journal of Infectious Diseases. 2000;**181**:261-272

[131] Escobar-Páramo P, Clermont O, Blanc-Potard AB, Bui H, Le Bouguénec C, Denamur E. A specific genetic background is required for acquisition and expression of virulence factors in *Escherichia coli*. Molecular Biology and Evolution. 2004;**21**:1085-1094

[132] Dobrindt U, Blum-Oehler G, Hartsch T, et al. S-fimbria-encoding determinant *sfa1* is located on pathogenicity island III_{536} of uropathogenic *Escherichia coli* strain 536. Infection and Immunity. 2001;**69**:4248-4256

[133] Guyer DM, Kao J-S, Mobley HLT. Genomic analysis of a pathogenicity island in uropathogenic *Escherichia coli* CFT 073: Distribution of homologous sequences among isolates from patients with pyelonephritis, cystitis, and catheter-associated bacteriuria and from fecal samples. Infection and Immunity. 1998;**66**:4411-4417

[134] Hacker J, Kaper JB. Pathogenicity islands and the evolution of microbes. Annual Review of Microbiology. 2000;**54**:641-679

[135] Barber AE, Norton JP, Spivak AM, and Mulvey MA. Urinary tract infections: Current and emerging management strategies. Clinical Infectious Diseases. 2013;**57**:719-724

[136] Goettsch W, van Pelt W, Nagelkerke N, et al. Increasing resistance of fluoroquinolones in *Escherichia coli* from urinary tract infections in The Netherlands. Journal of Antimicrobial Chemotherapy. 2000;**46**:223-228

[137] Gupta K, Hooton TM, Stamm WE. Increasing antimicrobial resistance and the management of uncomplicated community-acquired urinary tract infection. Annals of Internal Medicine. 2001;**135**:41-50

[138] Karlowsky JA, Hoban DJ, DeCorby MR, Liang NM, Zhanel GG. Fluoroquinolone resistant urinary isolates of *Escherichia coli* from outpatients are frequently multidrug resistant: Results from the North American Urinary Tract Infection Collaborative Alliance-Quinolone Resistance Study. Antimicrobial Agents and Chemotherapy. 2006;**50**:2251-2254

[139] Wong-Beringer A, Hindler J, Loeff M, et al. Molecular correlation for the treatment outcomes in bloodstream infections caused by *Escherichia coli* and *Klebsiella pneumoniae* with reduced susceptibility to ceftazidime. Clinical Infectious Diseases. 2002;**34**:135-146

[140] Foxman B. Epidemiology of urinary tract infections: Incidence, morbidity, and economic costs. American Journal of Medicine. 2002;**113**:5S-13S

[141] Drews SJ, Poutanen SM, Mazzulli T, et al. Decreased prevalence of virulence factors among ciprofloxacillin-resistant uropathogenic *Escherichia coli* isolates. Journal of Clinical Microbiology. 2005;**43**:4218-4220

[142] Vila J, Simon K, Ruiz J, et al. Are quinolone-resistant uropathogenic *Escherichia coli* less virulent? Journal of Infectious Diseases. 2002;**186**:1039-1042

[143] Velasco M, Horcajada JP, Mensa J, et al. Decreased invasive capacity of quinolone-resistant *Escherichia coli* in patients with urinary tract infections. Clinical Infectious Diseases. 2001;**33**:1682-1686

[144] Johnson JR, Van der Sche C, Kuskowski MA, Goessens W, Van Belkum A. Phylogenetic background and virulence profiles of fluoroquinolone-resistant clinical *Escherichia coli* isolates from the Netherlands. Journal of Infectious Diseases. 2002;**186**:1852-1856

[145] Platell JL, Cobbold RN, Johnson JR, et al. Commonality among fluoroquinolone-resistant sequence type ST131 extra-intestinal *Escherichia coli* isolates from humans and companion animals in Australia. Antimicrobial Agents and Chemotherapy. 2011;**55**:3782-3787

[146] Platell JL, Johnson JR, Cobbold RN, Trott DJ. Multidrug-resistant extra-intestinal *Escherichia coli* of sequence type ST131 in animals and foods. Veterinary Microbiology. 2011;**153**:99-108

[147] Rogers BA, Sidjabat HE, Paterson DL. *Escherichia coli* O25b-ST131: A pandemic, multi-resistant, community-associated strain. Journal of Antimicrobial Chemotherapy. 2011;**66**:1-14

[148] Johnson JR, Menard M, Johnston B, Kuskowski MA, Nichol K, Zhanel GG. Epidemic clonal groups of *Escherichia coli* as a cause of antimicrobial resistant urinary tract infections in Canada, 2002-2004. Journal of Antimicrobial Chemotherapy. 2009;**53**:2733-2739

[149] Cheng MF, Chen WL, Hung WY, et al. Emergence of extended spectrum-β-lactamase-producing *Escherichia coli* O25b-ST131: A major community-acquired uropathogen in infants. The Pediatric Infectious Disease. 2015;**4**:469-475

[150] Lavigne J-P, Vergunst A, Goret L. Virulence potential and genomic mapping of the worldwide clone *Escherichia coli* ST131. PLoS One. 2012;**7**:e34294

[151] Matsamura Y, Yamamoto M, Nagao M, Hotta H, et al. Emergence and spread of B2-ST131-O25b, B2-ST131-O16 and D-ST405 clonal groups among extended-spectrum-β-lactamase-producing *Escherichia coli* in Japan. Journal of Antimicrobial Chemotherapy. 2012;**67**:2612-2620

[152] Kudinha T, Johnson JR, Andrew SD, Kong F, Anderson P, Gilbert GL. *Escherichia coli* sequence type 131 (ST131) as a prominent cause of antimicrobial resistance among clinical and fecal *Escherichia coli* isolates from reproductive-age women. Journal of Clinical Microbiology. 2013;**51**:3270-3276

[153] Zhong YM, Liu WE, Liang XH, Li YM, Jian ZJ, Hawkey PM. Emergence and spread of O16-ST131 and O25b-ST131 clones among faecal CTX-M-producing *Escherichia coli* in healthy individuals in Hunan Province, China. Journal of Antimicrobial Chemotherapy. 2015;**70**:2223-2227

[154] Johnson JR, Johnston B, Clabots C, Kuskowski MA, Castanheira M. *Escherichia coli* sequence type ST131 as the major cause of serious multidrug-resistant *E. coli* infections in the United States. Clinical Infectious Diseases. 2010;**51**:286-294

[155] Cerquetti M, Giufre M, Garcia-Fernandez A, et al. Ciprofloxacin-resistant, CTX-M-15 producing *Escherichia coli* ST131 clone in extraintestinal infections in Italy. Clinical Microbiology and Infection. 2010;**16**:1555-1558

[156] Uchida Y, Mochiman T, Morokuma Y, et al. Clonal spread in Eastern Asia of ciprofloxacin-resistant *Escherichia coli* serogroup O25 strains, and associated virulence factors. International Journal of Antimicrobial Agents. 2010;**35**:444-450

[157] Zong Z, Partridge SR, Thomas L, Iredell JR. Dominance of *blaCTX-M* within an Australian extended-spectrum beta-lactamase gene pool. Antimicrobial Agents and Chemotherapy. 2008;**52**:4198-4202

5

Phenotypic and Genetic Diversity of Uropathogenic *Enterococcus faecalis* Strains Isolated in the Primorsky Region of Russia

Zaitseva Elena Aleksandrovna,
Komenkova Tatiana Sergeevna,
Melnikova Elena Aleksandrovna,
Shadrin Andrey Mikhailovich and
Luchaninova Valentina Nikolaevna

Abstract

Urinary tract infection (UTI) is a topical problem of the contemporary pediatrics, pediatric nephrology, and urology. *E. faecalis* isolated from urine of children was the most important factor in development of UTIs at departments for newborns in Primorsky region. The variability of biochemical and fermentation activities of pathogenicity factors and resistance to antibiotics suggested a phenotypic heterogeneity of *E. faecalis*. It was found that uropathogenic enterococci characterized with proteolytic activity are resistant to antibacterial agents with different action mechanisms. Clinical isolates of *E. faecalis* contained two and more studied pathogenicity genes. Eleven variants of genes combinations, which code pathogenicity factors of *E. faecalis*, were identified. Uropathogenic *E. faecalis* strains attributed to ST6, ST40, ST179, ST774, and ST116 are resistant to four and more groups of antimicrobial agents. Our research confirmed high virulence properties of *E. faecalis* isolated from urine of patients with and their manifestations depending on the patient's age. Clinically significant *E. faecalis* strains have a complex of virulent properties, which allow the bacteria to materialize their pathogenic potential on all stages of the inflammation process in urinary system.

Keywords: urinary tract infections, *Enterococcus faecalis*, virulent properties, phenotypes, genotypes, newborns

1. Introduction

Urinary tract infection (UTI) is a topical problem of the contemporary pediatrics, pediatric nephrology, and urology, which takes the second or third place in the structure of children's morbidity [1, 6, 9, 12]. Risk factors of UTI in children include neonatal period, in particular premature birth, family medical history, abnormalities of urinary tract development, disruptions of urodynamics, including vesicoureteric reflux, obstructive uropathy, neurogenic bladder malfunction, urolithiasis, constipation, fecal and perianal colonization, immunocompromising conditions, including AIDS, immunosuppression therapy, frequent bladder catheterization, diabetes, sexual activity in teenagers [1, 14, 15, 18]. Newborns and infants are under high risk of UTI development, among other factors, since their immune system is not yet sufficiently developed [7]. Among the many factors, which affect development and forecast of UTI, biological properties of microorganisms, which inhabit kidney tissue, are of no small importance [10, 22, 35, 43].

Etiological structure of UTI in children has changed recently. Many studies show the growing etiological significance of *Enterococcus faecalis* [1, 6, 8, 20, 37]. Clinical significance of enterococci, which were earlier considered in different saprophytes, is being reassessed currently [4, 10].

Increase in etiological significance of enterococci is caused by many reasons, including development of antibiotic resistance, in particular, resistance to cephalosporin, widely used for treating UTIs in children [8]. Enterococci can initiate the infectious process due to their genes coding many pathogenicity factors involved in adhesion and invasion processes, development of biofilms, and hystodamaging effect (Esp, Asa1, EfaA, CylA, CylM, GelE, FsrB, etc.) [6, 13, 16, 30, 35, 42]. It is known that virulence of microorganisms depends upon the quantity of these genes [17]. Scientists from Europe, England, America, India, and Japan are doing research in this area [21, 33, 38, 39, 41]. No research related to characteristics of intraspecific genetic variability, including pathogenicity factors, in uropathogenic *E. faecalis* isolates from children having UTI, has been done in Russia until now. All the above has been determined in the topic of the research, which was undertaken in the present paper.

The aim of this research was to identify genetic variability and phenotypic features of biologic properties in uropathogenic *E. faecalis* isolates from children having urinary tract infections to assess its virulent potential and clinical significance.

2. Materials and methods

At the first stage, bacterial tests of urine samples (n = 6438) isolated from patients in cases of UTI at the multispecialty regional children's hospital from 2008 to 2016 were analyzed. Patients were aged from 3 days to 17 years.

At the second stage, biological properties and genetic variability of enterococci were studied. *E. faecalis* (n = 71) were isolated from urine of children with urinary tract infections and age from 3 days to 17 years in the diagnostic titer from 10^4 CFU/ml and higher during from 2013 to 2016. *E. faecalis* NCTC 12697 was used as the typical culture. All strains of uropathogenic

Gene	Primer sequence	Product size (bp)	Reference
cylA	TGGATGATAGTGATAGGAAGT TCTACAGTAAATCTTTCGTCA	517	[11]
aggA	AAGAAAAAGTAGACCAAC AACGGCAAGACAAGTAAATA	1553	[11]
efaA	GACAGACCCTCACGAATA AGTTCATCATGCTGCTGTAGTA	705	[11]
eep	GAGCGGGTATTTTAGTTCGT TACTCCAGCATTGGATGCT	937	[5]
esp	TTGCTAATGCTAGTCCACGACC GCGTCAACACTTGCATTGCCGAA	933	[32]
gelE	ACCCCGTATCATTGGTTT ACGCATTGCTTTTCCATC	419	[34]

Table 1. Oligonucleotide primers used in the study.

E. faecalis were previously investigated using classical microbiological methods [22, 43]. Antimicrobial susceptibility was performed using disk diffusion method on the Muller-Hinton agar according to EUCAST.

Bacterial DNA of *E. faecalis* was isolated using DNA-express kit (Lytech, Russia). The testing of enterococci (n = 31) pathogenicity genes was made by polymerase chain reaction (PCR), using previously developed primer sets (**Table 1**) [5, 11, 32, 34], synthesized by Eurogen (Russia), on TProfessional 96 (Biometra, Germany). The amplification products were analyzed in a 1% agarose gel containing 1 μg/ml ethidium bromide in ultraviolet light using BioDocAnalyze (Biometra, Germany).

The obtained data were processed using the parametric analysis method. From the indicators of descriptive statistics, the relative values (P, %), their errors (m_p, %) were calculated. To evaluate the degree of interrelation, the Pearson correlation analysis (R) was performed with calculation of correlation coefficient (r) and reliability of correlation (p). At statistical processing of the received materials, the software package Statistica 10.0 is used in the operating environment Windows 2010.

The research was approved by Interdisciplinary Committee for Ethics of the Federal State Budgetary Educational Institution of Higher Education "Pacific State Medical University" of the Ministry of Healthcare of the Russian Federation (protocol no. 4, 26.12.2016).

3. Results

The most common uropathogen in children with UTI, who were treated at the multispecialty regional children's hospital, is *Escherichia coli*, for which specific gravity equals from 33.92 ± 1.7 to 62.96 ± 1.2%. Most frequently, it was pointed out in outpatients (in 62.96 ± 1.2% cases); less frequently, it was found at departments for newborns (33.92 ± 1.7%). The second significant etiological factor of UTI in children was *E. faecalis*, for which specific gravity ranged from 16.14 to 32.5% [22]. At the same time, *E. faecalis* was the most important factor in development of UTIs at departments for newborns: it was found in 57.2% of cases (**Figure 1**). Frequency of identifying *E. faecalis* in newborns diagnosed with UTI ranged from 30.8 to 74.5% of cases over 9 years.

The present study analyzed the features of phenotypic manifestations of biological properties, including antibiotic resistance of *E. faecalis* (n = 71) isolated from urine of children with UTI. All analyzed uropathogenic *E. faecalis* had typical properties—morphology (cocci or oval Gram-positive bacteria), biochemical activity against mannitol, methylene blue, its absence in rhamnose fermentation, variability in glucose, lactose, sucrose and 2,3,5-triphenyltetrazolium chloride (TTC), and lack of mobility and catalase (**Table 2**).

Most *E. faecalis* isolated from the urine of children with UTI had *in vitro* enzymatic activity associated with pathogenicity: hemolytic, proteolytic, lipolytic, and lecithinase. A capsule was found in 45.6 ± 6.6% of uropathogenic enterococci. An inverse relationship was established between the presence of a capsule in *E. faecalis* with α-type hemolysis ($r = 0.3$, $p = 0.0001$), fermentation of milk ($r = 0.31$, $p = 0.00$), and a positive correlation with the microorganism titer in the urine ($r = 0.33$, $p = 0.0332$).

A direct correlation was established among the lecithinase and DNAase activity of *E. faecalis* ($r = 0.31$, $p = 0.0438$), the manifestation of hemolytic activity (α- or β-type) in uropathogenic enterococci, and the presence of the gene *gel*E ($r = 0.49$; $p<0.05$).

The capsule ($p_{1-2}<0.001$; $p_{1-3}<0.01$), milk fermentation ($p_{1-2}<0.001$; $p_{1-3}<0.01$), gelatinous ($p_{1-2}<0.001$, $p_{1-3}<0.05$), and lipolytic activity with respect to the tween 60 ($p_{1-2}<0.01$, $p_{1-3}<0.01$) was determined more often in *E. faecalis*, isolated from the urine of newborn children (group 1) with UTI, than in other age groups.

E. faecalis, isolated from children under 1 year (group 2), have hemolytic activity more often than other age groups ($p_{2-1}<0.05$, $p_{2-3}<0.05$), but expressed less gelatinous activity ($p_{1-2}<0.001$;

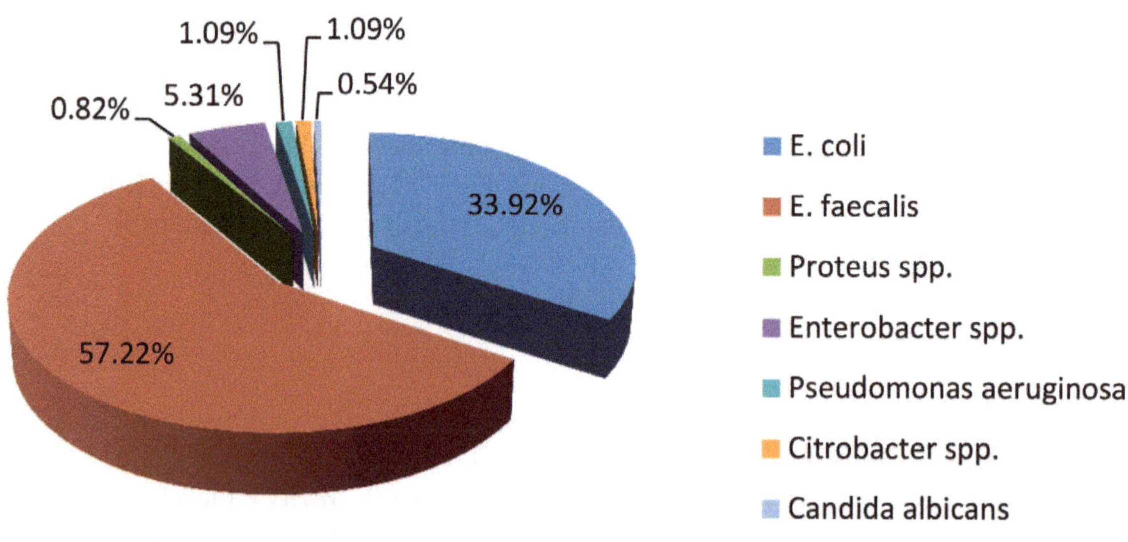

Figure 1. The etiological structure of UTI in newborn.

p_{2-3}<0.001). In this group, lipolytic activity against Tween 60 was less pronounced, but the differences were significant only between groups 1 and 2 (p<0.01).

E. faecalis isolated from patients older than 1 year (group 3) showed more lipolytic activity against Tween 80, compared to other age groups (p_{1-3}<0.001; p_{2-3}<0.01), gelatin's fermentation was determined more often than in enterococci of the group 2 (p<0.001). The hemolytic activity of enterococci in the group 3 differed little compared to the group of newborn children. The other biochemical properties associated with pathogenicity factors of *E. faecalis* strains of this age group were similar to enterococci isolated from children under 1 year of age (**Table 2**).

Assessment of antibiotics resistance revealed that all studied cultures of uropathogenic enterococci (n = 71) are sensitive to vancomycin and nitrofurantoin. We found that enterococci are

Biological properties	**Enzymatic activity of *E. faecalis***					
	Newborns (n = 21)		**Children from 29 days to 1 year (n = 18)**		**Children over 1 year old (n = 21)**	
	Number of examined cultures, n	**Abs. (P ± m_p, %)**	**Number of examined cultures, n**	**Abs. (P ± m_p, %)**	**Number of examined cultures, n**	**Abs. (P ± m_p, %)**
Reduction of TTC *■	19	18 (94.7 ± 5.1)	14	11 (78.6 ± 11.0)	21	20 (95.2 ± 4.7)
Reduction of methylene blue	19	19 (100)	14	14 (100)	21	21 (100)
Biochemical activity in relation to:						
Mannitol	20	20 (100)	13	13 (100)	19	19 (100)
Glucose ▲	20	19 (95.0 ± 4.9)	13	12 (92.3 ± 7.4)	19	19 (100)
Lactose ▲	20	19 (95.0 ± 4.9)	13	12 (92.3 ± 7.4)	19	16 (84.2 ± 8.4)
Rhamnose	21	0	13	0	19	0
Sucrose	20	17 (85.0 ± 8.0)	13	11 (84.6 ± 10.0)	19	16 (84.2 ± 8.4)
Presence of a capsule *▲	21	12 (57.1 ± 10.8)	17	6 (35.3 ± 11.6)	19	8 (42.1 ± 11.3)
Proteolytic activity in relation to:						
Milk *▲	21	18 (85.7 ± 7.6)	18	9 (50.0 ± 11.8)	21	10 (47.6 ± 10.9)
Gelatin *▲■	20	9 (45.0 ± 11.1)	17	2 (11.8 ± 7.8)	21	7 (33.3 ± 10.3)
Lecithinase activity	19	5 (26.3 ± 10.1)	15	4 (26.7 ± 11.4)	21	6 (28.6 ± 9.9)
Lipolytic activity in relation to:						
Tween 20	17	14 (82.4 ± 9.2)	12	11 (91.7 ± 7.9)	18	17 (94.4 ± 5.4)
Tween 60 *▲	8	4 (50.0 ± 17.2)	6	1 (16.7 ± 15.2)	11	3 (27.3 ± 13.4)
Tween 80 ▲■	21	14 (66.7 ± 10.3)	17	12 (70.6 ± 11.0)	19	16 (84.2 ± 8.4)

Note: *, p < 0.05 between 1 and 2 groups; ▲, p < 0.05 between 1 and 3 groups; ■, p < 0.05 between groups 2 and 3; Abs., absolute.

Table 2. Peculiarities of phenotypic manifestations biological properties of *E. faecalis* depending on the patient's age.

Id	ST	Isolate	Genotype						Total number of genes
			aggA	*esp*	*cylA*	*efaA*	*eep*	*gelE*	
1787	ST116	PR042	+	+	+	+	+	+	6
1789	ST179	PRV 052	+	+	+	+	+	+	6
1791	ST179	PRV100	+	+	+	+	+	+	6
1790	ST179	PRV105	+	+	+	+	+	+	6
	nd	PRV086	+	+	+	+	+	+	6
	nd	PR 230	+	+	+	+	+	+	6
1788	ST179	PRU047	+	—	+	+	+	+	5
	nd	PR 181	+	+	+	+	+	—	5
1781	ST16	PR050	+	+	+	+	+	—	5
1786	ST41	PRV049	+	+	—	+	+	+	5
	nd	PRL079	+	+	—	+	+	+	5
	nd	PRV080	+	+	—	+	+	+	5
1793	ST774	PRAs81	+	+	—	+	+	+	5
	nd	PR 198	+	—	—	+	+	+	4
	nd	PR 158	+	—	—	+	+	+	4
1780	ST6	PRV054	+	—	—	+	+	+	4
1779	ST6	PRN030	+	—	—	+	+	+	4
1795	ST774	PRA029	+	—	—	+	+	+	4
1792	ST774	PR51	+	—	—	+	+	+	4
1784	ST40	PR055	—	+	—	+	+	+	4
1785	ST40	PRA038	—	+	—	+	+	+	4
	nd	PR 228	+	—	+	+	+	—	4
1782	ST16	PRV092	+	—	+	+	+	—	4
	nd	PR 215	+	+	—	+	+	—	4
	nd	PR 223	+	+	—	+	+	—	4
1794	ST774	PR040	+	+	—	+	+	—	4
	nd	NCTC 12697	—	—	+	+	+	+	4
	nd	PR 97	—	—	+	+	+	+	4
	nd	PR 161	—	—	—	+	+	+	3
	nd	PR 206	—	—	—	+	+	+	3
1783	ST21	PRV082	—	—	—	+	+	—	2

Note: nd, not determined.

Table 3. Genotypes of uropathogenic *E. faecalis* in Primorsky region.

highly resistant to erythromycin (77.1 ± 5.02%), tetracycline (73.2 ± 5.3%), fluoroquinolones of the II and the III generations (ciprofloxacin (55.1 ± 5.9%), norfloxacin (48.6 ± 9.9%), and levofloxacin (46.5 ± 5.9%)). Were identified *E. faecalis* cultures, which are resistant (20.1 ± 4.9%) and mid-resistant (8.9 ± 3.5%) to the reserve drug linezolid. More than half (59.2 ± 5.8%) of the studied cultures of uropathogenic enterococci were resistant to several antibiotics (four or more antimicrobial agents).

It was found that enterococci, which are sensitive to penicillins, were characterized with lipolytic, lecithinase, and hemolytic (β-type) activity *in vitro*. Enterococci cultures which are resistant to fluoroquinolones, fermented sucrose, had proteolytic activity, and did not break down lactose. *E. faecalis*, which are resistant to gentamicin and erythromycin, had a capsule. Furthermore, *E. faecalis*, which are resistant to linezolid and chloramphenicol, had gelatinase, lecithinase, and lipolytic activities, as compared to other cultures (these data were not published).

In that way, analysis of biological properties of *E. faecalis*, isolated from urine of children with UTI in Primorsky region, showed that overwhelming majority of cultures had typical properties.

Id	Isolate	ST	Phenotype of antibiotic resistance	Genotype
1785	PRA038	40	TET-ERT-AmG-CHL-LZD	*esp-efaA-eep-gelE*
1784	PR055		TET-ERT-AmG-CHL	
1780	PRV054	6	TET-ERT-AmG-CHL-FLQ	*aggA-efaA-eep-gelE*
1779	PRN030		TET-ERT-AmG-CHL-FLQ	
1788	PRU047	179	TET-ERT-AmG-LZD	*aggA-cylA-efaA-eep-gelE*
1789	PRV052		TET-ERT-AmG	*aggA-esp-cylA-efaA-eep-gelE*
1791	PRV100		TET-ERT-AmG-CHL	
1790	PRV105		ERT-AmG-CHL-FLQ	
1787	PR042	116	TET-ERT-AmG-CHL-LZD	
1781	PR050	16	TET-ERT	*aggA-esp-cylA-efaA-eep*
1782	PRV092		TET-ERT-AmG	*aggA-cylA-efaA-eep*
1794	PR040	774	AmG-FX	*aggA-esp-efaA-eep*
1793	PRAs081		TET-ERT-PEN-AmG-FLQ	*aggA-esp-efaA-eep-gelE*
1795	PRA029		TET-ERT-PEN-FLQ	*aggA-efaA-eep-gelE*
1792	PR051		TET-ERT-AmG-FLQ	
1786	PRV049	41	TET	*aggA-esp-efaA-eep-gelE*
1783	PRV082	21	FLQ	*efaA-eep*

Note: TET, tetracycline; ERT, erythromycin; AmG, aminoglycosides; FLQ, fluoroquinolones; CHL, chloramphenicol; LZD, linezolid; PEN, penicillins.

Table 4. Antibiotic resistance of uropathogenic *E. faecalis* depending on the sequence type.

The mentioned variability of biochemical and fermentation activities of pathogenicity factors and resistance to antibiotics suggested a certain phenotypic heterogeneity of *E. faecalis.*

3.1. Molecular genetics typing of *E. faecalis*

E. faecalis was tested for genes, coding various pathogenicity factors, using PCR method. It was found that clinical strains (n = 30) of enterococci isolated from urine of children with UTI contained two and more studied pathogenicity genes. In this context, 27 out of 30 uropathogenic *E. faecalis* had four and more of the studied genes (**Table 3**).

Eleven variants of genes combinations, which code pathogenicity factors of *E. faecalis,* were identified. The most common variants are (*agg*A-*esp*-*cyl*A-*efa*A-*eep*-*gel*E) and (*agg*A, *efa*A, *eep*, *gel*E).

Multilocus sequence typing (MLST) divided 17 *E. faecalis* strains into eight (ST6, ST16, ST21, ST40, ST41, ST116, ST179, and ST774) sequence types (The results have not been published.) It was noticed that uropathogenic *E. faecalis* strains attributed to ST6, ST40, ST179, ST774, and ST116 are resistant to four and more groups of antimicrobial agents (**Table 4**).

The results demonstrate broad variability of the range of genes, which code pathogenicity factors and reveal sequence types with multiple resistances to antimicrobial agents among uropathogenic *E. faecalis* isolated from children with UTI in Primorsky region.

4. Discussion

Urinary tract infection is an inflammatory process in the organs of the urinary system without specifying the level of damage or growth of microorganisms in the urinary tract with possible development of local inflammatory changes. UTI refers to the factors that initiate the development of chronic kidney disease and depends on the age of the children [27]. Etiological multifactority is peculiarity of these infections. For a long time, commonly recognized pathogens of uroinfections are Gram-negative enterobacteria, among which *Escherichia coli* is prevalent [25, 26, 29, 31, 40, 44].

Interest to studying enterococci as participants of infectious diseases has increased in recent years. Our research has shown that *E. faecalis* are a common pathogen, which causes UTI in children, most often in newborns (from 30.8 up to 75% of cases). Perhaps this is not accidental, as according to some authors, this microorganism is detected in children from the first days of life and its amount exceeds the content of *E. coli* in the newborn period [19]. The reason for this microbial composition of urine appears to be functional immunodeficiency in this category of patients.

However, until now, the true etiological significance of these microorganisms in the development of the infectious process and unfavorable outcomes remains uncertain due to the ever-changing properties of *E. faecalis*. It is known that the ability of bacteria to affect the kidneys and urinary tract is determined not by one but by a complex of properties necessary for this process, that at the different stages of the infectious process in the urinary system organs from the microorganism, priority expression of certain pathogenetically significant traits and/or their combinations is required [6].

All analyzed uropathogenic *E. faecalis* had typical properties—morphology, biochemical activity against mannitol, methylene blue, its absence in rhamnose fermentation, variability in glucose, lactose, sucrose and 2,3,5-TTC, and lack of mobility and catalase.

At the same time, weak and delayed acid formation from lactose was in three cultures (only on the third day), and in 12 isolates during fermentation of sucrose (by day 10). The results obtained with respect to a number of carbohydrates differ from the literature data, as it is known that *E. faecalis* ferment lactose and sucrose, and in relation to other sugars can be variable (Berdzhi). Possibly, this is associated with the spread of certain *E. faecalis* biovars in the territory of Primorsky Krai or within a single multispecialty hospital.

According to results of research conducted in recent years, it was determined that enterococci produce many virulence factors, which conduce to development of the infectious process (hemolysin, gelatinase, enterococcal surface protein, aggregation substance, serine protease, capsule, etc.). The greatest number of virulence factors was found in *E. faecalis* isolated from urine. High proteolytic activity of *E. faecalis* (hydrolysis of gelatinase, casein, and collagen) causes toxic damage to tissues and conduce to cicatricial changes in kidney [6, 19, 43].

Moreover, the change in the properties of the microorganisms, causing the urinary tract infection, such as the development of resistance factors to antimicrobial drugs and the biofilm formation, makes it difficult to manage patients, especially with chronic persistent and often recurrent infection.

Our research confirmed high virulence properties of *E. faecalis* isolated from urine of patients with and their manifestations depending on the patient's age. For example, there is a negative correlation between the proteolytic activity of *E. faecalis* and the age of the children ($r = 0.28$, $p = 0.002$). Most *E. faecalis* isolated from the urine of children with UTI had *in vitro* enzymatic activity associated with pathogenicity: hemolytic, proteolytic, lipolytic, and lecithinase.

Currently, lipase is referred to understudied factors of enterococcal persistence, although it is known that lipase may be a potential virulence factor of *E. faecalis* [12]. Among the studied enterococci isolated from children with UTI, lipolytic activity was determined in $85.0 \pm 8.2\%$ of the cultures (more often with respect to Tween 20 and Tween 80). Enterococcus cultures showed heterogeneity in proteolytic and hemolytic activity. A reliable direct correlation between the phenotypic manifestation of β-type hemolytic activity with hydrolysis of gelatin ($r = 0.58$, $p = 0.0001$) and lecithinase activity ($r = 0.52$, $p = 0.0004$) of this uropathogen has been established. This confirms the combined effect of these pathogenic factors at a certain stage of the inflammatory process. A relationship was established between the phenotypic manifestation of pathogenicity factors and the age of patients.

The most common properties of *E. faecalis* isolated from urine of newborn children were a capsule, proteolytic, and lipolytic (in relation to Tween 60) activity. Enterococci isolated from 1-year-old children with UTI most frequently were characterized with hemolytic activity. Lipolytic (in relation to Tween 80) activity was most frequently found in cultures isolated from patients older than 1 year. The prevalence of these virulence factors suggests that they are associated with virulence of this species in UTI. Such features of the manifestation of biological properties *in vitro* indicate the selection of etiologically significant *E. faecalis* at the level of the macroorganism.

Furthermore, connection between sensitivity to antimicrobial drugs of *E. faecalis* and its biological properties was identified. It was found that uropathogenic enterococci characterized with proteolytic activity are resistant to antibacterial agents with different action mechanisms. In the work, it was found that *E. faecalis*, resistant to linezolid and chloramphenicol drugs that suppress protein synthesis at the level of the 50S subunit of the bacterial ribosome, possess a high pathogenic potential. These results require further research in this direction.

Interesting data were obtained with regard to the sensitivity of uropathogenic *E. faecalis* to the reserve drug linezolid, recommended for treatment of infections caused by strains, which are resistant to vancomycin, aminoglycosides, and betalactams. In Primorsky Krai, *E. faecalis* cultures were found resistant and intermediate sensitivity to linezolid. However, in Russia in the period from 2005 to 2013, there were isolated single enterococcal strains with reduced sensitivity to linezolid.

This way, the mentioned variability of biochemical and fermentation activity of factors related to pathogenicity demonstrated phenotypic heterogeneity of enterococci and might have a certain diagnostic significance.

Pathogenicity factors of bacteria are genetically determined by properties which are localized in genome of microorganisms in the form of "pathogenicity islands" [17]. These genetic elements can contain various sets of virulence genes, which are important for the development of the enterococcal infectious process, including genes of antibiotics resistance [17, 24]. At the present stage, the association of antibiotic resistance of *E. faecalis* with pathogenic factors is actively studied. It is known that strains of enterococci resistant to ampicillin, ciprofloxacin, and gentamicin, but sensitive to vancomycin and nitrofurantoin have more pathogenicity factors (hemolysin, gelatinase, hyaluronidase, form biofilms) than vancomycin resistant [2, 28]. *E. faecalis* having the *asa*1 gene are more resistant to fluoroquinolones (norfloxacin, ciprofloxacin, and levofloxacin) than isolates lacking this gene. Resistance to ciprofloxacin is significantly higher in *E. faecalis* having the genes *cyl*L and *cyl*S than in strains with their absence [23, 28]. *esp* gene-positive *E. faecalis* are more resistant to doxycycline than *esp* gene-negative cultures [3]. Among the strains with multidrug resistance, a high prevalence of genes *asa*1 and *esp was* observed [23, 36].

The research implemented using PCR method enabled to characterize in greater detail the structure of *E. faecalis* population isolated from children with UTI from Primorsky region. In our research, significant variability in occurrence frequency of the studied genes was found. Two of them—*efa*A (coding the surface antigen A (EfaA), which initiates the infectious process) and *eep* (coding Eep protein, which conduces to formation of a biofilm, making it resistant to various biological stress factors) were found in all studied uropathogenic *E. faecalis*, which proves their involvement in certain stages of the infectious process.

MLST analysis conducted earlier revealed eight sequence types, five of which were characterized by multidrug resistant.

This way, clinically significant *E. faecalis* strains have a complex of virulent properties, which allow the bacteria to materialize their pathogenic potential on all stages of the inflammation process in urinary system. This makes further research of the listed factors in clinical *E. faecalis* necessary to estimate objectively the contribution of these properties of the agent into pathophysiologic mechanism of infectious and inflammatory diseases.

5. Conclusions

1. Important role in the etiology of UTI is played not only by Gram-negative bacteria of the *Enterobacteriaceae* family, but also by gram-positive *E. faecalis*, which are of paramount importance in the development of UTI in newborns.

2. *E. faecalis*, isolated from the urine of children with UTI, have a complex of pathogenicity factors necessary for the development of the inflammatory process and their prolonged persistence in the urinary tract. The relationship between *E. faecalis* pathogenicity factors and the age of patients was determined.

3. Uropathogenic *E. faecalis* possess a polyantibiotic resistance, which is associated with its biological properties and belonging to a particular sequence type.

4. A set of phenotypic manifestations of the biological properties of *E. faecalis* (the presence/ absence of hemolytic, gelatinase, lecithinase, lipolytic activities) established in the study may determine its clinical significance and serve as an *in vitro* diagnostic marker of resistance of the studied uropathogen to certain groups of antibacterial drugs.

Acknowledgements

The research was supported with an internal grant from the university (registration No. AAAA-A18-118031390014-9).

Author details

Zaitseva Elena Aleksandrovna[1]*, Komenkova Tatiana Sergeevna[1], Melnikova Elena Aleksandrovna[1,2], Shadrin Andrey Mikhailovich[3,4] and Luchaninova Valentina Nikolaevna[5]

*Address all correspondence to: elza200707@mail.ru

1 Pacific State Medical University, Vladivostok, Russia

2 Regional Children's Clinical Hospital № 1, Vladivostok, Russia

3 G.K. Skryabin Institute of Biochemistry and Physiology of Microorganisms, Russian Academy of Sciences, Pushchino, Moscow Region, Russia

4 Pushchino State Institute of Life Sciences, Pushchino, Moscow Region, Russia

5 North-Western State Medical University named after I.I. Mechnikov, Saint-Petersburg, Russia

References

[1] Alberici I, Bayazit AK, Drozdz D, et al. Pathogens causing urinary tract infections in infants: A European overview by the ESCAPE study group. European Journal of Pediatrics. 2015;**174**(6):783-790. DOI: 10.1007/s00431-014-2459-3

[2] Banerjee T, Anupurba S. Prevalence of virulence factors and drug resistance in clinical isolates of *Enterococci*: A study from North India. Journal of Pathogens. 2015:7. ID 692612. DOI: 10.1155/2015/692612

[3] Baylan O, Nazik H, Bektöre B, Citil BE. The relationship between antibiotic resistance and virulence factors in urinary *Enterococcus* isolates. Mikrobiyoloji Bülteni. 2011;**45**(3):430-445

[4] Beganovic M, Luther MK, Rice LB, Arias CA, Rybak MJ, et al. A review of combination antimicrobial therapy for *Enterococcus faecalis* bloodstream infections and infective endocarditis. Clinical Infectious Diseases. 2018. DOI: 10.1093/cid/ciy064. [Epub ahead of print]

[5] Bittencourt ME, Suzart S. Occurrence of virulence-associated genes in clinical *Enterococcus faecalis* strains isolated in Londrina, Brazil. Journal of Medical Microbiology. 2004;**53**:1069-1073

[6] Bukharin OV, Gritsenko VA, Vyalkova AA. Factors of bacterial urotogenicity: A role in pathogenesis and importance in the diagnosis of pyelonephritis. Nephrology and Dialysis. 2001;**3**(4):469-475

[7] Chang SL, Shortliffe LD. Pediatric urinary tract infections. Pediatric Clinics of North America. 2006;**53**(3):379-400, vi. DOI: 10.1016/j.pcl.2006.02.011

[8] Chaschina IL, Tatochenko VK, Barkadze MK. The place of cephalosporins in the treatment of urinary tract infections in children. Current Pediatrics. 2012;**1**(1):158-161

[9] Chugunova OL, Shumikhina MV, Dumova SV. Current overview of the urinary system infection in newborns and infants. Effective Pharmacotherapy. 2013;**42**:38-47

[10] Diederich A-K, Wobser D, Spiess M, Sava IG, Huebner J, et al. Role of glycolipids in the pathogenesis of *Enterococcus faecalis* urinary tract infection. PLoS One. 2014;**9**(5):e96295. DOI: 10.1371/journal.pone.0096295

[11] Eaton TJ, Gasson MJ. Molecular screening of *Enterococcus* virulence determinants and potential for genetic exchange between food and medical isolates applied and environmental microbiology. 2001;**67**(4):1628-1635. DOI: 10.1128/AEM.67.4.1628-1635.2001

[12] Elsner H, Sobottka I, Mack D, Wirth R. Virulence factors of *Enterococcus faecalis* and *E. faecium* blood culture isolates. European Journal of Clinical Microbiology & Infectious Diseases. 2000;**19**:39-42

[13] Esther H, Bonten MJ, Willems Rob JL. Enterococcal surface protein Esp is important for biofilm formation of *Enterococcus faecium* E1162. Journal of Bacteriology. 2007;**189**(22): 8233-8240. DOI: 10.1128/JB.01205-07

[14] Flores-Mireles AL, Walker JN, Caparon M, Hultgren SJ. Urinary tract infections: Epidemiology, mechanisms of infection and treatment options. Nature Reviews. Microbiology. 2015;**13**(5):269-284. DOI: 10.1038/nrmicro3432

[15] Forster CS, Shaikh N, Hoberman A, Jackson E. Uropathogens and pyuria in children with neurogenic bladders. Pediatrics. 2018;**141**(5). DOI: 10.1542/peds.2017-3006

[16] Frank KL, Vergidis P, Brinkman CL, et al. Evaluation of the *Enterococcus faecalis* biofilm-associated virulence factors AhrC and Eep in rat foreign body osteomyelitis and in vitro biofilm-associated antimicrobial resistance. PLoS One. 2015;**10**(6):e0130187. DOI: 10.1371/journal.pone.0130187

[17] Gilmore MS, Clewell DB, Yasuyoshi I, Shankar N. Enterococci from commensals to leading causes of drug resistant infection [Internet]. Boston: Massachusetts Eye and Ear Infirmary; 2014. 668 pp

[18] Grazioli S, Parvex P, Merlini L. Antenatal and postnatal ultrasound in the evaluation of the risk of vesicoureteral reflux. Pediatric Nephrology. 2010;**25**(9):1687-1692

[19] Haid B, Pichler R, Becker T, Koen M, Berger C, et al. Late renal scarring and loss of kidney function despite successful therapy of vesicoureteral reflux in childhood: Case report and review of literature. International Journal of Case Reports in Medicine. 2015. DOI: 10.5171/2015.737441

[20] Kline KA, Lewis AL. Gram-positive uropathogens, polymicrobial urinary tract infection, and the emerging microbiota of the urinary tract. Microbiology Spectrum. 2016;**4**(2). DOI: 10.1128/microbiolspec.UTI-0012-2012

[21] Medeiros AW, Pereira RI, Oliveira DV, Martins PD. Molecular detection of virulence factors among food and clinical *Enterococcus faecalis* strains in South Brazil. Brazilian Journal of Microbiology. 2014;**45**(1):327-332. DOI: 10.1590/S1517-83822014005000031

[22] Melnikova EA, Zaitseva EA, Luchaninova VN. Features of urinary tract infection in children associated with *Enterococcus faecalis* in view of its biological properties. Nephrology. 2016;**20**(3):42-47

[23] Mete E, Kaleli I, Cevahir N, Demir M, et al. Evalution of virulence factors in *Enterococcus* species. Mikrobiyoloji Bülteni. 2017;**51**(2):101-114

[24] Miller WR, Munita JM, Arias CA. Mechanisms of antibiotic resistance in enterococci. Expert Review of Anti-Infective Therapy. 2014;**12**(10):1221-1236. DOI: 10.1586/14787210.2014.956092

[25] Naboka YL, Rymashevsky AN, Sviraeva EG, Bragina LE. Formation of the microflora of the digestive tract of newborns in dynamics. Journal of Microbiology, Epidemiology and Immunology. 2012;**3**:65-70

[26] Taneja N, Chatterjee SS, Singh M, Sharma M. Pediatric urinary tract infections in tertiary care center from north India. Indian Journal of Medical Research. 2010;**131**:101-105

[27] Osipovich SA. Immunological disorders, course and prognosis of recurrent infections of the urinary system in children. Pediatrics. Eastern Europe. 2013;**2**(2):42-55

[28] Padilla C, Lobos O. Virulence, bacteriocin genes and antibacterial susceptibility in *Enterococcus faecalis* strains isolated from water wells for human consuptision. Springerplus. 2013;**2**(1):43

[29] Petrosyan EK, Gavrilova VA, Reznikov AY. Treatment and prevention of recurrent urinary tract infection in children. Russian Herald of Perinatology and Pediatrics. 2010;**1**:85-88

[30] Preethee T, Kandaswamy D, Hannah R. Molecular identification of an *Enterococcus faecalis* endocarditis antigen *efa*A in root canals of therapy-resistant endodontic infections. Journal of Conservative Dentistry. 2012;**15**(4):319-322. DOI: 10.4103/0972-0707.101886

[31] Stein R, Dogan HS, Hoebeke P, Kocvara R, Nijman RJM, Radmayr C, Tekgul S. Urinary tract infections in children: EAU/ESPU Guidelines. European Urology. 2015;**67**:546-558

[32] Shankar V, Baghdayan AS, Huycke MM, et al. Infection-derived Enterococcus faecalis strains are enriched in esp, a gene encoding a novel surface protein. Infection and immunity. 1999;**67**(1):193-200

[33] Seno Y, Kariyama R, Mistuhata R, Monden K, Kumon H. Clinical implications of biofilm formation by *Enterococcus faecalis* in the urinary tract. Acta Medica Okayama. 2005;**59**(3): 79-87

[34] Soares RO, Fedi AC, Reiter KC, Caierão J, d'Azevedo PA. Correlation between biofilm formation and *gelE, esp*, and *agg* genes in *Enterococcus* spp. clinical isolates. Virulence. 2014;**5**(5):634-637. DOI: 10.4161/viru.28998

[35] Shankar N, Lockatell CV, Arto SB, Drachenberg C, Gilmore MS, Johnson DE. Role of *Enterococcus faecalis* surface protein Esp in the pathogenesis of ascending urinary tract infection. Infection and Immunity. 2001;**69**(7):4366-4372. DOI: 10.1128/IAI.69.7.4366-4372.2001

[36] Shahraki S, Nezhad Mousavi MR. Determination of virulence factors in clinical multidrug resistance *Enterococci* isolates at Southeast of Iran. Jundishapur Journal of Microbiology. 2017. DOI: 10.58.12/jim.45514

[37] Skepyan EN, Vasilevski IV, Toptun PD. Analysis of the spectrum of infections of the urinary tract and the characteristic their sensitivity to antimicrobial drugs the children's outpatient. Medical Panorama. 2013;**8**:35-38

[38] Stereva T, Atanasova D, Savov E, Petrova G, Mitov I. Incidence of virulence determinants in clinical *Enterococcus faecalis* and *Enterococcus faecium* isolates collected in Bulgaria. The Brazilian Journal of Infectious Diseases. 2016;**20**(2):127-133. DOI: 10.1016/j.bjid.2015.11.011

[39] Strezelecki Y, Hryniewicz W, Sadowy E. Gelatinase-associated phenotypes and genotypes among clinical isolates of *Enterococcus faecalis* in Poland. Polish Journal of Microbiology. 2011;**60**(4):287-292

[40] Vasilyeva LI, Kogan MI, Gudima IA, Naboka YL. Etiological structure and antibiotic susceptibility of pathogens of acute non-obstructive pyelonephritis in children. Attending Physician. 2009;**8**:8-11

[41] Upadhyaya PM, Ravikumar KL, Umapathy BL. Review of virulence factors of enterococci: An emerging nosocomial pathogen. Indian Journal of Medical Microbiology. 2009;**27**(4): 301-305. DOI: 10.4103/0255-0857.55437

[42] Upadhyaya PM, Umapathy BL, Ravikumar KL. Comparative study for the presence of enterococcal virulence factors gelatinase, hemolysin and biofilm among clinical and commensal isolates of *Enterococcus faecalis*. Journal of Laboratory Physicians. 2010;**2**(2):100-104. DOI: 10.4103/0974-2727.72159

[43] Zaitseva EA, Krukovich EV, Melnikova EA, Luchaninova VN, Komenkova TS, Vaysero NS. The role of pathogenicity factors of *Enterococcus faecalis* in the development of pyelonephritis in children. Pacific Medical Journal. 2017;**2**(68):58-61

[44] Zorc JJ, Kidoo DA, Shaw KN. Diagnosis and menagment of pediatric urinary tract infections. Clinical Microbiology Reviews. 2005;**18**:417-422

6

Management of Complicated Urinary Tract Infection

Ran Pang, Jianhua Deng and Xinyao Zhou

Abstract

The management of complicated urinary tract infection (UTI) remains a challenge since the coexisted conditions may significantly decrease the successful rate of treatment. In this chapter, the specific conditions including indwelling catheter, urolithiasis, neurogenic bladder, vesicoureteral reflux and pregnancy are listed. In terms of each condition, the potential influence on UTI and management strategy is discussed. Not only is the current evidence reviewed but also we present our experience on management of complicated UTI.

Keywords: urinary tract infection, catheter, urolithiasis, neurogenic bladder, vesicoureteral reflux, pregnancy

1. Introduction

Urinary tract infection (UTI), defined as an inflammatory response of the urothelium induced by a pathogenic organism, is one of the most common infectious diseases. It is estimated that one-third of the women may experience UTI by the age of 24, and half of the women suffer from at least one symptomatic UTI during their lifetime [1]. Basically, UTI can be classified as uncomplicated and complicated infection. The former is normally confined to bladder, which can be treated by short-course antibiotics. The latter refers to an infection associated with a condition which can increase the rate of therapy failures significantly. It is reported that 25–30% of adult women with UTI have at least one risk factor causing complicated UTI [2]. The common conditions which may result in complicated UTI are presented in **Table 1**. Not only do these factors decrease treatments' successful rate but also increase the recurrence risk of UTI. Therefore, when a complicated UTI is treated, management of the conditions needs to be taken into consideration.

Category	Specific conditions
Foreign bodies	Indwelling catheter
	Urolithiasis
Structural or functional abnormality of urinary tract	Neurogenic bladder
	Vesicoureteral reflux
	Obstructive uropathy
Others	Pregnancy
	Diabetes mellitus
	Renal failure
	Immunosuppression after kidney transplantation

Table 1. Specific conditions causing complicated UTI.

2. Catheter-associated UTI

Catheter-associated UTI is one of the most common complicated UTIs. It has been reported that catheter-associated UTI may lengthen the patients' hospital stay and increase the mortality and the direct medical cost [3, 4]. Typically, the microorganisms can enter urinary tract through the extraluminal or intraluminal route. The former means microbial pathogens can invade the bladder through the gap between the catheter and urethra, whereas the latter indicates that causative agents migrate to bladder along the internal lumen of the catheter. According to the data from National Healthcare Safety Network (NHSN), the top three pathogens causing catheter-associated UTI are *Escherichia coli* (21.4%), *Candida spp.* (21.0%) and *Enterococcus spp.* (14.9%), followed by *Pseudomonas aeruginosa* (10.0%), *Klebsiella pneumoniae* (7.7%) and *Enterobacter spp.* (4.1%) [5]. With the duration of catheterization prolonging, the pathogens may induce the formation of biofilm on the surface of the catheter, which causes the occurrence of antibiotic resistance [6]. Traditionally, antimicrobial therapy was considered as a prevention strategy for catheter-associated UTI. However, a survey in two Dutch district hospitals showed that the use of antibiotics was associated with the development of bacteriuria in patients catheterized for 3–14 days [7]. A recent cohort study further revealed that empirical antibiotic treatment had no effect on patients' prognosis [8]. Both European Association of Urology (EAU) and Infectious Diseases Society of America (IDSA) guidelines recommend against the use of systemic antimicrobial prophylaxis for catheter-associated UTI [9, 10]. By contrast, the consistent recommendation identified across guidelines is removal of the catheter as soon as possible. However, some patients have to be catheterized for a long time due to various disorders. For those patients, some practical strategies are developed to prevent and manage the catheter-associated UTI.

2.1. Alternatives to indwelling urethral catheter

Instead of indwelling urethral catheterization, some alternative approaches have been developed to minimize the catheter-associated UTI. Those approaches include use of external catheter, intermittent catheterization and suprapubic catheterization. Condom catheter is the most common external equipment, which is suitable for patients with severe storage lower urinary tract dysfunction such as urinary incontinence. It has been reported that condom catheter has a significant advantage in comparison with indwelling catheter. A randomized controlled trail (RCT) demonstrated that condom catheter might reduce 80% risks of catheter-associated UTI or death compared to indwelling catheter. Additionally, patients with condom catheter presented a significant higher satisfaction rate than ones with the indwelling catheter [11].

For patients with severe voiding lower urinary tract dysfunction, intermittent or suprapubic catheterization is an option to replace indwelling catheter. An early study investigated the incidence of bacteriuria in patients with intermittent or indwelling catheterization. Based on the results of urine culture, 32% of patients treated with intermittent catheterization had bacteriuria, which is significantly lower than 61% in ones with an indwelling catheter [12]. Another study revealed that patients with intermittent catheterization had less chance to suffer from pyelonephritis than the counterparts with indwelling catheterization (5 vs. 25%, $P < 0.01$) [13]. In a multicentered RCT, 87 patients with a postvoid residual (PVR) bladder volume of more than 150 ml were allocated to receive intermittent or indwelling catheterization. After 3 days, a significant lower risk of developing bacteriuria was found in the intermittent catheterization group compared with the indwelling catheterization group (14 vs. 38%, $P = 0.02$), so was the risk of UTI (12 vs. 33%, $P = 0.03$). In terms of patients' satisfaction, no marked difference was found between these two groups [14].

In general, intermittent catheterization can be practiced by a clean or sterile technique. Originally, sterile intermittent catheterization was applied as a standard method. In 1947, Guttman published the first report about sterile intermittent catheterization. In the report, he showed that this technique could decrease the risk of UTI and might be helpful for patients' recovery of micturition. About 19 years later, Guttman further reported his experience in the use of sterile intermittent catheterization. During 11 years, he applied this technique to manage a total of 476 patients. Based on the data from 409 males, the technique was related to an extremely low incidence in UTI, vesicoureteral reflux, hydronephrosis and urolithiasis. Although sterile intermittent catheterization has some advantages, it is costly and time-consuming. In 1970, Hence Lapides and Betty S. Lowe introduced another technique, that is, clean and intermittent self-catheterization. Subsequently, they published a series of articles in which they showed that this technique could not increase the incidence of UTI. Later, a number of emerged evidence suggested that sterile intermittent catheterization could not provide an extra benefit compared to clean techniques. Two RCTs demonstrated that different technique was associated neither with overgrowth of microorganisms in urinary tract nor with the symptomatic UTI [15, 16].

Suprapubic catheterization provides a treatment option for patients who are not suitable for intermittent catheterization such as those with low compliance bladder. Evidence has illustrated that suprapubic catheter may bring more benefits for patients compared to transurethral catheter. A retrospective cohort study showed that patients with suprapubic catheter had less clinical visits due to pain than ones with indwelling urethral catheter [17]. The result from a meta-analysis revealed that suprapubic catheterization was associated with a significant lower risk of bacteriuria and less discomfort compared with transurethral catheter [18]. A prospective open-labeled study presented that women with postoperative urinary retention favored suprapubic catheter due to a better catheter-specific quality of life [19]. According to the result from a network meta-analysis, indwelling urethral catheter did not increase the risk of UTI compared with either suprapubic tube or intermittent catheterization when duration of catheter was less than 5 days. In contrast, suprapubic tube or intermittent catheterization was associated with a lower rate of UTI when long-term catheterization is needed [20]. Based on our experience, suprapubic catheter has a significant advantage for male patients. We used suprapubic catheter to manage more than 20 male patients who suffered from recurrent acute bacterial prostatitis or epididymitis secondary to indwelling urethral catheter. We found that no one experienced these genitourinary infections again after the technique of catheterization was changed. Additionally, suprapubic catheter allows patients to observe their recovery of voiding function. We encourage patients to try to urinate with a closed suprapubic catheter if they have a low detrusor leak-point pressure (<40 cmH_20) assessed by urodynamics, which means patients' attempt of voiding cannot bring about upper urinary tract deterioration. After spontaneous voiding, patients need to open the suprapubic catheter and measure the PVR. Once the PVR is low enough, the removal of suprapubic catheter can be taken into consideration.

2.2. Catheter selection

To prevent the catheter-associated UTI, some special catheters have been designed and developed. They mainly include silver-coated, antibiotic-coated, hydrophilic and novel trefoil catheters.

As is known, silver is a kind of antiseptic. So it was hypothesized that catheter coated with silver could reduce the risk of UTI in patients treated by the indwelling catheter. Based on this hypothesis, a variety of silver-coated catheters have been developed. However, the efficacy of these catheters on UTI prevention varies from one to another. Evidence showed that silver alloy-coated catheter might reduce the incidence of UTI, but the silver oxide-coated one would not. A prospective single-center study conducted in Hong Kong investigated the incidence of UTI in patients with a silver alloy and hydrogel-coated catheter, which was compared with the counterparts with a standard catheter. The results showed that the incidence of UTI per 1000 catheter days was 6.4 and 9.4 in the silver-coated catheter group and standard catheter group, respectively. The silver-coated catheter group presented a 31% reduction in risk of UTI [21]. Lederer et al. reported the similar results in a retrospective cohort study in which 7 medical centers with 2778 active acute care beds in the United States were involved. They found that the silver alloy and hydrogel-coated catheter could cause a 47 and 58% relative reduction in UTI rate, respectively, compared to the conventional catheter when a different definition was applied [22]. In contrast, two clinical trials revealed that the use of silver oxide-coated catheter could not reduce the incidence of UTI and bacteriuria in comparison with standard catheter [23, 24]. Besides the two silver-coated catheters mentioned earlier, another silver nanoparticle-fabricated catheter has been developed. According to an experimental study, this silver nanoparticle catheter had significant antimicrobial and antibiofilm properties, as well as a remarkable ability to cause disorganization of bacterial cell membrane, which may prevent UTI effectively [25].

It has been shown that antibiotic-coated catheter has a significant antimicrobial activity. Desai et al. found that nitrofurazone-impregnated catheter could decrease the adherence of pathogenic microorganisms to catheter markedly, but the effect could only persist for 5 days after the catheterization [26]. Regev-Shoshani et al. further reported that both nitrofurazone- and nitric oxide-coated catheters had a great effect on the prevention of microbial growth and biofilm formation, which was more effective than silver-coated catheter [27]. Despite lack of available clinical data so far, the antibiotic-coated catheter may bring potential benefits for patients with indwelling catheter.

Hydrophilic catheter may decrease the friction between catheter and urethra during catheterization. Consequently, it reduces the potential mucosal trauma which can result in the bacterial colonization. A multicentered RCT showed that the use of hydrophilic catheter might decrease approximately one-third the risk of developing symptomatic UTI compared with standard catheter [28]. Similarly, the evidence from a meta-analysis supported marked benefits of hydrophilic catheter in terms of the incidence of UTI [29].

A novel trefoil catheter has been developed. Although it has not been reported for use in clinical practice, the preclinical study has shown its advantages. Sun et al. performed an experiment in which 66 rabbits were catheterized using either conventional or novel trefoil catheter randomly and reported that the novel catheter could decrease the incidence of bacteriuria. In addition, it was also found that the trefoil catheter caused a significant slighter mucosal inflammation than conventional catheter based on endoscopic assessment [30].

2.3. Catheter care

Catheter care is important for patients with an indwelling catheter since appropriate care can decrease the incidence of UTI. Both EAU and IDSA guidelines recommend maintaining a closed drainage system all the time [9, 10]. Once any breaks are detected, both the catheter and collecting system must be replaced as soon as possible. Besides, it is crucial to keep the drainage tubing being below the level of the patient's bladder and above the level of the collection bag, which can avoid the reflux of urine in drainage system. To minimize the risk of UTI, different types of collecting systems were developed. However, current evidence fails to show their different effects on prevention of UTI. Sullivan et al. conducted a RCT, in which 51 hospitalized dogs were catheterized with either an open or closed urine collection system. After analyzing the incidence of bacteriuria, they concluded that the type of urine collection system (open vs. closed) was not associated with the risk of developing bacteriuria [31].

In terms of the time point to change catheter, most guidelines recommend against changing catheter routinely. Instead, it is recommended to change the catheter before blockage occurs. Furthermore, some strategies including bladder irrigation with citric acid solution and oral acetohydroxamic acid have been proven to be effective for prevention of catheter blockage [32, 33]. By contrast, bladder washing with saline is not recommended due to lack of effectiveness [34].

3. Urolithiasis

Urolithiasis is one of the most common urological diseases with a rising incidence around the world. In general, UTI is usually considered as a complication of urolithiasis. Actually, it is also a potential pathogenic factor for a special urinary stone, struvite. Basically, the formation of struvite originates with the bacterial decomposition for urea. Some bacteria, including Proteus and Klebsiella, can decompose urea into ammonia and carbon dioxide, which can be further converted into ammonium and bicarbonate, respectively, and consequently, elevate the pH value of urine. With an alkaline urinary environment, the ammonium has a strong ability to combine with magnesium and phosphate. Once these chemical substances become supersaturated in urine, they will crystallize and deposit the struvite. The existence of urinary stone, especially struvite, may cause UTI difficult to treat because the stone may act as a nidus for microorganisms and result in obstruction in urinary tract.

According to our experience, when UTI and urolithiasis coexist, the individualized management strategy should be taken into consideration. If the stone causes a urinary tract obstruction, the initial treatment should focus on the decompression of the collecting system, which can avoid the infection being exacerbated. Normally, the best way of decompression is to remove the stone as soon as possible, which can be achieved either by ureteroscopic lithotripsy or by percutaneous nephrolithotripsy. However, if the patient cannot tolerate these minimally invasive surgeries, indwelling ureteral stent and percutaneous nephrostomy tube could be the optional treatment. Only with an unobstructed collecting system can the subsequent antibiotic therapy for UTI be efficient. For patients with coexistence of UTI and nonobstructive stone, empiric antibiotic therapy can be the initial treatment. Only when the UTI fails to manage, the invasive intervention is considered to remove the stone.

4. Neurogenic bladder

Neurogenic bladder refers to the bladder dysfunction secondary to a certain disease of the central nervous system or peripheral nerves. The specific conditions causing neurogenic bladder are various and the most common one is spinal cord injury, followed by multiple sclerosis, cerebral vascular events and Parkinson's disease [35]. Moreover, long-standing diabetes plays an important role in the development of neurogenic bladder. It is reported that patients with neurogenic bladder have a significant increased incidence of UTI. An observational study in which 46,000 patients with neurogenic bladder were investigated and followed up showed that 29.2–36.4% of patients were diagnosed with lower UTI annually [35]. Another study revealed that 81% of patients with spinal cord injury experienced at least one UTI during a period of 5 years [36]. The etiology of UTI caused by neurogenic bladder is diverse. It is reported that the bladder ischemia and defect of glycosaminoglycan layer induced by bladder overdistension reduce the barrier function of urothelium [37, 38]. Moreover, immunological impairment of bladder mucosa involving NK cell, B and T cell further decreases the bladder's ability to defend the pathogens [39, 40].

For patients with neurogenic bladder, the clean intermittent self-catheterization is the most common technique to avoid bladder overdistension. It remains a big issue whether prophylactic antibiotics can prevent bacteriuria and UTI in patients performing clean intermittent self-catheterization due to neurogenic bladder. Two double-blind, placebo-controlled, crossover trials showed that nitrofurantoin prophylaxis could reduce the risk of bacteriuria and UTI significantly [41, 42]. On the contrary, a Cochrane systematic review demonstrated that the evidence failed to prove the certain benefits of antibiotic prophylaxis in patients with clean intermittent self-catheterization [43]. In a recently published case series study, Cox L et al. described a successful treatment in reduction of UTI in patients with clean intermittent self-catheterization using intravesical instillations of gentamicin [44]. However, the treatment strategy needs to be further verified by well-designed RCTs.

5. Vesicoureteral reflux

Vesicoureteral reflux is the most common risk factor for UTI in children. It is reported that 30–40% of children with their first UTI episode are affected by this disorder [45, 46]. In general, vesicoureteral reflux is graded from I to V (mild to severe) according to the height of reflux up the ureter and degree of dilatation of the ureter. A high grade of vesicoureteral reflux, defined as grade IV and V, may lead to the renal scars due to UTI, which may further cause renal failure. Conventionally, antibiotic prophylaxis has been considered as the standard management for patients with vesicoureteral reflux. However, a large cohort study revealed that continuous antibiotic prophylaxis could not decrease the risk of recurrent UTI but might increase the risk of bacteria resistant to the antibiotic in children with vesicoureteral reflux [47]. As an approach to eliminate reflux, some invasive interventions including anti-reflux surgery and injection of bulking agent are used to reduce the breakthrough UTI. Basically, the surgical options include open or laparoscopic ureteral reimplantation. Based on clinical assessment, the reported successful rate for open and laparoscopic approach is 80–95% and 90–93%, respectively [48–50]. In contrast, the endoscopic injection presents a lower treatment successful rate in the range of 50–93% [48]. From our experience, surgical intervention may be an effective therapy for the patients who still suffer from UTI even on continuous antibiotic prophylaxis.

6. Pregnancy

It is reported that pregnant women have an increasing risk of UTI, especially upper UTI, because the physiological changes induced by pregnancy make them more likely to suffer from pyelonephritis. On the one hand, elevated level of progesterone during pregnancy can induce the relaxation of ureteric smooth muscles, which may lead to the urine retention in the renal collecting system and ureter. On the other hand, the noticeable increase in renal blood volume and glomerular filtration rate may contribute to the renal pelvic and ureteral dilation. The dilated upper urinary tract provides pathogens with a permissive environment to grow and reproduce. As a result, bacteriuria will develop pyelonephritis in 25–40% of pregnant women. The independent risk factors include history of UTI, low socioeconomic status, indigence, intercurrent diabetes and sickle cell trait. Therefore, short-course antibiotic therapy should be applied to prevent developing ascending UTI, once the bacteriuria is identified in pregnant women. It is investigated that the antibiotic therapy can reduce the incidence of pyelonephritis by 75% [51]. Generally, a three-day course of antibiotic therapy directed by urine culture is recommended for both symptomatic lower UTI and asymptomatic bacteriuria. When the result of culture is not available, an empiric therapy with a ß-lactam or nitrofurantoin can be used as the initial treatment. For patients with upper UTI, a 14- to 21-day course of intravenous antibiotic therapy should be adopted. The reported effective antibiotic includes a third-generation cephalosporin, gentamicin or aztreonam, which can be used as the initial treatment before the result of culture is available. In addition, it is crucial to identify whether an obstruction exists in every pregnant woman. Once the obstruction is diagnosed, it can be relieved by ureteral stent or percutaneous nephrostomy tube. For patients with ureteral stent or percutaneous nephrostomy tube, it is necessary to use the antibiotic continuously until after delivery.

7. Conclusion

The treatment of complicated UTI remains a challenge because the coexisted conditions are diverse. Appropriate management for these conditions is the prerequisite achieving a successful treatment for complicated UTI.

Acknowledgements

This work was supported by Beijing Municipal Science & Technology Commission No. Z161100000516156 and grant 2014S292 from Guang An Men Hospital, China Academy of Chinese Medical Sciences.

Author details

Ran Pang[1*], Jianhua Deng[2] and Xinyao Zhou[3]

*Address all correspondence to: pangran2002@gmail.com

1 Department of Urology, Guang An Men Hospital, China Academy of Chinese Medical Sciences, Beijing, P.R. China

2 Department of Urology, Peking Union Medical College Hospital, Chinese Academy of Medical Sciences and Peking Union Medical College, Beijing, P.R. China

3 Department of Rumatology, Guang An Men Hospital, China Academy of Chinese Medical Sciences, Beijing, P.R. China

References

[1] Foxman B. Epidemiology of urinary tract infections: Incidence, morbidity, and economic costs. Disease-a-Month. 2003;**49**(2):53-70

[2] Hooton TM. Recurrent urinary tract infection in women. International Journal of Antimicrobial Agents. 2001;**17**(4):259-268

[3] Chant C et al. Relationship of catheter-associated urinary tract infection to mortality and length of stay in critically ill patients: A systematic review and meta-analysis of observational studies. Critical Care Medicine. 2011;**39**(5):1167-1173

[4] Tambyah PA, Knasinski V, Maki DG. The direct costs of nosocomial catheter-associated urinary tract infection in the era of managed care. Infection Control and Hospital Epidemiology. 2002;**23**(1):27-31

[5] Hidron AI et al. NHSN annual update: Antimicrobial-resistant pathogens associated with healthcare-associated infections: Annual summary of data reported to the National Healthcare Safety Network at the Centers for Disease Control and Prevention, 2006-2007. Infection Control and Hospital Epidemiology. 2008;**29**(11):996-1011

[6] Kirmusaoglu S et al. The effect of urinary catheters on microbial biofilms and catheter associated urinary tract infections. Urology Journal. 2017;**14**(2):3028-3034

[7] Hustinx WN et al. Impact of concurrent antimicrobial therapy on catheter-associated urinary tract infection. The Journal of Hospital Infection. 1991;**18**(1):45-56

[8] Babich T et al. Empirical antibiotic treatment does not improve outcomes in catheter-associated urinary tract infection: Prospective cohort study. Clinical Infectious Diseases. 2017;**65**(11):1799-1805

[9] Hooton TM et al. Diagnosis, prevention, and treatment of catheter-associated urinary tract infection in adults: 2009 International clinical practice guidelines from the Infectious Diseases Society of America. Clinical Infectious Diseases. 2010;**50**(5):625-663

[10] Tenke P et al. European and Asian guidelines on management and prevention of catheter-associated urinary tract infections. International Journal of Antimicrobial Agents. 2008;**31**(Suppl 1):S68-S78

[11] Saint S et al. Condom versus indwelling urinary catheters: A randomized trial. Journal of the American Geriatrics Society. 2006;**54**(7):1055-1061

[12] Johansson I et al. Intermittent versus indwelling catheters for older patients with hip fractures. Journal of Clinical Nursing. 2002;**11**(5):651-656

[13] Turi MH et al. Proportion of complications in patients practicing clean intermittent self-catheterization (CISC) vs indwelling catheter. The Journal of the Pakistan Medical Association. 2006;**56**(9):401-404

[14] Hakvoort RA et al. Comparing clean intermittent catheterisation and transurethral indwelling catheterisation for incomplete voiding after vaginal prolapse surgery: A multicentre randomised trial. British Journal of Obstetrics and Gynaecology. 2011;**118**(9):1055-1060

[15] King RB et al. Clean and sterile intermittent catheterization methods in hospitalized patients with spinal cord injury. Archives of Physical Medicine and Rehabilitation. 1992; **73**(9):798-802

[16] Moore KN, Burt J, Voaklander DC. Intermittent catheterization in the rehabilitation setting: A comparison of clean and sterile technique. Clinical Rehabilitation. 2006; **20**(6):461-468

[17] Dunn TS, Figge J, Wolf D. A comparison of outcomes of transurethral versus suprapubic catheterization after Burch cystourethropexy. International Urogynecology Journal and Pelvic Floor Dysfunction. 2005;**16**(1):60-62. Discussion 62

[18] McPhail MJ, Abu-Hilal M, Johnson CD. A meta-analysis comparing suprapubic and transurethral catheterization for bladder drainage after abdominal surgery. The British Journal of Surgery. 2006;**93**(9):1038-1044

[19] Takase-Sanchez MM et al. Suprapubic versus transurethral bladder drainage following reconstructive pelvic surgery: A comparison of patient satisfaction and quality of life. International Urogynecology Journal. 2017;**28**(5):721-728

[20] Han CS et al. Comparison of urinary tract infection rates associated with transurethral catheterization, Suprapubic tube and clean intermittent catheterization in the postoperative setting: A network meta-analysis. The Journal of Urology. 2017;**198**(6):1353-1358

[21] Chung PH et al. A prospective interventional study to examine the effect of a silver alloy and hydrogel-coated catheter on the incidence of catheter-associated urinary tract infection. Hong Kong Medical Journal. 2017;**23**(3):239-245

[22] Lederer JW et al. Multicenter cohort study to assess the impact of a silver-alloy and hydrogel-coated urinary catheter on symptomatic catheter-associated urinary tract infections. Journal of Wound, Ostomy, and Continence Nursing. 2014;**41**(5):473-480

[23] Johnson JR et al. Prevention of catheter-associated urinary tract infection with a silver oxide-coated urinary catheter: Clinical and microbiologic correlates. The Journal of Infectious Diseases. 1990;**162**(5):1145-1150

[24] Riley DK et al. A large randomized clinical trial of a silver-impregnated urinary catheter: Lack of efficacy and staphylococcal superinfection. The American Journal of Medicine. 1995;**98**(4):349-356

[25] Thomas R et al. Inhibitory effect of silver nanoparticle fabricated urinary catheter on colonization efficiency of coagulase negative Staphylococci. Journal of Photochemistry and Photobiology. B. 2015;**149**:68-77

[26] Desai DG et al. Silver or nitrofurazone impregnation of urinary catheters has a minimal effect on uropathogen adherence. The Journal of Urology. 2010;**184**(6):2565-2571

[27] Regev-Shoshani G et al. Comparative efficacy of commercially available and emerging antimicrobial urinary catheters against bacteriuria caused by *E. coli* in vitro. Urology. 2011;**78**(2):334-339

[28] Cardenas DD et al. Intermittent catheterization with a hydrophilic-coated catheter delays urinary tract infections in acute spinal cord injury: A prospective, randomized, multicenter trial. Physical Medicine and Rehabilitation. 2011;**3**(5):408-417

[29] Chartier-Kastler E, Denys P. Intermittent catheterization with hydrophilic catheters as a treatment of chronic neurogenic urinary retention. Neurourology and Urodynamics. 2011;**30**(1):21-31

[30] Sun Y et al. Decreased urethral mucosal damage and delayed bacterial colonization during short-term urethral catheterization using a novel trefoil urethral catheter profile in rabbits. The Journal of Urology. 2011;**186**(4):1497-1501

[31] Sullivan LA, Campbell VL, Onuma SC. Evaluation of open versus closed urine collection systems and development of nosocomial bacteriuria in dogs. Journal of the American Veterinary Medical Association. 2010;**237**(2):187-190

[32] Burns JR, Gauthier JF. Prevention of urinary catheter incrustations by acetohydroxamic acid. The Journal of Urology. 1984;**132**(3):455-456

[33] Mayes J, Bliss J, Griffiths P. Preventing blockage of long-term indwelling catheters in adults: Are citric acid solutions effective? British Journal of Community Nursing. 2003; **8**(4):172-175

[34] Muncie Jr HL et al. Once-daily irrigation of long-term urethral catheters with normal saline. Lack of benefit. Archives of Internal Medicine. 1989;**149**(2):441-443

[35] Manack A et al. Epidemiology and healthcare utilization of neurogenic bladder patients in a US claims database. Neurourology and Urodynamics. 2011;**30**(3):395-401

[36] Biering-Sorensen F et al. Urological situation five years after spinal cord injury. Scandinavian Journal of Urology and Nephrology. 1999;**33**(3):157-161

[37] Perlow DL, Gikas PW, Horowitz EM. Effect of vesical overdistention on bladder mucin. Urology. 1981;**18**(4):380-383

[38] Vasudeva P, Madersbacher H. Factors implicated in pathogenesis of urinary tract infections in neurogenic bladders: Some revered, few forgotten, others ignored. Neurourology and Urodynamics. 2014;**33**(1):95-100

[39] Iversen PO et al. Depressed immunity and impaired proliferation of hematopoietic progenitor cells in patients with complete spinal cord injury. Blood. 2000;**96**(6):2081-2083

[40] Schlager TA et al. Bladder epithelium is abnormal in patients with neurogenic bladder due to myelomeningocele. Spinal Cord. 2004;**42**(3):163-168

[41] Johnson HW et al. A short-term study of nitrofurantoin prophylaxis in children managed with clean intermittent catheterization. Pediatrics. 1994;**93**(5):752-755

[42] Schlager TA et al. Nitrofurantoin prophylaxis for bacteriuria and urinary tract infection in children with neurogenic bladder on intermittent catheterization. The Journal of Pediatrics. 1998;**132**(4):704-708

[43] Niel-Weise BS et al. Urinary catheter policies for long-term bladder drainage. Cochrane Database of Systematic Reviews. 2012;**8**:CD004201

[44] Cox L et al. Gentamicin bladder instillations decrease symptomatic urinary tract infections in neurogenic bladder patients on intermittent catheterization. Canadian Urological Association Journal. 2017;**11**(9):350

[45] Marild S, Jodal U. Incidence rate of first-time symptomatic urinary tract infection in children under 6 years of age. Acta Paediatrica. 1998;**87**(5):549-552

[46] Jacobson SH, Hansson S, Jakobsson B. Vesico-ureteric reflux: Occurrence and long-term risks. Acta Paediatrica. Supplement. 1999;**88**(431):22-30

[47] Conway PH et al. Recurrent urinary tract infections in children: Risk factors and association with prophylactic antimicrobials. Journal of the American Medical Association. 2007;**298**(2):179-186

[48] Elmore JM et al. Incidence of urinary tract infections in children after successful ureteral reimplantation versus endoscopic dextranomer/hyaluronic acid implantation. Journal of Urology. 2008;**179**(6):2364-2367. Discussion 2367-8

[49] Akhavan A, Avery D, Lendvay TS. Robot-assisted extravesical ureteral reimplantation: Outcomes and conclusions from 78 ureters. Journal of Pediatric Urology. 2014; **10**(5):864-868

[50] Arlen AM et al. Outcomes of complex robot-assisted extravesical ureteral reimplantation in the pediatric population. Journal of Pediatric Urology. 2016;**12**(3):169e1-169e6

[51] Sweet RL. Bacteriuria and pyelonephritis during pregnancy. Seminars in Perinatology. 1977;**1**(1):25-40

7

Management of Urinary Tract Infections: Problems and Possible Solutions

Lorenza Murgia, Ottavia Stalio, Alyexandra Arienzo, Valeria Ferrante, Valentina Cellitti, Salvatore Di Somma, Paolo Visca and Giovanni Antonini

Abstract

In clinically suspected urinary tract infections (UTIs), empirical antibiotic treatment is usually started long before the laboratory results of urine culture and antibiogram are available. Although molecular diagnostic approaches are being applied to the diagnosis of many infections, UTIs are generally diagnosed by traditional culture methods. Patient care could greatly benefit from the development of a rapid, accurate, inexpensive test that could be done at patient's bedside, allowing the practitioner to plan targeted, more effective therapy. Such a test would potentially reduce incorrect or unnecessary use of antibacterial drugs and reduce the emergence of bacterial resistance. In response to this pressing and unmet clinical need, several methods have been developed in the last few years. Among these, the new point-of-care test (POCT) for detecting UTIs named Micro Biological Survey (MBS) UTI CHECK holds promise, as it allows semi-quantitative determination of bacterial load in urine leading to a fast detection of UTIs and to evaluation of bacterial antibiotic susceptibility. This new technology operates through a colorimetric survey performed in low-cost, ready-to-use, disposable vials, in which 1 ml of urine is inoculated without any preliminary treatment and requiring neither specialized personnel nor a specialized equipment.

Keywords: urinary tract infections, point-of-care test, clinical microbiology analysis, UTIs diagnosis, antimicrobial resistance

1. Introduction: definition and background over urinary tract infections (UTIs)

Urinary tract infections (UTIs) are caused by the presence and multiplication of microorganisms in the urinary tract, sometimes spreading to the bloodstream and possibly resulting in several clinical syndromes (e.g., pyelonephritis, cystitis, urethritis, epididymitis and prostatitis) [1].

Most UTIs are caused by bacteria, and when they occur in the urine without causing symptoms, this condition is called asymptomatic bacteriuria; when growth of bacteria leads to a panel of symptoms, this condition is referred to as symptomatic bacteriuria [1]. Urinary tract infections can manifest as bacteriuria with limited clinical symptoms and sepsis, depending on localized or systemic extension [2].

The onset of UTIs is mostly due to the ascent of microorganisms from the urethra, especially organisms of enteric origin, e.g., *Escherichia coli*, which is the causative pathogen in 70–95% of acute, uncomplicated UTIs in adults, followed by other Enterobacteriaceae, such as *Proteus mirabilis* and *Klebsiella* spp., and by *Staphylococcus saprophyticus* in 5–10% of cases [2]; hence, the higher frequency of UTIs in women than men, depending on anatomic structure, and the increased risk of infection following bladder catheterization, which compromises natural defense mechanisms. A small fraction of UTIs can have hematogenous origin, and usually involve a few relatively uncommon microorganisms (e.g., *Staphylococcus aureus*, *Candida* spp., *Salmonella* spp. and *Mycobacterium tuberculosis*), which cause primary infections elsewhere in the body and thus reach the urinary tract [2].

UTIs are among the most prevailing infectious diseases with a substantial financial burden on society [3]. The incidence of community-acquired UTIs is highest in young women [1]: almost half of all women will experience at least one episode of UTI during their lifetime, and nearly 1 in 3 women will have had at least one episode of UTI by the age of 24 years [2]. Urinary tract infection incidence increases with age for both sexes. It is estimated that 10% of men and 20% of women over the age of 65 years have asymptomatic bacteriuria [1].

Reports from European countries and the USA show that ca. 15% of all community-prescribed antibiotics are dispensed for UTIs [3]. UTIs account for many annual hospital admissions, especially among the elderly: in the UK, the number of emergency admissions of older people with a primary diagnosis of UTI showed a 200% increase from 2001/2002 to 2012/2013, parallel to a related increase in bed days, which both are the second highest increase (in absolute terms) among groups of conditions [4]. Nevertheless, UTIs are believed to have been greatly overcoded in recent years: part of the increase may be due to changes in coding practice, part to increased emergence of antibiotic resistance [4]. Moreover, UTIs represent at least 40% of all hospital acquired infections and most of them occur following catheterization, which is considered one of the main risk factors associated to onset of UTIs [3].

2. Current laboratory standards in UTI diagnosis

The clinical evidence of UTI is based on a number of basic criteria, including clinical symptoms, and laboratory data which should provide evidence of the presence of microorganisms by culturing of urine samples, or other specific tests [2]. However, the diagnosis of UTIs is primarily based on symptoms and signs. Tests that suggest or prove the presence of bacteria or white cells in the urine may contribute additional information to inform management but rarely have important implications for diagnosis, also considering the long time often required for obtaining results with traditional methods [5].

The gold standard for diagnosis of bacteriuria is culture of appropriate urine sample [6, 7]. Sampling by needle aspiration minimizes the risk of contamination, while catheter and midstream sampling show a higher risk of contamination and therefore yield more false positive results [5]. However, needle aspiration is invasive and midstream sampling is preferred in clinical practice [8]. Routine culture is generally carried out streaking 10 μl of urine sample on agar plates containing selective or differential media and reading results after at least 24–48hours of incubation, considering characteristic colony morphologies and average quantitation. If there is the need for more accurate quantitative results, 100 μl plating following serial dilutions of urine sample must be performed [9]. The main value of urine culture is to identify microorganisms, most often bacteria; indirect indicators of the presence of bacteria (for example, urinary nitrites) are much less valuable than urine culture [5].

The number of bacteria in urine has been considered relevant for the diagnosis of UTIs since the Sixties, when Kass developed the concept of significant bacteriuria (10^5 CFU/ml) opening up to quantitative microbiology for the diagnosis of infectious diseases; his notion is still generally used to help diagnosis. Nevertheless, it has recently become clear that no fixed bacterial count can be applied to all kinds of UTIs and all circumstances, and even low bacterial concentrations are considered clinically relevant considering specific clinical pictures, sampling protocols and patient's sex. The problem of counting low numbers must then be considered [2].

Along with pathogen identification, outlining its antimicrobial susceptibility profile is considered to be crucial to ensure an appropriate treatment [10]. Antimicrobial susceptibility testing is routinely performed using the Kirby-Bauer disk diffusion technique according to Clinical and Laboratory Standards Institute (CLSI) guidelines, meaning culturing bacteria from urine samples on agar plates in presence of disks containing selected antibiotics; interpretation of results requires the measurement of halos of inhibition around disks according to reference tables [11].

As with most bacterial infections, diagnosis of UTI depends on culturing the clinical sample in the clinical laboratory, and results are typically delayed of two to three days from sample acquisition [10]. This is due to the need for sample transport to the laboratory and the time required for bacteria to grow on culture media [10]. Thus, the standard method for UTI diagnosis is time consuming and logistically difficult [6].

Since the patient cannot remain untreated during this rather prolonged period before definitive diagnosis is obtained, physicians usually prescribe broad spectrum antibiotics prior to antibiogram results. This practice has many undesirable consequences in the short and long terms, such as treatment failure leading to spread or chronicization of infection, increased health care costs, and increased antibiotic resistance by a growing number of bacterial strains. Given these drawbacks, it is obvious that a rapid and accurate method of UTI diagnosis and bacterial antibiotic susceptibility assessment would offer significant health benefits [12].

The introduction of partial and complete automation in clinical diagnostic in the 2000s has allowed the management of large-scale sample volumes and workflows optimization still providing reliable results for both pathogen identification and antibiotic susceptibility testing [10, 13].

Large-scale systems, anyway, are expensive and require more dedicate space, equipment and more personnel competence, which makes them applicable to a large hospital setting, but are difficult to establish in a small hospital, or in a limited-resource setting (e.g., developing countries). These high-throughput culture-based instruments, moreover, remain relatively slow and are not amenable for point-of-care use [10].

The introduction of matrix-assisted laser desorption/ionization time-of-flight mass spectrometry (MALDI-TOF) technology in microbiology has allowed rapid and reliable bacterial identification, featuring both high sensitivity and specificity, improving efficiency and saving consumables and labor [14, 15]. MALDI-TOF technique is usually coupled with culture of urine samples, to allow isolation of bacteria and therefore obtain pure cultures, which will undergo MALDI-TOF analysis after some sample treatment. Recently, extensive databases have been developed that include protein profiles of main microorganisms involved in infections; some studies have therefore investigated the possibility to apply MALDI-TOF analysis directly to urine samples, yielding promising results also when coupling such analysis with screening methods, such as automated microscopic urine sediment analysis [16, 17]. It must be considered, however, that such high-throughput technology has high installation and maintenance costs, and requires dedicated spaces, limiting its use in routine analyses to centralized laboratories. Moreover, the technique cannot currently identify two species of bacteria when present simultaneously, and cannot determine antibiotic susceptibility; thus, traditional culture of urine samples is still necessary [18].

Nevertheless, the occurrence of more than one bacterial strain in urine samples participating in the infection should not be overlooked. Polymicrobic infections are more often associated with catheterization and aging, reaching 10% incidence rates in the community and 30% in hospital setting among elderly people [19]. Bacterial strains recovered from polymicrobic infection show metabolic alterations and altered virulence traits, such as antibiotic resistance [19]. However, relationships between coinfecting strains are not yet fully understood [20], although some studies are exploiting such infections' mechanisms [21, 22]. As clinical laboratories tend to report cultures showing single or clearly predominant bacteria and will not routinely report occurrence of polymicrobic associations, unless significant numbers of each species are detected, quite a large portion of UTIs are not correctly diagnosed nor treated, threatening patient's safety [19, 23–25]. Therefore, an improvement of diagnosis and clinical pathways is needed in order to enhance not only detection of pathogens in urine, but also profiling the whole microflora and determining the antimicrobial susceptibility of individual components.

3. When a urine culture followed by antibiogram is needed

Even though the incidence of UTIs is higher in women [6], also related pathologies in men, such as epididymitis and prostatitis, may be caused by migration of pathogens from the urethra or bladder, the most common pathogens isolated being *Chlamydia trachomatis*, Enterobacteriaceae (typically *E. coli*) and *Neisseria gonorrhoeae*. For this last species, to reach correct diagnosis and plan following treatment, culture of mid-stream urine should be performed, together with nucleic acid amplification test (NAAT) on first voided urine or Gram staining in order to specifically detect *Neisseria gonorrhoeae* or *Chlamydia trachomatis* [6, 26].

Urine culture is recommended to determine the presence or absence of clinically significant bacteriuria in patients prior to urological interventions (e.g., surgery) and the presence of bacteriuria is controlled by directed pre-operative treatment of the detected pathogen [2, 6].

Urine culture is considered a valuable tool during patients' follow-up: in women whose symptoms do not resolve or recur within 2–4 weeks after the completion of treatment, urine culture and antimicrobial susceptibility test should be performed and a new antibiotic regimen should be considered. Afterward, in patients who underwent antibiotic treatment, a follow-up with subsequent urine culture should verify the treatment efficacy [2]. Urine culture is also recommended in women who present with atypical symptoms, pregnant women and males with suspected UTI [2].

In case of complicated UTIs, a broader range of bacteria is expected to be involved (often within the Enterobacteriaceae family), and these are more likely to show antibiotic resistance. Moreover, patients with a complicated UTI are more prone to have recurrent infections (more than 3 episodes/year) [2, 8, 27, 28]. Therefore, the choice of a therapy for these conditions must be supported by urine culture and antimicrobial susceptibility testing to avoid ineffective antibiotics administration.

Urine culture is also required in pediatric settings, where UTIs are the most common infections in children and infants, together with upper respiratory and gastrointestinal ones, with 30% recurrence rate reported within a year after initial UTI [2, 29]. Diagnosing pediatric UTIs may be difficult, because of communication difficulties in describing symptoms and vagueness of signs in small children; therefore, the definitive diagnosis of infection in children requires a positive urine culture [2].

In febrile patients with negative results on dipstick, microscopic, or automated urinalysis, urine culture is unnecessary if there is an alternative cause of the fever or inflammatory signs. However, if the dipstick and/or urinalysis are positive, confirmation of UTI by urine culture is mandatory [29]. In febrile children with signs of UTI (clinical signs, positive dipstick and/or positive microscopy, better if urine culture is available), antibiotic treatment should be initiated as soon as possible to eradicate the infection, prevent bacteremia, improve clinical outcome, diminish the likelihood of renal involvement during the acute phase of infection, and reduce the risk of immediate and long-term complications, including renal scarring and renal failure [29, 30].

4. Empirical treatment of UTIs

The gold standard for diagnosis and successful management of UTIs is to obtain identification and quantification of the infecting agents, along with antibiotic susceptibility assessment to direct a specific therapy [31]. The use of microbiological culture method is well established in the diagnosis of infectious diseases [32]; however, such reference method is time-consuming, requiring on average 24–48hours, thus laboratory results are not immediately available, especially at patient's presentation in the Emergency Department [32, 33]. For this reason, in order to avoid even serious complications (e.g., sepsis) and mitigate patients' discomfort, the initial treatment specified by international guidelines as first step in UTIs management is most often empirical [32]. Nevertheless, this empirical approach contributes to mis- and overuse of antibiotics [10], resulting from unnecessary or inappropriate antimicrobial therapy, participating in recent arise in bacterial resistance. In fact, for people with symptoms of UTI and bacteriuria the main aim of treatment is relief of symptoms, but in case of unsuccessful treatment it could cause some alteration of urinary tract microflora, leading to an increased risk of clinical adverse events, including infections with multi-drug-resistant organisms and the development of antibiotic-resistant UTIs [1]. Infections caused by multi-drug-resistant pathogens, such as extended-spectrum beta-lactamase (ESBL) and carbapenemase producing Gram-negative bacteria, methicillin-resistant *Staphylococcus aureus* (MRSA), and bacteria resistant to broad-spectrum antibiotics, such as fluoroquinolones and cephalosporins, are indeed increasingly recorded among UTIs and are the cause of a serious challenge to the public health system today [2, 10, 34].

The spread of antibiotic resistance is a threat to patients undergoing urological surgery in general [2], and multi-drug-resistant bacterial infections can limit the availability of effective treatment options, especially in low-income countries, rendering some UTIs difficult to treat and increasing healthcare costs [30].

This situation is generally promoted by several factors, including the overuse and misuse of antimicrobials in human and veterinary medicine and, indirectly, in agriculture. Measures to prevent and control the increase of antimicrobial resistance as well as the dissemination of resistance genes are crucial [35]. Prudent prescribing and rational use of antibiotics is a key component of action plans for reducing antimicrobial resistance [1, 2, 35, 36]. Antimicrobial stewardship programs have become a priority to optimize the outcome of prevention and treatment of infection while limiting overuse and misuse of antimicrobial agents [6], also following a systematic audit approach [37, 38]. In addition, non-antibiotic strategies are being explored [6]. There are many non-antimicrobial measures recommended, especially for recurrent UTIs [2, 28, 39, 40], but only a few results from well-designed studies are available for evidence-based recommendations [2, 41].

In general, the choice of antibiotics should be based, among other factors, upon identification and susceptibility pattern of the organism causing the UTI and the ecological collateral effects including selection of resistant bacteria by the chosen antimicrobial [2].

It must be considered, though, that the in vitro susceptibility of community-acquired uropathogens varies according to age and geographic region, and, as magnitude and variability of antimicrobial resistance patterns in the community grow, so does the need for continuous large-scale surveillance systems, in order to create databases linking epidemiological, clinical and laboratory data [42].

Therefore, the development and implementation of new clinical tools in routine medical practice could help optimizing antibiotic administration, leading to a more prudent and rational use of antibiotics. A rapid screen may be a more practical approach to yield benefits for the patient, the physician, and the laboratory [43].

The advent of new innovative diagnostic devices for UTI management, complementary to the reference culture-based methods, may lead to a new deal improving routine practice. Immunocompromised patients (e.g., diabetes mellitus, chronic kidney disease, and kidney transplant) with UTIs could particularly benefit from such diagnostic improvements. Clinical diagnosis of UTIs in this category of patients is challenging, because causative pathogens may be slightly different to those in the general population, and because of patients' clinical picture complexity. Early diagnosis is imperative in this group, and treatment of UTIs should be tailored according to individual patient characteristics [44].

5. Alternative and non-culture-based methods for the detection of UTIs

Because of the clinical importance of early UTI diagnosis, alternative rapid near-patient urine tests have been developed, such as urine dipsticks, which are widely used [31] in spite of their uncertain diagnostic accuracy [6]. The urine dipsticks test is commonly used for presumptive diagnosis of UTIs: it detects the presence of biochemical markers in urine samples which may be useful to establish the diagnosis of UTI [2]. Although many urine biomarkers for UTIs have recently been considered [45], markers that showed best results in diagnostic accuracy are nitrite and leukocyte esterase [6]. Although being cost-effective [46], such test shows low sensitivity that limits its clinical usefulness, [6] and analysis may be biased since a number of bacterial species are unreactive in these tests (e.g., no reduction of nitrates) [47, 48]. Furthermore, urine dipstick test does not detect bacteria, nor their concentration, which is essential to diagnose UTIs according to guidelines, and provides no information about antimicrobial susceptibility. Urine dipsticks are, anyway, cheap, easy to use, can be performed at doctor's office, in pharmacies or at home (even though urine dipstick test is not intended for self-diagnosis purposes [49], are available without prescription and provide results of easy interpretation within minutes.

Among hospital tests routinely used for urine analysis, microscopy examination of urine sediment has since long time been used, also undergoing automation to improve results. Although sensitivity is high, specificity is too low for exclusive use in clinical settings. Moreover, such technique requires sample centrifugation, and experienced personnel is needed to avoid errors in microscopic examination [6].

Flow cytometry found applications in many fields, also including medical disciplines [50]. Automated platforms of urinary flow cytometry have been widely adopted by centralized laboratories [10]. Flow cytometry allows of rapid detection of bacteria, white blood cells, red blood cells, epithelial cells, casts, crystals, yeasts and spermatozoa. They offer the benefit of standardize urine sediment analysis and reduce the error associated with subjective interpretation of results [51]. Nevertheless, the poor quality of available studies was confirmed in a recent meta-analysis, which also showed current low accuracy and specificity of such method that should not be used as the sole screening tool for UTIs ([51], and references therein).

Dipslide technology has been proposed to simplify traditional culture-based methods: the test allows the detection of bacteria in liquid matrices by observing growth on different agar media (e.g., CLED agar and MacConkey agar) after immersion into sample and following 24-hour incubation. Overall, despite being simple to use and cost-effective, dipslide technology can only be considered as a guide to support further analyses: such test shows low accuracy when compared to the reference culture method [6], and no reliable detection of $<10^4$ CFU/ml can be obtained [7]. For this reason, dipslides are currently unsuited to routine use in clinical setting with further studies required to determine the best combination of culture media [6].

For the short term, molecular biology techniques such as real-time PCR could be used to complement conventional culture-based methods for pathogens identification, especially with regard to shortening the time to obtain results, shortening the time to decision of antibiotic therapy [32]. However, this method is limited by the broadness of the panel of pathogens included in the test, and both sensibility and specificity are low when compared to urine culture. Moreover, such technology requires many steps for sample preparation and does not allow a viable count, also considering that up to now the clearance of bacterial DNA from urine is unclear. The need for quantification in UTI diagnosis should drive future developments of commercial real-time PCR pathogen detection tools to include a quantification option [32].

In addition, possible new routes have been explored aiming to develop new clinical tools to help rapidly identify uropathogens, such as: the detection of volatile organic compounds in urine by gas chromatography and mass spectrometry and following comparison between profiles using compounds databases [52]; the use of Raman and Surface Enhanced Raman Spectroscopy, which can provide quantification and identification of bacteria populations and possibly assessment of antibiotic susceptibility, although results are still preliminary and must be significantly expanded [12]; the use of impedance spectroscopy to detect ultra-low concentrations of *E. coli* in human urine and provide quantification for UTI diagnosis [53].

Although rapid, these technologies do not provide microbiological diagnosis nor susceptibility information, which remain the cornerstone of diagnosis, particularly in settings of complicated UTI [10].

In summary, laboratory urine culture remains the gold standard investigation for UTI diagnosis [6].

6. The importance of point-of-care tests in UTI diagnosis

Some tests have been developed aiming to provide rapid and accurate diagnostic information to direct treatment decisions at the patient's bedside, which seem to have yielded good consent among practitioners [54].

Rapid and definitive near-the-patient diagnosis of UTI would have a favorable impact on its management [10]: a rapid turnaround of results could influence clinical decisions such as triage, referral, and decision to discharge the patient. Prompt clinical interventions could be provided by caregivers, meaning timely antibiotic treatment could be initiated and imprecise empirical treatment avoided [10, 55]. This would improve health outcome also providing diagnostics tools for limited-resource settings [55]. Point-of-care tests (POCTs) can provide considerable savings in health care costs by reducing the number of patients visiting health centers simultaneously improving the quality of life for patients by reducing their number of visits to health care facilities [55]. An early diagnosis based on POCTs can also enable clinicians to start antibiotic administration earlier and thereby increase chances of successfully treating the disease. In future, innovation through rapid and reliable POCTs is advisable, updating technologies to ensure efficient data management and simplify use by healthcare professionals, eventually lowering medical costs [55]. POCTs could allow a better screening and follow-up of patients not only by hospitals, but also by pharmacies and general practitioners, helping decentralize diagnosis and therefore reduce the workload of laboratories, with consequent reduction of costs related to urine analysis and management of UTIs and reduction of human errors leading to mix-ups of patient samples sent to off-site laboratories [55].

Several POCT for UTIs have been developed and are currently commercially available. They can be distinguished in: (*i*) culture-based devices, (*ii*) (semi-)automated urine analyzers and (*iii*) enzymatic assays [56]. All culture-based devices allow semi-quantification of bacterial growth and evaluation of the infecting bacterial species. Most often, samples need to be cultured and appreciable bacterial growth can be achieved in not less than 16–24 hours. The (semi-)automated urine analyzers have the same read-out as the urine dipstick test and UTI diagnosis is based on the presence of markers such as nitrites and leukocytes. Although the human error involved in visual interpretation can be eliminated and results can be obtained in 1–2 minutes, these tests do not significantly improve current practice exhibiting very low sensitivity and limited positive predictive value. The same problem has been reported for enzymatic assays [57–61].

Biosensors offer a promising approach for improving molecular diagnostic in POC settings [10]. Biosensors are binary systems composed of a recognition and a transducer element that can generate a measurable proportional signal following binding of the target analyte to the recognition element (e.g., antibody, enzyme), which allows quantitative detection of a biological entity [10]. Even though biosensors technology has been applied successfully to the field of clinical diagnostic (e.g., blood glucose and pregnancy tests), no such tests have been implemented to date to improve routine diagnosis of UTIs [55]. Indeed, key features of biosensors, such as portability, rapidity, and cost-effectiveness in comparison with their macro-scale counterparts, could be crucial for the development of a POCT for UTI pathogens identification and antimicrobial susceptibility assessment. Nevertheless, considering the urine matrix, such biosensors would require multistep sample preparation with amplification/enrichment steps to improve target detection, and such biological matrix could impair sensor performance with its variations in biochemical parameters (e.g., inhibitors, non-specific binding). Moreover, such tests should have a multiplex approach to ensure identification of a broad panel of pathogens in different clinical scenarios, and should provide antimicrobial susceptibility testing to drive treatment, but genetic non-culture based approaches are limited by the fast evolution rate of defense mechanisms among bacteria. Biosensors POCTs could anyway complement reference methods helping saving resources in terms of materials, money and time, because rapid, simple and cost-effective tests could optimize further analyses therefore reducing the burden on laboratories [10].

The Micro Biological Survey (MBS) POCT "UTI CHECK" appears to hold good promise for early detection and antimicrobial susceptibility profiling of uropathogens. The MBS method allows rapid and accurate bacterial quantification through an automated colorimetric culture-based test; urine samples are inoculated into disposable ready-to-use reaction vials, which color will change thanks to redox indicators following bacterial growth after incubation (see **Figure 1**). Results of preliminary *in vitro* validation studies [62, 63] showed that the results obtained with this method are comparable to the reference culture-based methods.

Such findings encouraged further research in hospital settings, and clinical trials have been carried out [31] in which the efficacy of the MBS POCT was compared to the reference method, used in hospital routine, and other methods, such as urine dipsticks: the MBS POCT

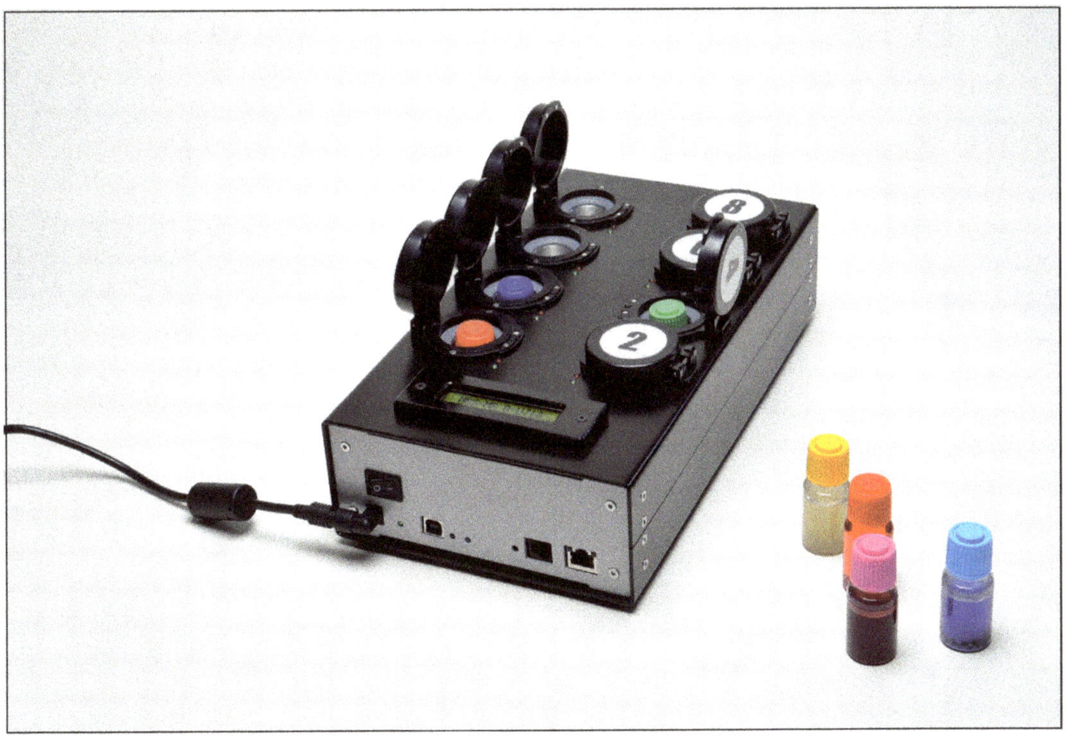

Figure 1. MBS "UTI CHECK." MBS "UTI CHECK" is an automated colorimetric culture-based test. It is composed by mono-use, disposable and ready-to-use reaction vials (right) in which 1 ml of urine can be inoculated without any preliminary treatment. Up to eight urine-inoculated reaction vials can be independently allocated in an automatic thermostated optical reader (left) that it is able to detect color change induced by the growth of bacteria and automatically correlates the time required for color change with the number of bacteria present in the urine samples. Different vials contain selected antibiotics and the occurrence of the color change in the presence of antibiotics indicates antibiotic resistance of bacteria present into the urine sample.

Product	Manufacturer/ location	Description of device	Analysis time	Additional equipment required	Positive result outcomes	Method principle	Number of samples tested; Test population	Threshold for significant growth	Accuracy	Sensitivity (%) (95% CI)	Specificity (%) (95% CI)	Ref
FLEXICULT™	Statens Serum Institut Diagnostica/ Denmark	Chromogenic agar plate with 6 segments – 5 evaluating anti-biotic sensitivities and 1 control segment	24 hours	Incubator	Semi-quantification of bacterial growth, evaluation of the species present, and assessment of sensitivity to the antibiotics in each of the plate segments	Microbial culture and susceptibility testing	N = 200/124 (outpatient setting)/76 (secondary care setting)	≥10^5 CFU/ml	—	87.0% (67.9–95.5)	83.2% (74.7–89.2)	[23]
Uricult Trio	Orion Diagnostics/ Finland	Plastic slide with two opposing agar media	16–24 hours when incubated at 36.8 °C or 1–3 days at room temperature	Incubator	Semi-quantification of bacterial growth, evaluation of the species present	Microbial culture	198 (pediatric patients aged 0–7)	≥10^4 CFU/ml	—	68%	82%	[26]
							434 (primary health care setting)	≥10^3 to ≥10^5 CFU/ml for doubtful uropathogens	88%	88%	90%	[27]
DipStreak (Chromostreak)	Novamed/ Israel	Plastic paddle with two opposing agar media, housed in a closed transparent plastic tube	18–24 hours	Incubator	Semi-quantification of bacterial growth, evaluation of the species present	Microbial culture	N = 1070 (251 hospitalized patients and 819 outpatients)	>10^5 CFU/ ml (single organism + mixed culture)	98%	95.7%	99.2%	[28]

Product	Manufacturer/ location	Description of device	Analysis time	Additional equipment required	Positive result outcomes	Method principle	Number of samples tested; Test population	Threshold for significant growth	Accuracy	Sensitivity (%) (95% CI)	Specificity (%) (95% CI)	Ref
DiaSlide	Novamed/ Israel	Hinged plastic case containing two opposing agar media	24 hours	Incubator	Semi-quantification of bacterial growth	Microbial culture	473 (prescreened hospital urine specimens using UriScreen)	$\geq 10^4$ CFU/ml	—	98.3%	97.5%	[29]
onSite	Trek Diagnostics System/USA	Hinged plastic case containing two opposing agar media	Not specified	Incubator	Semi-quantification of bacterial growth, evaluation of the species present	Microbial culture						
MBS UTI CHECK	MBS srl/Italy	Mono-use disposable vials for chromogenic analysis	3–5 hours	MBS Multireader	Semi-quantification of bacterial load, assessment of sensitivity to selected antibiotics	Measure of the catalytic activity of redox enzymes of bacteria	N = 223 (emergency department)	$\geq 10^5$ CFU/ ml (single organism + mixed culture)	99%	92.6% (75.7–99.1)	100% (94.9–100)	[17]

Table 1. Features of main POCTs for UTI diagnosis.

showed high accuracy, sensitivity and specificity, comparable to the reference method's and higher than urine dipsticks' [31]. Although not providing bacterial identification, MBS "UTI CHECK" allows bacteria detection and quantification in urine samples. Preliminary results showed that this POCT can provide uropathogens' susceptibility pattern to a panel of antibiotics. The analytical time required for UTI diagnosis is usually less than 3 hours (up to 5–6 hours when the bacterial load is equal or less than 1×10^5 CFU/ml) and antimicrobial susceptibility assessment is obtained in less than 10 hours, which could guide downstream medical decisions with crucial information within few hours. Notably, this method features cost-effectiveness, user-friendliness, portability, easy interpretation of results, which all can lead to successful use at the patient's bedside [31]. The MBS point-of-care testing device could be developed into a valuable aid for the management of UTIs, possibly addressing more precise diagnosis and appropriate therapy also proving useful in treatment outcome evaluation. Features of main POCTs available on market, including MBS "UTI CHECK," are summarized in **Table 1**.

7. Conclusions

To date, hospital settings rely mainly on laboratory analysis following urine culture reference method; this approach requires a considerable effort in terms of workload and up to 3 days to achieve results. Furthermore, it can lead to unnecessary antimicrobial overuse which ultimately promotes the emergence of resistance [31].

The unnecessary use of antibiotic treatment may be minimized following two roads: on one hand by the establishment of antibiotic stewardship programs which require healthcare staff involvement in regular training in best use of antimicrobial agents for an improved adherence to local, national or international guidelines and regular consultation with infectious diseases physicians, with audit [6]; on the other hand by improving diagnostic pathways [1], possibly relying on use of POCTs that feature incorporation of pathogen identification with antimicrobial susceptibility testing, sufficiently versatile to be adaptable for different pathogen profiles in different clinical scenarios [10]. The advent of accurate and robust POCTs could allow a more rational screening before treatment or admission and to improve follow-up of patients for treatment outcome evaluation and for monitoring of antimicrobial prescribing performance and local pathogen resistance profiles [6].

Such approach could ultimately lead to treatment customization according to individual patients' characteristics through fast antibiotic susceptibility testing results [44], with the ultimate aim of improving patients' welfare and reduce healthcare costs.

Acknowledgements

Prof. Vincenzo Ziparo (Istituto Dermopatico dell'Immacolata – IRCCS, Rome, Italy) is gratefully acknowledged for helpful discussions.

Author details

Lorenza Murgia[1], Ottavia Stalio[1], Alyexandra Arienzo[1], Valeria Ferrante[2], Valentina Cellitti[2], Salvatore Di Somma[3], Paolo Visca[1] and Giovanni Antonini[1,2]*

*Address all correspondence to: giovanni.antonini@uniroma3.it

1 Department of Sciences, Roma Tre University, Rome, Italy

2 Interuniversity Consortium "Biostructures and Biosystems National Institute", Rome, Italy

3 Emergency Medicine, Department of Medical-Surgery Sciences and Translational Medicine, Sapienza University of Rome, Sant'Andrea Hospital, Rome, Italy

References

[1] National Institute for Health and Care Excellence. Urinary Tract Infections in Adults – Quality Standard. 2015. Available from: http://nice.org.uk/guidance/qs90

[2] Grabe M, Bartoletti R, Bjerklund Johansen TE, Cai T, Çek M, Köves B, Naber KG, Pickard RS, Tenke P, Wagenlehner F, Wullt B. Guidelines on urological infections. 2015. Available from: http://uroweb.org/ [Accessed 31st October 2017]

[3] Grabe M, Bartoletti R, Bjerklund Johansen TE, Çek HM, Pickard RS, Tenke P, Wagenlehner F, Wullt B. Guidelines on urological infections. 2014. Available from: http://uroweb.org/ [Accessed 31st October 2017]

[4] Wittenberg R, Sharpin L, McCormick B, Hurst J. Understanding emergency hospital admissions of older people. Report No. 6. Oxford: Centre for Health Service Economics & Organisation (CHSEO); 2014

[5] Scottish Intercollegiate Guidelines Network (SIGN). Management of Suspected Bacterial Urinary Tract Infection in Adults. Edinburgh: SIGN (SIGN Publication No. 88); 2012 Available from: http://www.sign.ac.uk

[6] Pickard R, Bartoletti R, Bjerklund-Johansen TE, Bonkat G, Bruyère F, Çek M, Grabe M, Tenke P, Wagenlehner F, Wullt B, Guidelines Associates: Cai T, Köves B, Pilatz A, Pradere B, Veeratterapillay R. Guidelines on urological infections. 2016. Available from: http://uroweb.org/ [Accessed 31st October 2017]

[7] Schmiemann G, Kniehl E, Gebhardt K, Matejczyk MM, Hummers-Pradier E. The diagnosis of urinary tract infection. Deutsches Ärzteblatt International. 2010;**107**(21):361-367. DOI: 10.3238/arztebl.2010.0361

[8] Takhar SS, Moran GJ. Diagnosis and management of urinary tract infection in the emergency department and outpatient settings. Infectious Disease Clinics of North America 2014;**28**:33-48. DOI: http://dx.doi.Org/10.1016/j.idc.2013.10.003

[9] European Confederation of Laboratory Medicine. European urinalysis guidelines. Scandinavian Journal of Clinical and Laboratory Investigation. Supplementum. 2000;**231**:1-86

[10] Mach KE, Wong PK, Liao JC. Biosensor diagnosis of urinary tract infections: A path to better treatment? Trends in Pharmacological Sciences. 2011;**32**(6):330-336

[11] Clinical and Laboratory Standards Institute. Supplemental Tables. Performance Standards for Antimicrobial Susceptibility Testing; Fifteenth Informational Supplement. CLSI Publication M100-S15, M2-A8 and M7-A6. Pennsylvania: CLSI; 2005

[12] Kastanos E, Kyriakides A, Hadjigeorgiou K, Pitris C. A novel method for bacterial UTI diagnosis using Raman Spectroscopy. International Journal of Spectroscopy. 2012; Article ID: 195317, 13 pages. DOI: 10.1155/2012/195317

[13] Croxatto A, Prod'hom G, Faverjon F, Rochais Y, Greub G. Laboratory automation in clinical bacteriology: what system to choose? Clinical Microbiology and Infection 2016; **22**:217-235. DOI: http://dx.doi.org/10.1016/j.cmi.2015.09.030

[14] Gaillot O, Blondiaux N, Loïez C, Wallet F, Lemaître N, Herwegh S, Courcol RJ. Cost-effectiveness of switch to matrix-assisted laser desorption ionization–time of flight mass spectrometry for routine bacterial identification. Journal of Clinical Microbiology. 2011;**39**(12):4412. DOI: 10.1128/JCM.05429-11

[15] Neville SA, LeCordier A, Ziochos H, Chater MJ, Gosbell IB, Maley MW, van Hal SJ. Utility of matrix-assisted laser desorption ionization–time of flight mass spectrometry following introduction for routine laboratory bacterial identification. Journal of Clinical Microbiology 2011;**49**(8):2980-2984. DOI:10.1128/JCM.00431-11

[16] Ferreira L, Sánchez-Juanes F, González-Ávila M, Cembrero-Fuciños D, Herrero-Hernández A, Manuel González-Buitrago J, Muñoz-Bellido JL. Direct identification of urinary tract pathogens from urine samples by matrix-assisted laser desorption ionization–time of flight mass spectrometry. Journal of Clinical Microbiology. 2010;**48**(6):2110-2115. DOI: 10.1128/JCM.02215-09

[17] Íñigo M, Coello A, Fernández-Rivas G, Rivaya B, Hidalgo J, Quesada MD, Ausina V. Direct identification of urinary tract pathogens from urine samples, combining urine screening methods and matrix-assisted laser desorption ionization–time of flight mass spectrometry. Journal of Clinical Microbiology. 2016;**54**(4):988-993. DOI: 10.1128/JCM.02832-15

[18] Wang X-H, Zhang G, Fan Y-Y, Yang X, Sui W-J, Lu X-X. Direct identification of bacteria causing urinary tract infections by combining matrix-assisted laser desorption ionization–time of flight mass spectrometry with UF-1000i urine flow cytometry. Journal of Microbiological Methods. 2013;**92**(3):231-235. DOI: https://doi.org/10.1016/j.mimet.2012.12.016

[19] Croxall G, Weston V, Joseph S, Manning G, Cheetham P, McNally A. Increased human pathogenic potential of *Escherichia coli* from polymicrobial urinary tract infections in comparison to isolates from monomicrobial culture samples. Journal of Medical Microbiology. 2011;**60**:102-109. DOI: 10.1099/jmm.0.020602-0

[20] Mach KE, CB D, Phull H, Haake DA, Shih M-C, Baron EJ, Liao JC. Multiplex pathogen identification for polymicrobial urinary tract infections using biosensor technology: A prospective clinical study. The Journal of Urology. 2009;**182**:2735-2741. DOI: 10.1016/j.juro.2009.08.028

[21] Alteri CJ, Mobley HLT. Metabolism and fitness of urinary tract pathogens. Microbiology Spectrum. 2015;**3**(3). DOI: 10.1128/microbiolspec.MBP-0016-2015

[22] Armbruster CE, Smith SN, Johnson AO, DeOrnellas V, Eaton KA, Yep A, Mody L, Wu W, Mobley HLT. The pathogenic potential of Proteus mirabilis is enhanced by other uropathogens during polymicrobial urinary tract infection. Infection and Immunity. 2017;**85**:e00808

[23] Alteri CJ, Himpsl SD, Mobley HLT. Preferential use of central metabolism in vivo reveals a nutritional basis for polymicrobial infection. PLoS Pathogens. 2015;**11**(1):e1004601. DOI: 10.1371/journal.ppat.1004601

[24] Kline KA, Lewis AL. Gram-positive uropathogens, polymicrobial urinary tract infection, and the emerging microbiota of the urinary tract. Microbiology Spectrum. 2016;**4**(2). DOI: 10.1128/microbiolspec.UTI-0012-2012

[25] Mann R, Mediati DG, Duggin IG, Harry EJ, Bottomley AL. Metabolic adaptations of uropathogenic *E. coli* in the urinary tract. Frontiers in Cellular and Infection Microbiology. 2017;**7**:241. DOI: 10.3389/fcimb.2017.00241

[26] Zanella MC, Schoofs F, Huttner B, Huttner A. Infections urinaires basses non associées aux sondes urinaires chez l'homme. Urétrite, cystite et prostatite. Revue Médicale Suisse. 2017;**13**:808-814

[27] Wang A, Nizran P, Malone MA, Riley T. Urinary tract infections. Primary Care: Clinics in Office Practice, DOI. 2013;**40**:687-706 http://dx.doi.Org/10.1016/j.pop.2013.06.005

[28] Osamwonyi B, Foley C. Management of recurrent urinary tract infections in adults. Surgery (Oxford). 2017;**35**(6):299-305 ISSN 0263-9319. DOI: http://dx.doi.org/10.1016/j.mpsur.2017.03.004

[29] Stein R, et al. Urinary tract infections in children: EAU/ESPU guidelines. European Urology. 2015;**67**(3):546-558

[30] Bryce A, Hay AD, Lane IF, Thornton HV, Wootton M, Costelloe C. Global prevalence of antibiotic resistance in paediatric urinary tract infections caused by *Escherichia coli* and association with routine use of antibiotics in primary care: systematic review and meta-analysis. British Medical Journal 2016;352:i939. DOI: http://dx.doi.org/10.1136/bmj.i939

[31] Arienzo A, Cellitti V, Ferrante V, Losito F, Stalio O, Cristofano F, Marino R, Magrini L, Santino I, Mari A, Visca P, Di Somma S and Antonini G on behalf of GREAT Network A pilot clinical trial on a new point-of-care test for the diagnosis and fast management of urinary tract infections in the emergency department. International Journal of Clinical & Medical Microbiology. 2016;**1**:107. DOI: http://dx.doi.org/10.15344/ijcmm/2016/107

[32] Lehmann LE, Hauser S, Malinka T, et al. Rapid qualitative urinary tract infection pathogen identification by SeptiFast® real-time PCR. Bereswill S, ed. PLoS One 2011;**6**(2):e17146. DOI:10.1371/journal.pone.0017146

[33] Stalenhoefa JE, van Dissel JT, van Nieuwkoop C. Febrile urinary tract infection in the emergency room. Current Opinion in Infectious Diseases 2015;**28**:106-111. DOI: 10.1097/QCO.0000000000000121

[34] Routh JC, et al. Increasing prevalence and associated risk factors for methicillin resistant Staphylococcus aureus bacteriuria. The Journal of Urology. 2009;**181**:1694-1698

[35] Linhares I, Raposo T, Rodrigues A, Almeida A. Incidence and diversity of antimicrobial multidrug resistance profiles of uropathogenic bacteria. BioMed Research International. 2015; Article ID: 354084, 11 pages. DOI: 10.1155/2015/354084

[36] Mandal J, Acharya NS, Buddhapriya D, Parija SC. Antibiotic resistance pattern among common bacterial uropathogens with a special reference to ciprofloxacin resistant *Escherichia coli*. The Indian Journal of Medical Research. 2012;**136**(5):842-849

[37] Malmartel A, Dutron M, Ghasarossian C. Tracking unnecessary negative urinalyses to reduce healthcare costs: a transversal study. European Journal of Clinical Microbiology & Infectious Diseases. 2017;**36**(9):1559-1563. DOI: 10.1007/s10096-017-2968-x

[38] Sobolewski K, Costello J, Miller L. Development of antibiotic stewardship practices targeting urinary tract infections in a hospital with consultant-based infectious disease services. Physical Therapy. 2017;**42**(8):527-532

[39] Barrons R, Tassone D. Use of Lactobacillus probiotics for bacterial genitourinary infections in women: a review. Clinical Therapeutics. 2008;**30**(3):453-468. DOI: 10.1016/j.clinthera.2008.03.013

[40] Tsai CC, Lai TM, Lin PP, Hsieh YM. Evaluation of lactic acid bacteria isolated from fermented plant products for antagonistic activity against urinary tract pathogen Staphylococcus saprophyticus. Probiotics Antimicrob Proteins. 2017. DOI: 10.1007/s12602-017-9302-x

[41] Beerepoot MA, et al. Nonantibiotic prophylaxis for recurrent urinary tract infections: A systematic review and meta-analysis of randomized controlled trials. The Journal of Urology. 2013;**190**(6):1981-1989

[42] Gupta K, Sahm DF, Mayfield D, Stamm WE. Antimicrobial resistance among uropathogens that cause community-acquired urinary tract infections in women: A nationwide analysis. Clinical Infectious Diseases. 2001;**33**(1):89-94. DOI: https://doi.org/10.1086/320880

[43] Pezzlo M. Detection of urinary tract infections by rapid methods. Clinical Microbiology Reviews. 1988;**1**(3):268-280. DOI: 10.1128/CMR.1.3.268

[44] Tandogdu Z, Cai T, Koves B, Wagenlehner F, Bjerklund-Johansen TE. Urinary tract infections in immunocompromised patients with diabetes, chronic kidney disease, and kidney transplant. European Urology Focus. 2016;**2**(4):394-399. DOI: 10.1016/j.euf.2016.08.006

[45] Masajtis-Zagajewska A, Nowicki M. New markers of urinary tract infection. Clinica Chimica Acta. 2017;**471**:286-291. DOI: 10.1016/j.cca.2017.06.003

[46] Turner D, Little P, Raftery J, Turner S, Smith H, Rumsby K, Mullee M. Cost effectiveness of management strategies for urinary tract infections: results from randomised controlled trial. British Medical Journal. 2010;**340**:c346. DOI: 10.1136/bmj.c346

[47] Demilie T, Beyene G, Melaku S, Tsegaye W. Diagnostic accuracy of rapid urine dipstick test to predict urinary tract infection among pregnant women in Felege Hiwot Referral Hospital, Bahir Dar, North West Ethiopia. BMC Research Notes. 2014;**7**:481. DOI: 10.1186/1756-0500-7-481

[48] Mambatta AK, Jayarajan J, Rashme VL, Harini S, Menon S, Kuppusamy J. Reliability of dipstick assay in predicting urinary tract infection. Journal of Family Medicine and Primary Care. 2015;**4**(2):265-268. DOI: 10.4103/2249-4863.154672

[49] Understanding Urine Tests, PubMed Health [Internet]. Dec 30, 2016. Available from: https://www.ncbi.nlm.nih.gov/pubmedhealth/PMH0072534/ [Accessed Aug 20, 2017]

[50] Jarzembowski T, Daca A, Witkowski J, Rutkowski B, Gołębiewska J, Dębska-Ślizień A. Changes of PBP5 gene expression in enterococcal isolates from renal transplantation recipients. BioMed Research International. 2013;**2013**:687156. DOI: 10.1155/2013/687156

[51] Shang Y, et al. Systematic review and meta-analysis of flow cytometry in urinary tract infection screening. Clinica Chimica Acta. 2013;**424**:90-95. DOI: 10.1016/j.cca.2013.05.014

[52] Johnson EU, Probert CSJ, Persad R, Khalid T, Ratcliffe N. Urinary volatile organic compounds: Novel approach to rapid UTI diagnosis. European Urology Supplements. 2014; **13**:e676

[53] Settu K, Chen C-J, Liu J-T, Chen C-L, Tsai J-Z. Impedimetric method for measuring ultralow concentrations in human urine. Biosensors and Bioelectronics. 2015;**66**:244-250 ISSN 0956-5663. DOI: http://dx.doi.org/10.1016/j.bios.2014.11.027

[54] Howick J, Cals JWL, Jones C, et al. Current and future use of point-of-care tests in primary care: an international survey in Australia, Belgium, The Netherlands, the UK and the USA. BMJ Open. 2014;**4**(8):e005611. DOI: 10.1136/ bmjopen-2014-005611

[55] Srinivasan B, Tung S. Development and applications of portable biosensors. Journal of Laboratory Automation. 2015;**20**(4):365-389. DOI: 10.1177/2211068215581349

[56] Baerheim A. Empirical treatment of uncomplicated cystitis. Scandinavian Journal of Primary Health Care. 2012;**30**(1):1-2. DOI: 10.3109/02813432.2012.649629

[57] Waisman Y, Zerem E, Amir L, Mimouni M. The validity of the uriscreen test for early detection of urinary tract infection in children. Pediatrics. 1999;**104**(4):e41

[58] Bongard E, Frimodt-Møller N, Gal M, Wootton M, Howe R, Francis N, Goossens H, Butler CC. Analytic laboratory performance of a point of care urine culture kit for diagnosis and antibiotic susceptibility testing. European Journal of Clinical Microbiology & Infectious Diseases. 2015;**34**:2111-2119. DOI: 10.1007/s10096-015-2460-4

[59] Holm A, Cordoba G, Sørensen TM, Jessen LR, Siersma V, Bjerrum L. Point of care susceptibility testing in primary care – does it lead to a more appropriate prescription of antibiotics in patients with uncomplicated urinary tract infections? Protocol for a randomized controlled trial. BMC Family Practice. 2015;**16**:106. DOI: 10.1186/s12875-015-0322-x

[60] Schot MJC, Van Delft S, Kooijman-Buiting AMJ, de Wit NJ, Hopstaken RM. Analytical performance, agreement and user-friendliness of six point-of-care testing urine analysers for urinary tract infection in general practice. BMJ Open 2015;5(5):e006857. DOI: 10.1136/bmjopen-2014-006857

[61] National Institute for Health Research (NIHR), Diagnostic Evidence Cooperative Oxford. Point-of-Care Testing for Urinary Tract Infections. Horizon. Scan Report number: 0045, 2016

[62] Bottini G, Losito F, Arienzo A, Priolisi FR, Mari A, Visca P, Antonini G. A new method for microbiological analysis that could be used for point-of-care testing (POCT). The Open Emergency Medicine Journal. 2013;**5**:13-15. DOI: 10.2174/1876542401305010013

[63] Arienzo A, Losito F, Bottini G, Priolisi FR, Mari A, Visca P, Antonini G. A new device for the prompt diagnosis of urinary tract infections. Clinical Chemistry and Laboratory Medicine. 2014;**52**(10):1507-1511. DOI: 10.1515/cclm-2014-0294

8

Virulence Factors of Uropathogenic *E. coli*

Sorwer Alam Parvez and Dolilur Rahman

Abstract

In order for a successful infection and creating a satisfactory environment inside the host, strains of uropathogenic *Escherichia coli* (UPEC) need some special features that are achieved by expressing particular genes, called virulence factors. Two of the most important surface virulence factors of UPEC are type 1 fimbriae and P fimbriae that are crucial for the colonization process inside the urinary tract. Expression of these virulence factors converts a commensal strain into an uropathogen. Beside these factors, outer membrane proteins also contribute to virulence being involved in the secretory machinery; an example of such type is TolC protein that transfers α-hemolysin across the outer membrane of *E. coli*. However, α-hemolysin along with many other toxins serves various pathogenic roles during UTIs including adhesion, colonization, cytotoxic activity, etc. Moreover, virulence factors located on bacterial surface including capsule and lipopolysaccharides may also have the contribution to UTIs providing antiphagocytosis and antibactericidal complement activity.

Keywords: virulent factors, *E. coli*, UPEC, urinary tract infection, type 1 fimbriae, P fimbriae, α-hemolysin, cytotoxic necrotizing factor 1 (CNF1), siderophores, hemin uptake system, flagellar motility

1. Introduction

The most commonly living microorganism of the human gastrointestinal tract and also the most common causative agent of bacterial urinary tract infection is *E. coli* [1]. Though they remain in a good relationship with their hosts, they might appear as a subject of consideration in immunocompromised hosts. This common inhabitant of the gastrointestinal tract usually remains in a symbiotic relationship with the host and plays a role in maintaining the homeostasis of the intestinal tract. Though most of the strains of *E. coli* are harmless, some serotypes can cause food poisoning. *E. coli* present in the normal human microbiota produces vitamin

K_2. Strains of *E coli*, however, obtaining ability to colonize inside the urinary tract and to make themselves safe from the host immune system, become uropathogenic *E. coli*. UPEC causes >80% of UTI [2]. Urinary tract infections are very common, and approximately 10% of people [3] and half of all women (at least one time) become infected throughout their life. According to a study, more than 100,000 patients in the United States are hospitalized annually due to urinary tract infections [4], and in the year 2011, 400,000 patients were hospitalized, and the estimated cost was about 2.8 billion USD [5]. Infections can occur in both upper and lower urinary tracts. Lower urinary tract infection is known as cystitis, and in the case of upper urinary tract infection, it is called pyelonephritis. Without distinction of site, in order to cause infection, the causative agent must at first dodge the host's immune system and colonize in the urinary tract [6]. Several different virulent factors are needed for the bacterial population to cause infections [7]; for instance, pathogenic strains of *E. coli* express adherence factors which form pili or fimbriae of different types for their attachment in the sites where they usually do not live [7]; these are structural virulence factors and predominantly include P fimbriae and type 1 fimbriae [1]. Fimbrial adhesins such as PapG and CsgA are virulence factors that facilitate the attachment of *E. coli* [8]. In animal models, type 1 fimbriae aggrandize the chance survival of *E. coli* [9]. Beside these, UPEC can impair host immune system by a variety of ways [10], such as toxins and iron acquisition systems, and these are called secreted virulence factors. The production of these virulence factors by UPEC may cause an inflammatory response which makes a possible pathway for UTI symptoms [1]. However, both the host and the uropathogenic *E. coli* strain have different roles in the establishment and colonization process in the urinary tract [11]. Here in this chapter, different types of important virulence factors of uropathogenic *E. coli* will be discussed.

In Gram-negative and some Gram-positive bacteria, virulence genes are allocated in particular segments (about 10–200 kilo bases in size) of their genome which have different G + C content than the other parts of the genome that are termed as pathogenicity islands. They are present in the virulent strains but present rarely in the nonpathogenic strains of the same species. These sequences can be transferred horizontally from species to species [12]. Pathogenicity islands encode virulence factors such as adherence factors, toxins, and iron acquisition systems which are important virulence factors of UPEC.

2. Adhesion

Urine of uninfected person is sterile due to urinary flow and antimicrobial activity of uric acid. Regular flow of urine does not allow microorganism to colonize inside the urinary tract. However, attachment of *E. coli* to uroepithelial cells allows them to overwhelm the effect of urine flow. For many pathogenic microorganisms, it is considered as the first step in the colonization process [13, 14], and both the host and *E. coli* function in this process. The ability of UPEC to colonize depends upon the expression of different fimbrial adhesins. For a successful adherence to the host cell surface, UPEC expresses many adherence factors which are crucial for attachment and thus regarded as virulence factors. Many bacterial adhesins are organized in a thin filamentous structure called fimbriae or pili although there are evidences of presence of adhesins in the cell surface of bacteria. Adhesins of fimbrial nature are important during attachment process [15]. Fimbriae, also known as pili, are long hair-like structures contained in the cell surface of bacteria that recognize specific compounds usually carbohydrates of the target host cells [11]. Pili are the short form of fimbriae and might be used interchangeably with fimbriae. Fimbriae consist of oligomeric pilin proteins. These proteins are arranged in such a manner that they form a helical cylindrical structure and are both thinner and shorter than flagellum. These proteinaceous structures are expressed in uropathogenic strains of *E. coli* and are considered as virulence factors [11]. Most of the receptors for these fimbriae are carbohydrates. They include type 1 fimbriae, P fimbriae, and thin aggregative fimbriae [16]. Many bacterial pathogens can produce an array of these adhesins, and often inhibition of a single adhesin may cost enough to a bacterium to lose its virulence. Functions of pili or fimbriae are not limited only to adhesion and can help in many other crucial pathways for the microbe to survive and evade the immune system of the host. Evolution of different types of adhesins plays a role in tissue tropism.

In gram-negative bacteria like UPEC, adhesins are unveiled by chaperone-usher-assisted pathway. This pathway involves two proteins, one is a periplasmic chaperone, and the other is a protein called usher. Usher act as the base of the structure, and the function of chaperone is folding and recruitment of the subunits [17, 18]. In absence of the chaperone, pilin proteins are degraded and misfolded and thus cannot be assembled in the form of a mature pilus. On the other hand, usher helps to mature the fimbriae and its transportation through the outer assuring integrity of the outer membrane. The constituents of usher proteins are an N-terminal domain (NTD), 24-stranded beta-barrel channel, a plug domain, and two C-terminal domains (CTD). In uropathogenic *E. coli* strains, chaperone-usher family fimbriae are more abundant.

2.1. Type 1 fimbriae

In 99% of *E. coli* strains, genes to encode type 1 fimbriae are present [19], and during urinary tract infections, they damage urinary tract cells by mediating an increased inflammation [20]. In order to enter into the host cells of the urinary tract, type 1 fimbriae play a great role. Type 1 fimbriae are remarkably versatile virulence factors of UPEC that can stabilize the attachment of the bacteria to different type of cells throughout the urinary tract. Though in Bowman's capsules and glomerulus their binding sites could not be identified, a strong affinity of type 1 fimbriae was found in proximal tubules and vessel walls. In the bladder, they bind strongly to muscular layers and moderately to vessel walls. Receptors for type 1 fimbriae were also found in the distal tubules and collecting ducts. They can also induce their binding to the surface of macrophages [9]. These fimbriae recognize uroplakin from bladder epithelial cells and mannoside-containing host proteins. Unlike many other important types of adhesins, these are encoded by the bacterial backbone DNA [21] and are mainly composed of FimA proteins along with FimF, FimG, and FimH [17]. FimA proteins are most in number but are not pivotal for virulence. Among other subunits of type 1 fimbriae, allelic variations of FimH determine the sugar specificity and deletion of *fimH* results in less amount of colonization in mouse models of ascending UTI, and colonization could be restored by expression of plasmid with *fimH* gene [20]. FimH alone or in association with LPS can stimulate toll-like receptor 4 (TLR4) to initiate particular signaling cascade that may activate the humoral immune response. Many studies revealed that expression of type 1 fimbriae results in virulence and loss of expression results in loss of expression but their presence cannot be correlated with UTI as normal fecal strains also have equally expressed type 1 fimbriae [22]. However, type 1 fimbriae-mediated attachment is a crucial stage for cystitis. Adhesins of these fimbriae are mannose sensitive.

2.2. P fimbriae

P-fimbriated *E. coli* are pyelonephritogenic and attach to the carbohydrate structure alpha-D-Galp-(1-4)-beta-D-Galp. In the kidney, they bind strongly to Bowman's capsule, glomerulus, and endothelial cells of vessel walls. This highly organized composite structure is composed of six subunits at least. Once P fimbriae expressed *E. coli* enter the urinary tract, they establish bacteriuria and help to cross the epithelial barrier to enter the bloodstream and can cause hemagglutination of erythrocytes [14]. This type of fimbriae is encoded by *pap* gene cluster (also known as *fso* and *fst*), and *pap* + strains remain longer in the intestinal flora than pap-strains [23]. P antigens are expressed in the cell surface of red blood cells and in various cells lining in the urinary tract. P1 (present in glycoproteins in human), P, P^K, and LKE antigens act as the receptors for P-fimbriated UPEC. P-fimbriated *E. coli* cannot agglutinate red blood cells that lack P antigen. Isolated P fimbriae can bind to a synthetic analogue of its receptor, and experimental application of that analogue impedes infection process.

There are at least nine genes in the pap gene cluster with two restriction sites at two ends. The regulatory part starts the following Eco R1 consisting of papI and papB. Then papA, papH, papC, papD, papE, papF, and papG are situated, and after these, Bam HI is present. Approximately 1000 of subunits form a P fimbria, being united in a helical manner. Among them the major constituent is the protein subunit PapA (19.5 KD), and minor subunits are PapE (16.5 KD), PapF (15 KD), and PapG (35 KD). In the periplasmic space, PapD (27.5 KD) may be present and can also be incorporated in the structure. Another protein PapC, which is the largest one with 80 KD of mass, assists the process by transporting the subunits outside the part of the cell. Though PapA is the major constituent, it is not mandatory for attachment, and among many serotypes, PapA molecules show high homology with the amino acids of N and C termini. PapA also has an average level of similarity with structural subunits of other *E. coli* fimbriae including type 1 fimbriae. The minor subunits at the tip of fimbria determine the specificity to the receptor. Many mutational analyses revealed that mutation in PapA does not affect the adherence, while mutation in other genes (i.e. *papEFG*) does not hamper fimbrial structural appearance. In the fine structure of P fimbriae, a PapF-PapG complex is formed which is attached to PapA (bulk potion of the structure) subunits through PapE subunits. Finally, PapH terminates the assembly of the fimbriae and attaches thereby [16]. An important thing is that the amino acid sequence of PapG is approximately similar to that of Shiga toxin. Shiga toxin is found in some serotypes of *E. coli*. Another role of PapG was found in some variants of P fimbriae which is they can initiate subunit polymerization [14].

Many experiments show that expression of these fimbriae is not relevant to urinary tract infection, while more sophisticated other experiments have concluded about their role in pathogenesis. However, during infection in immunocompromised patients, less expression of P fimbriae is observed, which indicated that P fimbriae are needed to overcome certain types of host immune attacks. Although P fimbriae can initiate inflammatory responses by activating TLR4 [24], it protects UPEC from human polymorphonuclear leukocytes (hPMNLs). In the rapidly changing environment through the urinary tract, environmental influences affect the expression of P fimbriae. Expression of P fimbriae is favored at 37°C and inhibited at a range of 18–22 °C, but there are some variations in this phenomenon. The temperature-dependent expression is controlled by a region close to *papB* of the pap gene cluster.

2.3. Dr/Afa adhesins

Dr blood group antigen is a membrane protein of red blood cells and located on the decay accelerating factor (DAF) that protects red blood cells from being degraded or lysed by autologous complements. Another important function of DAF is to regulate complement cascade [25]. These antigens are recognized by Dr and Afa adhesin family of uropathogenic *E. coli.* There are both fimbrial (F1845 and O75X) and non-fimbrial (AFA I and AFA II) types of adhesins. Immuno-invasion of UPEC by hiding from the host humoral immune response is somehow mediated by Dr family of adhesins [26]. These microscopically invisible fimbriae are present in the cell wall, and their structural and organization properties are quite different from other types of fimbriae [13]. Chloramphenicol can inhibit O75X binding to a specific part of the Dr antigen, but it cannot inhibit other adhesins of this family which indicates that Dr family adhesins can recognize specific sites at the Dr [25]. For years, several studies were conducted to identify specific sites for binging of Dr family hemagglutinins. For instance, a strong affinity of O75X was found to Bowman's capsule, proximal and distal tubules, and the collecting duct basement membranes. In the bladder, they strongly bind to connective tissues.

2.4. Other fimbriae as virulence factors

F1C is a virulence factor responsible for urinary tract infections, which is encoded by an operon of seven genes, i.e., *focAICDFGH,* where FocA is the major subunit and FocH is the tip adhesin [26]. F1C receptors are present in bladder endothelium and muscular layer. They cannot bind to the epithelium. They bind to glomeruli, distal tubules, collecting ducts, and vascular endothelial cells. Studies show that F1C fimbriae and pyelonephritis are correlated though there is a little difference in the prevalence of type 1 fimbriae in UTI strains and normal fecal isolates. Prevalence of F1C fimbriae in normal fecal isolates is 10% which is 16% in UTI strains [26]. S fimbriae are genetically identical to F1C fimbriae and differ only by the tip adhesin SfaS. Criteria that are needed to be recognized as a virulence factor were determined by different studies regarding S fimbriae. There are some other adhesins that are not crucial for the survival of UPEC strains such as F9 fimbriae.

3. Toxins

Several toxic substances or proteins secreted by uropathogenic strains of *E. coli* play a consequential role as virulence factors in UTIs. However, toxins have the ability to alter the host cell signaling cascade and modulate inflammatory responses. Several in vitro and in vivo studies showed that toxins also contribute to the stimulation of the host cell death and releasing of necessary nutrients, which provide the ability to access deeper tissues within the urinary tract [27]. In 1987, CDT toxin (cyclomodulins) was first reported as virulent toxin in UPEC [28] which opened a new door in the study of the pathogenesis of UTIs, and then many other toxins in UPEC were reported including α-hemolysin (HlyA), cytotoxic necrotizing factor 1 (CNF1), secreted autotransporter toxin (SAT), cytolysin A, plasmid-encoded toxin (PET), vacuolating autotransporter toxin (VAT), Shigella enterotoxin-1 (ShET-1), arginine succinyltransferase (AST), etc.

3.1. α-hemolysin

Among all the toxins, α-hemolysin (HlyA) is very important which is a lipoprotein and belongs to the RTX (repeats in toxin) toxins family [13, 29, 30]. HlyA is a pore-forming toxin and causes inducible nitric-oxide-synthase (iNOS)-mediated cell membrane injury and apoptosis [31]. However, HlyA can lyse erythrocytes and nucleated host cells at high concentration by a process enabling UPEC which may damage the host immune effector cells for gaining enhanced access to the host nutrients and iron stores. But when the concentration is low, HlyA can induce the apoptosis of target host cells and promote the exfoliation of bladder epithelial cells [13, 32, 33]. Besides, HlyA can also contribute to nephropathogenicity, which was proved by infecting mice transurethrally or intravesically with toxin producer and nonproducer isogenic clone pairs of *E. coli* [34]. A recent study showed that HlyA regulates the dephosphorylation of Akt, which is a multifunctional signaling regulator and responsible for controlling inflammatory responses in the host, as well as the cell cycle control [35]. Moreover, HlyA has the role in the increased production of IL-6 and IL-8 by inducing Ca^{2+} oscillations in renal epithelial cells [36].

3.2. Cytotoxic necrotizing factor 1 (CNF1)

Another virulence factor secreted by *E. coli* named cytotoxic necrotizing factor 1 (CNF1) is also involved in UTIs and stimulates actin stress fiber formation and membrane ruffle formation in a Rho GTPase-dependent manner that results in the entry of *E. coli* into the cells [37]. The toxin has a remarkable effect on the actin skeletal of HEp-2 cells and produces large vacuoles in HEp-2 cells [28]. However, several in vitro and in vivo studies showed that this protein interferes with polymorphonuclear phagocytosis and evokes apoptotic death of bladder epithelial cells and may lead to bladder cell exfoliation and to enhanced bacterial access to underlying tissue [38, 39]. In addition, there is also a possibility of the association of CNF1 with the hemolysin in the virulence mechanism, which is beneficial for the bacteria [28].

3.3. Secreted autotransporter toxin (SAT)

Secreted autotransporter toxin (SAT) may also be important as a virulence factor for the pathogenesis of UTIs being had a toxin activity against cell lines of bladder or kidney origin. SAT is a serine protease autotransporter which falls within one subgroup of autotransporters recently classified as the SPATE (serine protease autotransporters of *Enterobacteriaceae*) family and associated with pyelonephritic *E. coli* strains [40, 41]. SAT may have the cytopathic activity that results in the damage of the host tissue and may increase the propagation ability of the UPEC. However, this toxin may facilitate entry of pyelonephritogenic strains into the bloodstream resulting from specific damage to the glomeruli and proximal tubules [40].

3.4. Cytolethal distending toxin (CDT)

Cytolethal distending toxin, having a unique property of damaging the DNA of the target cell, was first reported in pathogenic *E. coli* in 1987 [28, 42]. This toxin has the ability to arrest the cell cycle and contributes to the pathogenesis of UTIs [43, 44]. However, CDT is an operon product encoding three proteins including CdtA, CdtB, and CdtC proteins which are encoded by cdtA, cdtB, and cdtC genes, respectively [28]. CDT has DNase I-like enzymatic activity and attacks DNA, while the other bacterial toxins attack the cell membrane or different targets within the cytoplasm [45]. This unique property of attacking DNA damages the target cell DNA which results in progressive cell distending leading to cell death [27].

3.5. Other toxins

Some others including cytolysin A and toll/interleukin (IL-1) receptor (TIR) domain-containing protein (Tcp) are also considered as virulence factors in UTIs [46, 47]. The former causes apoptosis of the host cells [47], while the other has the ability to subvert TLR signaling that gives a survival advantage during UTIs [46]. However, Tcp is associated with pyelonephritis but rare in environmental *E. coli*, in fecal flora of healthy children and in less severe forms of UTI [27]. Besides these, Tcp has also the role in the human avoidance system and cytopathic effect on the kidney [48].

In addition to these toxins, vacuolating autotransporter toxin (VAT), Shigella enterotoxin-1 (ShET-1) and arginine succinyltransferase (AST) may also contribute to UTIs. VAT has the cytotoxic effect on the bladder and kidney, while the two others are involved in the invasion of the infections [48]. However, VAT is a highly protected immunogenic protein that belongs to the protease family of SPATE [28].

4. Siderophores

Iron is a very important molecule for all living beings, and *E. coli* uses iron for transporting and storing oxygen, DNA synthesis, electron transport, and metabolism of peroxides. But the amount of iron availability is reduced in the host urinary tract during UTIs [49]. In response to this, *E. coli* possesses some multiple functionally redundant systems that mediate iron uptake by secreting low-molecular-weight Fe^{3+}-chelating molecules which are known as siderophores [50]. Iron utilization, mediated by these siderophores, is critical for colonization of the urinary tract by UPEC [51]. There are four distinct siderophore systems found in *E. coli* such as yersiniabactin, aerobactin, enterobactin, and salmochelin [52]. These systems also include some genes such as ent genes encoding enterobactin, iuc genes encoding aerobactin, and iro genes encoding an ent-like system. However, all these systems are expressed under low-iron conditions and are negatively regulated by ferrous iron and the ferric uptake regulator Fur [53].

4.1. Aerobactin

Aerobactin is a low-weight molecule and a hydroxamate siderophore with a higher Fe^{3+}-binding stability in acidic environments and is maximally produced at low pH [44, 53]. This siderophore extracts Fe^{3+} from host iron-binding proteins and is taken up through an outer membrane receptor protein [44]. However, aerobactin has many advantages over other siderophores and is formed from the condensation of two lysine molecules and one citrate catalyzed by an enzyme named aerobactin synthase [13, 25, 30].

4.2. Enterobactin

Enterobactin is another specialized highly prevalent catecholate siderophore which is less soluble and less stable than aerobactin [53–55]. But this siderophore has a higher iron affinity and can deferrate transferrin more rapidly than aerobactin in aqueous solution [13, 54]. However, iron is released from enterobactin through the hydrolysis of this siderophore [13]. Besides these, enterobactin may afford UPEC the ability to colonize within an iron-limiting environment such as the urinary tract [56]. But this siderophore has a limitation that it can be inactivated by host proteins such as serum albumin and siderocalin [25].

4.3. Yersiniabactin

Yersiniabactin, a mixed-type siderophore, is widespread in *Enterobacteriaceae* including *E. coli* and encoded on the high-pathogenicity island [53]. Yersiniabactin has a high iron affinity and produced yersiniabactin-Fe^{3+} complex binding to the iron molecule which recognizes the specific bacterial outer membrane TonB-dependent receptor and Fyu (Psn). The iron molecule is released from yersiniabactin in the cytosol with the help of membrane-embedded proteins [57]. In addition, this siderophore increases resistance to copper stress by chelating Cu^{2+} [10].

4.4. Salmochelin

Salmochelin is a glucosylated derivative of enterobactin which is not recognized by siderocalin and thus escapes from the host immune response [53]. However, siderocalin, neutrophil gelatinase-associated lipocalin is also known as lipocalin 2 that binds enterobactin and prevents its uptake [53, 56]. To overcome this, enterobactin is modified to salmochelin by glucosylation via the action of glucosyltransferase and is not recognized by lipocalin 2 [56]. However, a recent study found that salmochelin siderophore receptor IroN is involved in the invasion of urothelial cells, and thus IroN may play both an iron uptake receptor and an internalization factor in the establishment of urinary tract infections [26].

4.5. Hemin uptake system

There is another iron acquisition system called hemin uptake system including ChuA and Hma, which involves direct upregulation of haem receptors. This system uptakes free iron during UTIs, and several studies found its role in bacterial growth and biofilm formation [48, 58, 59]. ChuA expression is regulated by other regulatory proteins, for instance, in uropathogenic *E. coli* strain 536, increase in RfaH level induces the expression of ChuA [60]. But the other receptor Hma functions independently of ChuA, and a residue, Tyr-126, is necessary for its function. However, both ChuA and Hma contribute to haem utilization which is required for the maximum kidney colonization [51].

5. Capsule

The main role of a capsule is to cover and protect the bacterium from various unfavorable conditions as well as the host immune system, which is mainly constituted of polysaccharide [1].

The capsule provides protection against engulfment and complement-mediated bactericidal effect in the host, also including antimicrobial resistance and antiserum activity [1, 48]. Certain capsulars, such as K1 and K5, prevent a proper humoral immune response of the infected host by showing a molecular mimicry to tissue components [1]. The K1 polysaccharide, a linear α2–8-linked sialic acid homopolymer, has a very important role in IBC development as well as in the multiple stages of UTI pathogenesis [27, 50].

6. Lipopolysaccharide

Lipopolysaccharide (LPS) is an integral component of the cell wall and consists of the highly conserved lipid A-core and repeating O-antigen subunits that differ greatly between strains based on the sugar residues and their linkage patterns within the repeating subunits [37, 61]. LPS is very well known to activate host response and to induce nitric oxide and cytokine (IL-1, TNF-α) production which enhances the inflammatory response [1, 15]. It also induces the synthesis of specific antibodies to the somatic antigen and exerts an immune-adjuvant effect that promotes the humoral immune response to other antigens of the pathogen. However, certain antigenic types of LPS are also involved in resistance of the pathogen to the killing effect of the normal human serum [46]. According to study upon animal models, acute renal failure due to LPS depends on the systemic response to LPS and does not depend on expression of functional LPS receptor, TLR4, in the kidney. But it is not clear whether LPS plays a role in mediating a renal failure and acute allograft injury in patients with ascending UTIs [1].

7. Motility

Flagellum is an organelle that is responsible for bacterial motility and plays a role in the initial adhesion phase of biofilm formation [1, 62]. A recent study showed that motility is involved in the migration of the infection from the bladder to the kidneys [63]. About 70–90% of all urinary tract infections is caused by flagellated UPEC, and pathogenesis involves contact between the bacteria and epithelial cell surface of the urinary tract [1]. However, flagellar motility enhances the ability of *E. coli* by adaptive responses to attractive or repellent environmental stimuli [15].

8. Mechanism of immune escape

Toll-like receptor 4 (TLR4) in the epithelial cells of the mammalian bladder can recognize lipopolysaccharides (LPS) of bacterial cell wall, and the downstream signaling cascade produces IL-6 and IL-8, of which IL-8 is well known as an important chemoattractant for neutrophils. Urinary levels of IL-6 and IL-8 are measurable in UPEC-infected human and murine models. There is another pathway parallel to this one that is responsible for increased levels of IL-6 and IL-8 in urine. Upon TLR-4 activation by LPS, intracellular level of cAMP is increased and results in of Ca^{2+} influx. Later, cAMP response element-binding protein (CREB) becomes phosphorylated.

Phosphorylation of CREB results in the expression of IL-6 and IL-8 [24]. Mutation in TLR4 in murine models revealed its role on bacterial pathogenesis. There are other receptors related to UTI pathogenesis. One of such is CXCR1, but there are both types of evidences that demonstrate the positive and "no correlation" of CXCR1 with recurrent UTIs. Polymorphisms in IL-8 genes were found to have a correlation with pyelonephritis in the case of no correlation with CXCR1 mutation [19, 64]. TLR4 can be activated by the presence of type 1 fimbriae and P fimbriae.

As there are enough studies to evidence the activation of immune response against UPEC strains, there must be some ways that are used by these bacteria to overcome unfavorable situations early in the infection. Incubation of human urothelial cells with type 1-fimbriated UPEC strains resulted in increased apoptosis. In the case of a nonpathogenic type 1-fimbriated strain (HB101) of *E. coli*, rate of apoptosis was approximately 50% of that of pathogenic strains of UPEC [65]. UPEC blocks NF-κB, and this results in apoptosis and a decreased cytokine secretion.

Another indispensable way is the expression of toll/IL-1 receptor domain-containing protein (TcpC), which was discovered in UPEC strain CFT073. TcpC interacts with myeloid differentiation primary response 88 (MyD88), a protein that, in human, is encoded by *MYD88* gene. Interaction of TcpC and MyD88 subsequently stops downstream signaling pathways mediated by TLRs.

Modification of capsular lipopolysaccharides specific to the pathogenic strain can cause the failure of TLR4 to recognize the pathogen. However, LPS biosynthetic genes encoded by *rfa, rfb* operons, and *surA* are the factors responsible for the suppression of TLR-initiated signaling cascades. Biosynthesis of a number of outer membrane proteins and fimbriae is facilitated by the protein encoded by surA, which is a periplasmic cis-trans prolyl isomerase [66, 67].

9. Conclusions

Several epidemiological, serological, and bacteriological studies revealed that uropathogenic *E. coli* is the pathogen most frequently associated with UTIs. In recent years, our understanding of virulence factors and behavior of this pathogen is increased remarkably. Several studies showed that *E. coli* colonizes the urinary tract and may ascend toward the bladder to cause cystitis. If it is left untreated, UPEC may ascend the ureters to the kidney and establish a secondary infection. Our increased understanding of its virulence factors can uncover novel approaches to control UPEC-mediated UTIs. However, accumulation of theoretical knowledge through virulence studies allows practical applications and may facilitate the application of more precise approaches in phenotypic or molecular diagnosis and epidemiology.

Author details

Sorwer Alam Parvez* and Dolilur Rahman

*Address all correspondence to: sorwersust@yahoo.com

Shahjalal University of Science and Technology, Sylhet, Bangladesh

References

[1] Bien J, Sokolova O, Bozko P. Role of uropathogenic *Escherichia coli* virulence factors in development of urinary tract infection and kidney damage. International Journal of Nephrology. 2012:e681473

[2] Wurpel DJ, Beatson SA, Totsika M, Petty NK, Schembri MA. Chaperone-usher fimbriae of *Escherichia coli*. PLoS One. 2013;**8**(1):e52835

[3] Farajnia S, Alikhani MY, Ghotaslou R, Naghili B, Nakhlband A. Causative agents and antimicrobial susceptibilities of urinary tract infections in the northwest of Iran. International Journal of Infectious Diseases. 2009;**13**(2):140-144

[4] Johnson JR, Stamm WE. Urinary tract infections in women: Diagnosis and treatment. Annals of Internal Medicine. 1989;**111**(11):906-917

[5] Simmering JE, Tang F, Cavanaugh JE, Polgreen LA, Polgreen PM. The increase in hospitalizations for urinary tract infections and the associated costs in the United States, 1998-2011. Open Forum Infectious Diseases. Oxford University Press. 2017;**4**(1):e281

[6] Müller CM, Åberg A, Straseviçiene J, Emődy L, Uhlin BE, Balsalobre C. Type 1 fimbriae, a colonization factor of uropathogenic *Escherichia coli*, are controlled by the metabolic sensor CRP-cAMP. PLoS Pathogens. 2009;**5**(2):e1000303

[7] Kaper JB, Nataro JP, Mobley HL. Pathogenic *Escherichia coli*. Nature Reviews Microbiology. 2004;**2**(2):123

[8] Luna-Pineda VM, Ochoa S, Cruz-Córdova A, Cázares-Domínguez V, Vélez-González F, Hernández-Castro R, et al. Urinary tract infections, immunity, and vaccination. Boletín Médico del Hospital Infantil de México. 2018;**75**(2):67-78

[9] Vizcarra IA, Hosseini V, Kollmannsberger P, Meier S, Weber SS, Arnoldini M, et al. How type 1 fimbriae help *Escherichia coli* to evade extracellular antibiotics. Scientific Reports. 2016;**6**:18109

[10] Olson PD, Hunstad DA. Subversion of host innate immunity by uropathogenic *Escherichia coli*. Pathogens. 2016;**5**(1):2

[11] Winberg J. P-fimbriae, bacterial adhesion, and pyelonephritis. Archives of Disease in Childhood. 1984;**59**(2):180

[12] Hacker J, Blum-Oehler G, Mühldorfer I, Tschäpe H. Pathogenicity islands of virulent bacteria: Structure, function and impact on microbial evolution. Molecular Microbiology. 1997;**23**(6):1089-1097

[13] Johnson JR. Virulence factors in *Escherichia coli* urinary tract infection. Clinical Microbiology Reviews. 1991;**4**(1):80-128

[14] Riegman N, Die I, Leunissen J, Hoekstra W, Bergmans H. Biogenesis of F71 and F72 fimbriae of uropathogenic *Escherichia coli*: Influence of the FsoF and FstFG proteins and localization of the Fso/FstE protein. Molecular Microbiology. 1988;**2**(1):73-80

[15] Emody L, Kerenyi M, Nagy G. Virulence factors of uropathogenic *Escherichia coli*. International Journal of Antimicrobial Agents. 2003;**22**:29-33

[16] Collinson SK, Emödy L, Kay WW. Thin aggregative fimbriae from diarrheagenic *Escherichia coli*. Journal of Bacteriology. 1992;**174**(13):4490-4495

[17] Klemm P, Schembri MA. Bacterial adhesins: Function and structure. International Journal of Medical Microbiology. 2000;**290**(1):27-35

[18] Volkan E, Kalas V, Hultgren S. Pili and fimbriae of gram-negative bacteria. Molecular Medical Microbiology. 2nd ed. London: Academic Press. 2015:147-162

[19] Vigil PD, Alteri CJ, Mobley HL. Identification of in vivo-induced antigens including an RTX family exoprotein required for uropathogenic *Escherichia coli* virulence. Infection and Immunity. 2011;**79**(6):2335-2344

[20] Connell I, Agace W, Klemm P, Schembri M, Mărild S, Svanborg C. Type 1 fimbrial expression enhances *Escherichia coli* virulence for the urinary tract. Proceedings of the National Academy of Sciences. 1996;**93**(18):9827-9832

[21] Hallstrom KN, McCormick BA. Pathogenicity islands: Origins, structure, and roles in bacterial pathogenesis. Molecular Medical Microbiology. 2nd ed. London: Academic Press; 2015:303-314

[22] Nielubowicz GR, Mobley HL. Host–pathogen interactions in urinary tract infection. Nature Reviews Urology. 2010;**7**(8):430

[23] Wullt B, Bergsten G, Connell H, RoÈllano P, Gebretsadik N, Hull R, et al. P fimbriae enhance the early establishment of *Escherichia coli* in the human urinary tract. Molecular Microbiology. 2000;**38**(3):456-464

[24] Hunstad DA, Justice SS. Intracellular lifestyles and immune evasion strategies of uropathogenic *Escherichia coli*. Annual Review of Microbiology. 2010;**64**:203-221

[25] Nowicki B, Labigne A, Moseley S, Hull R, Hull S, Moulds J. The Dr hemagglutinin, afimbrial adhesins AFA-I and AFA-III, and F1845 fimbriae of uropathogenic and diarrhea-associated *Escherichia coli* belong to a family of hemagglutinins with Dr receptor recognition. Infection and Immunity. 1990;**58**(1):279-281

[26] Spurbeck RR, Mobley HL. Uropathogenic *Escherichia coli*. *Escherichia Coli*. 2nd ed. London: Academic Press; 2013:275-304

[27] Agarwal J, Srivastava S, Singh M. Pathogenomics of uropathogenic *Escherichia coli*. Indian Journal of Medical Microbiology. 2012;**30**(2):141

[28] Soltani S, Emamie AD, Dastranj M, Farahani A, Davoodabadi A, Mohajeri P. Role of toxins of uropathogenic *Escherichia coli* in development of urinary tract infection. British Journal of Pharmaceutical Research. 2018;**21**(1):e.JPRI.39188

[29] Eberspächer B, Hugo F, Bhakdi S. Quantitative study of the binding and hemolytic efficiency of *Escherichia coli* hemolysin. Infection and Immunity. 1989;**57**(3):983-988

[30] Bhakdi SUCHARIT, Mackman N, Nicaud JM, Holland IB. *Escherichia coli* hemolysin may damage target cell membranes by generating transmembrane pores. Infection and Immunity. 1986;**52**(1):63-69

[31] Chen M, Jahnukainen T, Bao W, Daré E, Ceccatelli S, Celsi G. Uropathogenic *Escherichia coli* toxins induce caspase-independent apoptosis in renal proximal tubular cells via ERK signaling. American Journal of Nephrology. 2003;**23**(3):140-151

[32] Russo TA, Davidson BA, Genagon SA, Warholic NM, MacDonald U, Pawlicki PD, et al. *E. coli* virulence factor hemolysin induces neutrophil apoptosis and necrosis/lysis in vitro and necrosis/lysis and lung injury in a rat pneumonia model. American Journal of Physiology. Lung Cellular and Molecular Physiology. 2005;**289**(2):L207-L216

[33] Cavalieri SJ, Bohach GA, Snyder IS. *Escherichia coli* α-hemolysin: Characteristics and probable role in pathogenicity. Microbiological Reviews. 1984;**48**(4):326-343

[34] Den Bosch JF, Emödy L, Kétyi I. Virulence of haemolytic strains of *Escherichia coli* in various animal models. FEMS Microbiology Letters. 1982;**13**(4):427-430

[35] Ristow LC, Welch RA. Hemolysin of uropathogenic *Escherichia coli*: A cloak or a dagger? Biochimica et Biophysica Acta (BBA) - Biomembranes. 2016;**1858**(3):538-545

[36] Uhlen P, Laestadius A, Jahnukalnen T. α-Haemolysin of uropathogenic *E. coli* induces Ca^{2+} oscillations in renal epithelial cells. Nature. 2000;**405**(6787):694-697

[37] Bower JM, Eto DS, Mulvey MA. Covert operations of uropathogenic *Escherichia coli* within the urinary tract. Traffic. 2005;**6**(1):18-31

[38] Mills M, Meysick KC, O'Brien AD. Cytotoxic necrotizing factor type 1 of uropathogenic *Escherichia coli* kills cultured human uroepithelial 5637 cells by an apoptotic mechanism. Infection and Immunity. 2000;**68**(10):5869-5880

[39] Fiorentini C, Fabbri A, Matarrese P, Falzano L, Boquet P, Malorni W. Hinderance of apoptosis and phagocytic behaviour induced by *Escherichia coli* cytotoxic necrotizing factor 1: Two related activities in epithelial cells. Biochemical and Biophysical Research Communications. 1997;**241**(2):341-346

[40] Guyer DM, Radulovic S, Jones FE, Mobley HL. Sat, the secreted autotransporter toxin of uropathogenic *Escherichia coli*, is a vacuolating cytotoxin for bladder and kidney epithelial cells. Infection and Immunity. 2002;**70**(8):4539-4546

[41] Guyer DM, Henderson IR, Nataro JP, Mobley HL. Identification of sat, an autotransporter toxin produced by uropathogenic *Escherichia coli*. Molecular Microbiology. 2000; **38**(1):53-66

[42] Guerra L, Cortes-Bratti X, Guidi R, Frisan T. The biology of the cytolethal distending toxins. Toxins. 2011;**3**(3):172-190

[43] Féria CP, Correia JD, Gonçalves J, Machado J. Detection of virulence factors in uropathogenic *Escherichia coli* isolated from humans, dogs and cats in Portugal. In: Genes and Proteins Underlying Microbial Urinary Tract Virulence. Boston, MA: Springer; 2002. pp. 305-308

[44] Tóth I, Hérault F, Beutin L, Oswald E. Production of cytolethal distending toxins by pathogenic *Escherichia coli* strains isolated from human and animal sources: Establishment of the existence of a new cdt variant (type IV). Journal of Clinical Microbiology. 2003; **41**(9):4285-4291

[45] Ladant D, Alouf JE, Popoff MR. The Comprehensive Sourcebook of Bacterial Protein Toxins. London: Academic Press; 2005

[46] Cirl C, Wieser A, Yadav M, Duerr S, Schubert S, Fischer H, et al. Subversion of toll-like receptor signaling by a unique family of bacterial toll/interleukin-1 receptor domain–containing proteins. Nature Medicine. 2008;**14**(4):399

[47] Lai XH, Arencibia I, Johansson A, Wai SN, Oscarsson J, Kalfas S, et al. Cytocidal and apoptotic effects of the ClyA protein from *Escherichia coli* on primary and cultured monocytes and macrophages. Infection and Immunity. 2000;**68**(7):4363-4367

[48] Jahandeh N, Ranjbar R, Behzadi P, Behzadi E. Uropathogenic *Escherichia coli* virulence genes: Invaluable approaches for designing DNA microarray probes. Central European Journal of Urology. 2015;**68**(4):452

[49] Henderson JP, Crowley JR, Pinkner JS, Walker JN, Tsukayama P, Stamm WE, et al. Quanti tative metabolomics reveals an epigenetic blueprint for iron acquisition in uropathogenic *Escherichia coli*. PLoS Pathogens. 2009;**5**(2):e1000305

[50] Olson PD, Justice SS, Hunstad D. *Escherichia coli* in urinary tract infections. Molecular Medical Microbiology. 2nd ed. London: Academic Press; 2015;**76**(7):1373-1387

[51] Hagan EC, Mobley HLT. Haem acquisition is facilitated by a novel receptor Hma and required by uropathogenic *Escherichia coli* for kidney infection. Molecular Microbiology. 2008;**71**(1):79-91

[52] Neilands JB, Bindereif A, Montgomery JZ. Genetic basis of iron assimilation in pathogenic *Escherichia coli*. In: Genetic Approaches to Microbial Pathogenicity. Berlin, Heidelberg: Springer; 1985. pp. 179-195

[53] Hagberg L, Jodal U, Korhonen TK, Lidin-Janson G, Lindberg U, Eden CS. Adhesion, hemagglutination, and virulence of *Escherichia coli* causing urinary tract infections. Infection and Immunity. 1981;**31**(2):564-570

[54] Warner PJ, Williams PH, Bindereif A, Neilands JB. ColV plasmid-specific aerobactin synthesis by invasive strains of *Escherichia coli*. Infection and Immunity. 1981;**33**(2):540-545

[55] De Lorenzo V, Martinez JL. Aerobactin production as a virulence factor: A reevaluation. European Journal of Clinical Microbiology and Infectious Diseases. 1988;**7**(5):621-629

[56] Wiles TJ, Kulesus RR, Mulvey MA. Origins and virulence mechanisms of uropathogenic *Escherichia coli*. Experimental and Molecular Pathology. 2008;**85**(1):11-19

[57] Billips BK, Forrestal SG, Rycyk MT, Johnson JR, Klumpp DJ, Schaeffer AJ. Modulation of host innate immune response in the bladder by uropathogenic *Escherichia coli*. Infection and Immunity. 2007;**75**(11):5353-5360

[58] Reigstad CS, Hultgren SJ, Gordon JI. Functional genomic studies of uropathogenic *Esche richia coli* and host urothelial cells when intracellular bacterial communities are assembled. Journal of Biological Chemistry. 2007;**282**(29):21259-21267

[59] Garcia EC, Brumbaugh AR, Mobley HL. Redundancy and specificity of *Escherichia coli* iron acquisition systems during urinary tract infection. Infection and Immunity. 2011; **79**(3):1225-1235

[60] Nagy G, Dobrindt U, Emody L, Karch H, Hacker J. Expression of hemin receptor molecule ChuA is influenced by RfaH in Uropathogenic *Escherichia coli* strain 536. Infection and Immunity. 2001;**69**(3):1924-1928

[61] Sarkar S, Ulett GC, Totsika M, Phan MD, Schembri MA. Role of capsule and O antigen in the virulence of uropathogenic *Escherichia coli*. PLoS One. 2014;**9**(4):e94786

[62] Ong CLY, Ulett GC, Mabbett AN, Beatson SA, Webb RI, Monaghan W, et al. Identification of type 3 fimbriae in uropathogenic *Escherichia coli* reveals a role in biofilm formation. Journal of Bacteriology. 2008;**190**(3):1054-1063

[63] Lane MC, Alteri CJ, Smith SN, Mobley HL. Expression of flagella is coincident with uropathogenic *Escherichia coli* ascension to the upper urinary tract. Proceedings of the National Academy of Sciences. 2007;**104**(42):16669-16674

[64] Lundstedt AC, McCarthy S, Gustafsson MC, Godaly G, Jodal U, Karpman D, et al. A genetic basis of susceptibility to acute pyelonephritis. PLoS One. 2007;**2**(9):e825

[65] Klumpp DJ, Weiser AC, Sengupta S, Forrestal SG, Batler RA, Schaeffer AJ. Uropathogenic *Escherichia coli* potentiates type 1 pilus-induced apoptosis by suppressing NF-κB. Infection and Immunity. 2001;**69**(11):6689-6695

[66] Justice SS, Hunstad DA, Harper JR, Duguay AR, Pinkner JS, Bann J, et al. Periplasmic peptidyl prolyl cis-trans isomerases are not essential for viability, but SurA is required for pilus biogenesis in *Escherichia coli*. Journal of Bacteriology. 2005;**187**(22):7680-7686

[67] Klemm P. Fimbrial adhesins of *Escherichia coli*. Reviews of Infectious Diseases. May-Jun 1985;**7**(3):321-340

9

Uropathogenic *Escherichia coli* and Fimbrial Adhesins Virulome

Payam Behzadi

Abstract

Urinary tract infections (UTIs) rank second among infectious diseases around the world, and this makes them significant. There are many microbial agents which may cause UTIs. *Enterobacteriaceae* family members are recognized as important UTI bacterial causative agents. Among them, uropathogenic *Escherichia coli* (UPEC) pathotypes are considered as the most important bacterial agents of UTIs. Today, genomics and bioinformatics explain us why UPEC strains are so considerable pathogens regarding UTIs. There is a diversity of *E. coli* strains involving commensal and pathogenic strains. Genomics shows that commensal strains of *E. coli* encompass the minimal amount of genome and genetic elements among *E. coli* populations, whereas the pathotypes of *E. coli* possess the maximal or a big portion of genomic elements. Previous studies confirm the presence of a vast range of virulence genes within the pool of *E. coli* pathotypes like UPEC. So, the pool of virulence genes (virulome) belonging to UPEC enables UPEC pathotypes to have huge genomes with the ability of different levels of pathogenesis. The more virulence factors, the more pathogenicity. Due to the presence of a mass of virulence factors within UPEC cellular structures, well-known fimbrial adhesins in UPEC pathotypes are discussed in this chapter.

Keywords: uropathogenic *Escherichia coli*, genomics, fimbriae, adhesins, virulence factors, urinary tract infections

1. Introduction

Every year, several million people suffer from urinary tract infections (UTIs), and of course it costs expensive for governments and healthcare medicine centres [1, 2].

UTIs with second ranking are one of the most dominant infectious diseases around the world. Although UTIs include vast etiological microbial agents, two pathogenic microorganisms such as *Escherichia coli* (*E. coli*) (as a predominant pioneer bacterial agent) and Candida albicans (C. albicans) (as a predominant pioneer fungal agent) are the most recognized UTI etiologic pathogens [3–6].

The pangenomic and phylogenetic studies have revealed five different categories within the species of *E. coli*. These five categories involve A, B1, B2, D and E, which depending on their strains can cause extra- and intra-intestinal infections. The extra-intestinal pathogenic *E. coli* (ExPEC) may lead to a vast range of infectious diseases. So, uropathogenic *E. coli* (UPEC) represents one of the most important causative bacterial pathotypes of UTIs. Three phylogroups of A, B1 and E encompass intra-intestinal commensal and/or pathotypes of *E. coli*, whereas the B2 and D phylogroups involve, respectively, the most and the least numbers of UPEC pathotypes [7, 8].

1.1. Biology of urinary tract infections

There are different types of UTIs with a diversity of clinical demonstrations. Today, we know that the UTI syndromes are completely in association with hosts' immune system activities, type of causative microbial agent and the contributed microbial virulence factors. UTIs may be appeared as acute or chronic lower (typically known as cystitis) and/or upper (typically known as pyelonephritis) urinary tract infections, with symptomatic or asymptomatic manifestations and complicated or uncomplicated demonstrations. So, asymptomatic bacteriuria and simple cystitis with some ignorable irritations may be recognized as light and mild UTIs, respectively; while the urosepsis is known as a serious deathful type of UTI. Generally, the uncomplicated UTIs are recognized in patients with no previous background for UTIs, whereas the complicated UTIs normally happen in patients with previous problems in their urinary tracts. The remarkable point of view is the association between predisposing factors of diabetes, sexual intercourse, gender, catheterization, pregnancy, overweight, genetic factors, host's immune system responses and the type of UTIs and their severities [3, 5, 8–12].

In accordance with previous surveys, there are several numbers of microbial pathogens which can be identified as UTI pathogenic microorganisms. The microbial pathogens depending on the type of UTIs involve a vast number of pathogenic causative agents including Gram-negative bacteria, e.g. UPEC, *Klebsiella* spp., *Enterobacter* spp., *Proteus* spp., *Citrobacter* spp., *Morganella morganii*, *Acinetobacter* spp., *Salmonella* spp. and *Pseudomonas aeruginosa*; Gram-positive bacteria such as Staphylococcus aureus (*methicillin-sensitive* S. aureus (*MSSA*) and/or *methicillin-resistant* S. aureus (*MRSA*)), Staphylococcus epidermidis (*methicillin-sensitive* S. epidermidis (*MSSE*) *and/or methicillin-resistant* S. epidermidis (*MRSE*)), *Staphylococcus saprophyticus*, *Streptococcus* spp., *Enterococcus faecium*, *Enterococcus faecalis*, diphtheroids and *Corynebacterium urealyticum* and fungal agents like C. albicans, Candida glabrata and Candida tropicalis. As aforementioned, some pathogens are predominant in complicated UTIs, and some others are responsible for uncomplicated UTIs; however, the UPEC strains are common causative agents in both types of complicated and uncomplicated UTIs. Moreover, the presence of living microbial cells determines the condition of UTIs. The usual threshold for UTI pathogens is estimated $\geq 10^5$ living cells per urine millilitre (ml). As each living cell can grow and create its own colony, the 10^5 cells can be construed as 10^5 colony-forming units (CFUs). But we have to notice that, in some cases, the aforementioned threshold must be counted less than 10^5 CFUs/ml [3, 6, 10–14].

1.2. The genus of *Escherichia*: A great bacterial empire

The genus of *Escherichia* includes *E. albertii, E. coli, E. fergusonii, E. hermannii, E. marmotae* and *E. vulneris*. The familiarity of these species is shown in **Figure 1**. In addition to these species, there are some *Escherichia* strains which have no differences in their phenotypes; but from the genotypic aspects, they have different characteristics. These strains are named as cryptic clades, which are branched into five strains of C-I to C-V [15–18].

E. coli is the most famous member of Gram-negative bacterial family of *Enterobacteriaceae* which was identified by Theodor *Escherich*. This non-spore forming and generally motile (with a peritrichous flagellated arrangement) facultative anaerobic rod-shaped bacterium was named *E. coli* by the suggestion of Castellani and Chalmers in 1919 [7, 19, 20]. There are a diversity of *E. coli* strains which are divided into commensal types (intra-intestinal non-pathogenic strains) and pathotypes (intra-intestinal pathogenic *E. coli* (InPEC) and extra-intestinal pathogenic *E. coli* (ExPEC)). The commensal types of *E. coli* are able to be settled within the infants' alimentary canal just in some hours after birth as beneficial normal flora populations [21, 22].

The *E. coli* pathotypes are divided into a vast range of strains which may cause different types of infectious diseases. **Table 1** indicates the pathotypes and their related infections. In accordance with the table, the pathotypes have been divided into three groups: ExPEC, InPEC and ShiToPInPEC. Phylogenetic studies show a close relationship between *Shigella* spp. and *E. coli*. A close genetic similarity is recognized between *Shigella* spp. and enteroinvasive *E. coli* (EIEC) pathotypes [4, 7, 23–30].

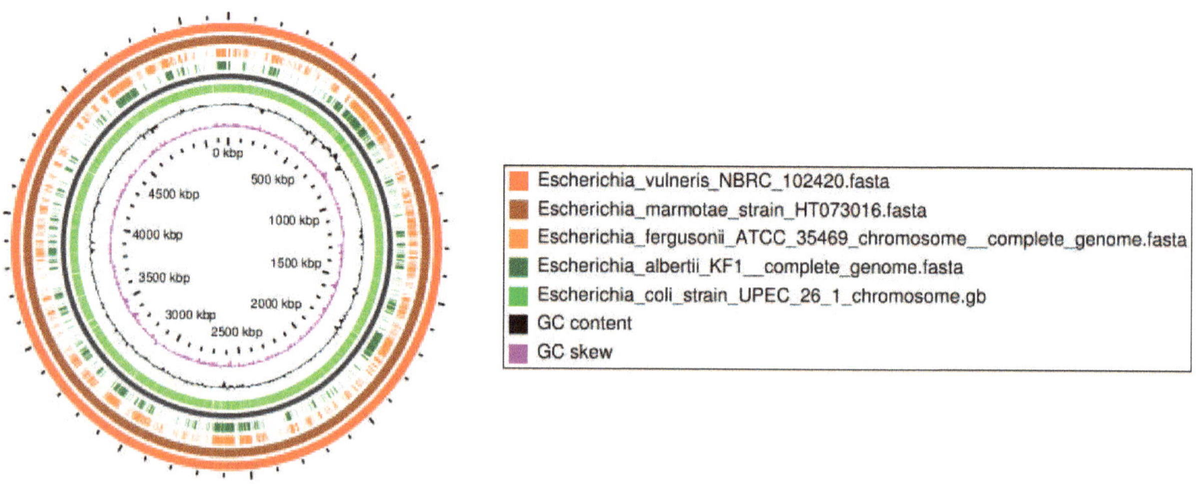

Figure 1. The genome of uropathogenic *E. coli* (UPEC) has been compared with *E. albertii, E. fergusonii, E. marmotae* and *E. vulneris* by the online GView Server system. The figure indicates genomic familiarities between the *Escherichia* species. As shown, the species of *E. marmotae* and *E. vulneris* have very close genomic similarities with UPEC, whereas there is some dissimilarity between genomic treasures of *E. albertii, E. fergusonii* and UPEC (GView Server; https://server.gview.ca/).

Category	Pathotype	Type of infection	Appearance	Phylogroup
ExPEC	Neonatal Meningitis E.coli (NEMEC)	Meningitis in neonates	Opportunistic	D, E
	Septic E.coli (SEPEC)	Sepsis	Opportunistic	B1
	Uropathogenic E.coli (UPEC)	Urogenital tract infections	Opportunistic	B2, D
InPEC	Entero -Aggregative E.coli (EAEC)	Diarrhoea (bloody)	Pathogenic	
	Entero -Pathogenic E.coli (EPEC)	Diarrhoea (bloody)	Pathogenic	A, B1, D, E
	Entero -Toxigenic E.coli (ETEC)	Diarrhoea (bloody)	Pathogenic	
Shigella Toxin Producer InPEC (ShiToPInPEC)	Entero -Hemorrhagic E.coli (EHEC)	Bloody Diarrhoea	Pathogenic	B1, D, E
	Entero -Invasive E.coli (EIEC)	Bloody Diarrhoea	Pathogenic	A, B1, E
	Adhesive -Invasive E. coli (AIEC)	Bloody Diarrhoea	Pathogenic	B2
	Diffused -Adhesive E.coli (DAEC)	Bloody Diarrhoea	Pathogenic	A, B2, D

Table 1. The categorization of *E. coli* pathotypes, the related infections and the condition of appearance.

2. *Escherichia coli* and pangenomics

E. coli is a quite diverse genus which involves a vast range of strains with different metabolic properties, pathogenesis, genomic treasure, virulence factors and ecological varieties. These characteristics make *E. coli* an important case in association with infectious diseases. The *E. coli* strains range from commensal strains (useful normal flora) to AIEC, DAEC, EAEC, EHEC, EIEC, EPEC, ETEC, NEMEC, SEPEC and UPEC pathotypes. The characteristic diversities among *E. coli* strains are completely pertaining to their specific pangenomes. The type of genes and the gene pool of microorganisms determine the quality and the quantity of genetic evolutionary properties [4, 7, 22].

The term pangenome was applied by Sigaux for a database with the content of tissues and tumour genomic data; but the application of pangenome with its microbial content was used by Tettelin and colleagues for the first time, and this refers to a collection of genes and genetic elements in a family group which can be recognized among species of a genus. According to genomic studies, each microbial genus encompasses a main genomic pool which is known as core genome. The core genome contains all those vital genes belonging to different species of a microbial genus. In addition to core genome, there is a group of genomic materials pertaining to species members of a genus which is named as extra genome (flexible or accessory genome). Sometimes some accessory genome pools contain unique genes which are completely related to specific strain. The extra genome possesses genes that are vital but varies in different genome pools. Some genera bear closed pangenomes, whereas the others contain open pangenomes. The open pangenomic microbial organisms involve a vast range of strains. In parallel with molecular techniques, bioinformatics has a key role in pangenomics. Computational analyses give us brilliant information regarding chromosomal genes and motile genetic elements such as plasmids, transposons and phages. Today, the bacterial genus of *E. coli* is known as the most progressive prokaryote with the highest detected genomic sets [7, 31–34].

The complete genomic data regarding *E. coli* (K12 strain) was reported in 1997 for the first time. Due to the recent aforementioned information regarding *E. coli* genomics, we now know that each strain comprises core genome, accessory genome (extra genome and/or flexible genome) and some unique genes which are specific for each strain. Furthermore, the accessory genomic pool which is flexible may contain integrons, pathogenicity islands (PAIs), phages, plasmids, prophages and transposons. The presence of these genomic elements is related to the nature of the environment in which bacterial cells exist. So, the size of genome is completely dependent on the habitat of bacteria. In another word, the condition of genomic pool and sequence of the genome determine the biological characteristics of the bacteria. Therefore, genomics of *E. coli* strains reveal the needs of them in their own habitats [7, 23, 35].

The reported results from previous studies show that the commensal strains of *E. coli* bear the smallest pangenome (with no virulence genes or with minimal capacity), whereas the pathogenic strains of *E. coli* like UPEC pathotypes encompass large pangenomes (because of the presence of a mass of virulence genes). So, the added genes in pathotype pangenomes are recognized as virulence genes (virulome). It is estimated that UPEC pathotypes carry 10^5 bp much more than commensal strains within their pangenomes. This property gives a high plasticity to UPEC pathotype pangenomes. As shown in published reports, the pangenome of *E. coli* strains involve 4.6–5.9 Mbp and the chromosomal genomes are consisted of limited number of genes [7, 23, 26, 36].

Table 2 shows a number of well-known databases in which the genomic data regarding *E. coli* genomes are accessible.

Database	The main subject	URL	Reference
EcoCyc *E. coli* Database	*Escherichia coli* K-12 MG1655	https://ecocyc.org/	[37, 38]
EcoGene 3.0	*Escherichia coli* K-12	http://ecogene.org/	[39]
Kyoto Encyclopedia of Genes and Genomes (KEGG)	Genes, genomes, etc.	http://www.genome.jp/kegg/ http://www.genome.jp/kegg/	[40]
SHared Information of GENetic Resources (SHIGEN)	The profiling of *Escherichia coli* chromosome (PEC) database	https://shigen.nig.ac.jp/ecoli/pec/	[41]
Pfam 31.0	Protein family database	http://pfam.xfam.org/	[42]
Ensembl Genomes (The European Bioinformatics Institute (EMBL-EBI))	Genomes	http://ensemblgenomes.org/	[43]
The DNA Data Bank of Japan (DDBJ)	Nucleotide sequence database	http://www.ddbj.nig.ac.jp/	[44]
GenBank (National Center for Biotechnology Information (NCBI))	Nucleotide sequence database	http://www.ncbi.nlm.nih.gov/genbank/	[45]

Table 2. Some useful and helpful databases which can be used for *Escherichia coli* pangenome.

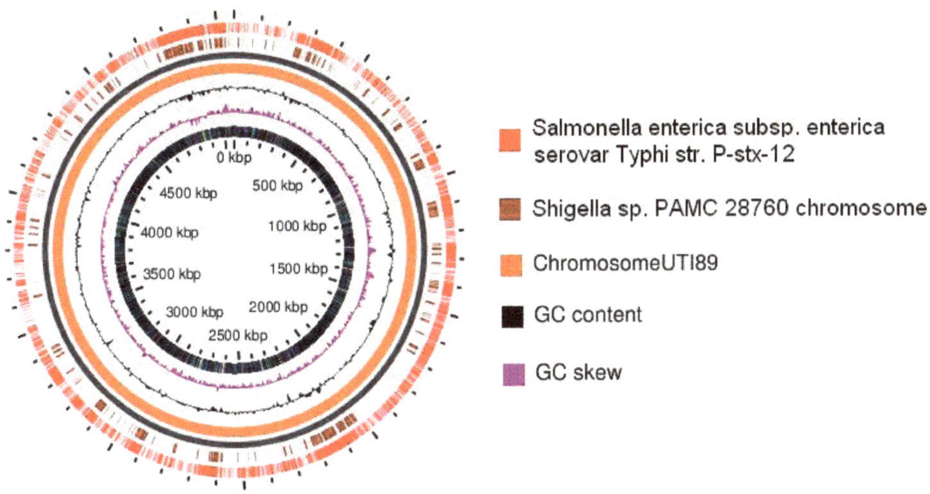

Figure 2. A chromosomal comparison between UPEC (UTI89), *Shigella* sp. and *Salmonella enterica*. The GC content and GC skew are shown, too (GView Server; https://server.gview.ca/).

The pangenomic studies reveal an interesting evolutionary relationship between *E. coli*, *Shigella* spp. and *Salmonella enterica*. It seems that *E. coli* is the ancestor of *Shigella* spp. The *Shigella* spp. have derivated from *E. coli* pathotypes within a duration of 270,000–35,000 years, whereas the origination of *E. coli* and *S. enterica* bacteria from a common progenitor goes back to 100,000,000 years ago [4, 46] (**Figure 2**).

3. Uropathogenic *Escherichia coli* (UPEC)

The UTIs are divided into community-acquired and nosocomial infectious diseases. The UPEC pathotypes are the most dominant causative bacterial agents of UTIs. As previous investigations show, about 50% of nosocomial and up to 95% of community-acquired UTIs are occurred by UPEC strains. So, the UPEC pathotypes are one of the most considered UTI causative agents worldwide. These reports lead us to a wide variety of virulence factors in UPEC pathotypes. Besides, the bioinformatic approaches and pangenomics confirm the presence of a giant treasure of virulence genes within the pangenome of UPEC [7, 8, 35, 47].

The spread of virulence genes among UPEC pathotypes is quite different. The range of UTIs varies from ignorable cases like asymptomatic bacteriuria to deathful cases like urosepsis. The severity of UTIs is completely in association with the UPEC virulence gene pool (virulome). Sometimes, pathotypes undergo mutations in their hosts' bodies which may lead to lose their own virulence genes. It seems that the UPEC pathotypes, which may cause asymptomatic bacteriuria, have undergone virulence gene deletions. On the other hand, strong uropathogenic strains encompass a mass of virulence genes which enable them to occur severe UTIs within their hosts' bodies. The occurrence of UTIs is associated with the host's genetic predisposing factors, immune system, gender, hospitalization, catheterization, social behaviour, sexual activities, personal hygiene and the presence of virulence factors in uropathogenic microbial agents [3, 7, 11, 13, 22, 48–50].

The outcomes of several studies reveal the presence of a huge number of virulence factors which have been expanded among different strains of UPEC. Here, the most considerable virulence factors are mentioned and the most considerable filamentous adhesins are explained one by one.

4. Uropathogenic *Escherichia coli* (UPEC) virulome

The severity of UPEC pathogenesis is completely in association with diversity of virulence genes in their pangenomes. **Figure 3** shows the pangenome of UTI89. The virulence genes may be located on chromosomes (added through vertical gene transfer) or plasmids, transposons, integrons and phages (added via horizontal gene transfers). Previous studies indicate that the majority of virulence genes belonging to UPEC are located on pathogenicity islands (PAIs) where many of genes are transferred from other species rather than *E. coli* through the feature of horizontal genomic exchange. UPEC pathotypes are effective pathogens due to their high capacity of virulome. The diversity of virulence factors enables UPEC to manifest different types of UTIs in their human hosts. Adhesion, immune system escape mechanisms, iron uptake systems, protease enzymes and toxins are the most significant mechanisms that UPEC pathotypes should utilize them to survive in the human host urinary tract [22, 51–53].

Because of the vast variety of pathogenicity potentials in UPEC strains, only hair-like structures of afimbrial adhesins (including curli and Afa) and fimbrial adhesins (comprising Dr, Type 1 fimbriae, Type 3 fimbriae, F1C fimbriae, S fimbriae, P fimbriae, Auf and F9 fimbriae) are discussed in this chapter. There are some useful databases such as Center for Genomic Epidemiology (https://cge.cbs.dtu.dk/services/VirulenceFinder/) and Virulence Factors of Pathogenic Bacteria (http://www.mgc.ac.cn/VFs/) which may be used for detection and identification virulence genes within the *E. coli* strain populations' genomes [54].

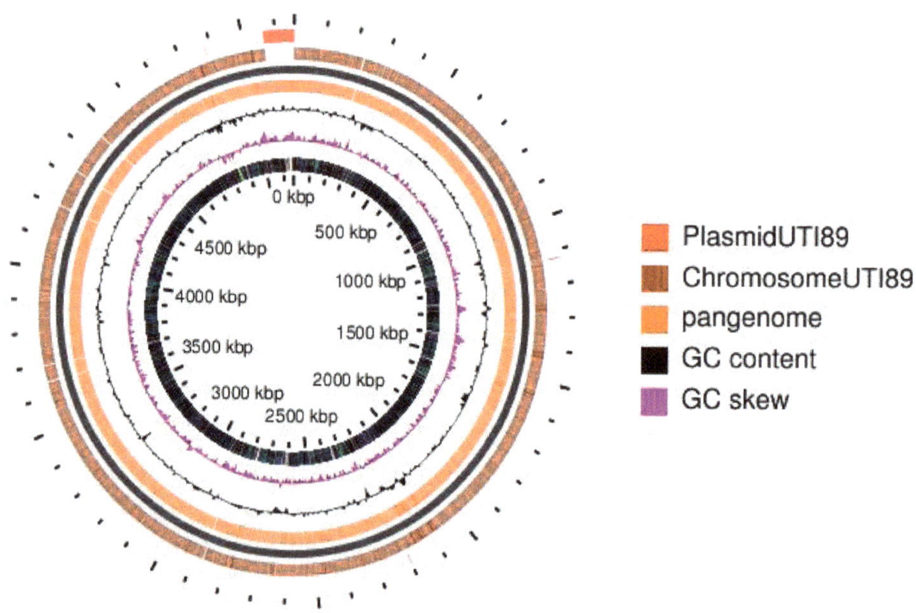

Figure 3. The pangenome map (chromosomal and plasmid genomes) of UPEC (UTI89). The GC content and GC skew are shown, too (GView Server; https://server.gview.ca/).

4.1. Filamentous adhesin virulome

Each microorganism either pathogen or non-pathogen needs to be adhered for colonization. Indeed, colonization of pathogenic microorganisms results in pathogenesis within human body's host. For this reason, UPEC has a range of superficial proteins and adhesins (**Table 3**). However the hair-like structured fimbriae are invaluable virulence factors which enable UPEC pathotypes to have successful attachment, colonization, biofilm formation and virulence [7, 22, 53, 55–65].

Fimbrial adhesins are superficial peritrichous arranged exterior proteinaceous appendages which target special motifs upon the cell surface receptors to join them in the manner of key-and-lock operation. These adhesins are able to attach onto biotic (e.g. host cells) and abiotic (e.g. catheter) surfaces. The aforementioned characteristics make UPEC bacteria functional and effective pathogenic microorganisms. The attachment of bacterial cells of UPEC onto the host cells is a complicated process which may be caused by important proteinaceous molecules of adhesins. Adhesins prepare suitable condition for a successful signalling controlled communication between UPEC cells and human body cells. In other words, the fimbrial adhesins act as signal molecules. As shown in **Table 3**, the most studied and recognized superficial filamentous adhesins are Curli, Dr, AFA, Type 1 fimbriae, Type 3 fimbriae, F1C fimbriae, S fimbriae, P fimbriae, F9 fimbriae and Auf. Some of these superficial fimbrial organelles involving F1C, P, S, Auf, Type 1, Type 3 and F9 fimbriae are categorized into chaperone-usher (CU) proteins [8, 27, 53, 59, 62, 66].

4.1.1. Curli adhesins

Curli adhesins of UPEC are known as types of fragile exterior proteinous coiled fibrous appendages which contribute in linking the UPEC cells onto related receptors situated upon the human body cells such as endothelial cells, epithelial cells, matrix proteins, urothelial cells, mucosal cells, blood cells, etc. In addition to UPEC pathotypes, curli adhesins are recognized in *Salmonella* spp. too. The affinity between curli organelles and Congo red makes it easy to observe these tiny adhesins by microscope. Curli adhesins with up to 12 nm width and 1 μm length are made of CsgA (curlin as major content with amyloid property) and CsgB (as minor content with amyloid property and nucleator activity) proteins. The highly conserved curli gene clusters in UPEC pathotypes are organized into *csgBAC* and *csgDEFG* operons. Curli molecules are effective structures to adhere UPEC cells onto the urine bladder and kidney urothelial cells within human bodies [50, 52, 53, 57, 67–69] (**Table 3**).

4.1.2. Dr/Afa adhesins

The Dr and Afa adhesins are the members of DR family. Dr adhesins (with a homology rate of ≥70%) and Afa molecules are able to bind to the Dr^a blood group antigen molecules situated onto the decay-accelerating factors (DAFs). The DAF molecules are located upon the surface of different types of cells such as urothelial cells. The Dr gene operons consisted of five genes, including *draA–draE,* which are detectable in 7% of the UPEC populations. The *draE* gene is responsible for Dr haemagglutinin production, which is contributed in type IV collagen attachment. *draA–draG* genes are highly conserved and produce the accessory proteins, whereas the *draE* genes with lower conserved sequences are responsible for adhesin structural subunits. Moreover, the AFA adhesins are encoded by a five-member gene operon including *afaA, afaE, afaD, afaB* and *afaC*. The proteins of AFAI and AFAIII are known as Dr family members. In accordance with previous studies, some of Dr and AFA adhesins have close similarities with chaperone-usher pathway adhesins. The AFA adhesins are recognized in up to 65% of UPEC pathotypes causing cystitis, 26% causing pyelonephritis and 6% asymptomatic bacteriuria (ABU) [7, 8, 22, 55, 61, 70, 71] (**Table 3**).

4.2. Chaperone-usher fimbrial adhesins

There are varieties of fimbriae which are produced by Gram-negative bacteria such as *Enterobacteriaceae* family members. The subunits of these fimbriae are assembled by different pathways like CU pathway. Those fimbriae produced via CU pathway are the most frequent filamentous organelles among Gram-negative bacteria populations. The CU pathway is a kind of common bacterial secretion system with a high conservancy. In a fimbrial CU pathway, chaperone (a periplasmic protein molecule) together with a pore-forming protein of usher (situated within bacterial outer membrane) orchestrate this secretion system. So through the CU pathway, the usher protein plays its role as platform assembler by employing a chaperone to produce and secrete subunits of CU fimbriae class. F1C, P, S, Auf, Type 1, Type 3 and F9 fimbriae in UPEC pathotypes are known as CU pathway proteinaceous adhesins [62, 66, 72–75] (**Table 3**).

4.2.1. *Type 1 fimbriae*

Type 1 fimbriae as mannose-sensitive adhesins (belonging to chaperone-usher class) are able to attach to those receptors with mannose residues. Uroplakin molecules with high frequency in human urine bladder are known as one of the most important Type 1 fimbriae receptors. Furthermore, there are different types of Type 1 fimbriae receptors which are located on human ureter and Henle's tubules. These fimbriae are encoded in 99% of commensal and pathogenic strains of *E. coli* including UPEC pathotypes. As important virulence factors, Type 1 fimbriae have peripheral arrangement upon the microorganisms' surfaces with a number of 1–5 hundred. Type 1 fimbriae with up to 10 nm width and up to 2 μm length are able to perform haemagglutination. The Type 1 fimbriae are encoded by the highly conserved gene operon consisted of nine genes of *fimBEAICDFGH*. The FimH protein which is located on the top of Type 1 fimbria is recognized as the main adhesin. FimG, Fim F and FimA protein molecules are, respectively, situated under the FimH molecule. FimC and FimD play their roles as chaperone and usher proteins, respectively. The recombinase enzymes of FimB and FimE activate as bidirectional switching molecules for turning on and/or turning off the cluster gene expression. The activities of FimB and FimE are directly associated with environmental factors [7, 22, 50, 53, 55, 60, 62, 68, 71, 74, 76, 77] (**Table 3**).

4.2.2. *Type 3 fimbriae*

Type 3 fimbriae are encoded by *mrk* gene operon of *mrkABCDEF* in UPEC and other members of *Enterobacteriaceae* family such as Klebsiella pneumoniae. The highly conserved gene of *mrkB* encodes chaperone protein of MrkB, whereas the MrkC plays role as usher protein. MrkA and MrkF are the major and minor subunits in Type 3 fimbriae, respectively. The adhesin molecule of Type 3 fimbria is recognized as MrkD and MrkE plays its role as a regulator protein. It seems that *mrk* gene cluster originally belongs to K. pneumoniae which has been horizontally transferred into UPEC pathotypes by plasmids. The role of Type 3 fimbriae in biofilm formation regarding catheter-associated urinary tract infections (CAUTs) is significantly considered [53, 56] (**Table 3**).

4.2.3. F1C fimbriae

The F1C fimbriae are encoded by a gene operon consisting of seven genes of *focAICDFGH*. F1C fimbriae are expressed by up to 30% of UPEC pathotypes. The F1C fimbria is composed of FocA (major fimbrin subunits), FocF and FocG (minor fimbrin subunits) proteins. On the top of F1C fimbria, FocH monomer is located which acts as an adhesin. So, F1C fimbriae adhere onto the receptors with galactosylceramide (situated on the surfaces of urothelial cells of the urinary bladder, kidneys and ureters) and globotriaosylceramide (located in kidneys) residues. Previous surveys indicate a strong attraction between F1C fimbriae and Gal-NAc-beta-1-4-Gal-beta structure of glycolipids. FocC and FocD proteins are recognized as chaperone and usher molecules, respectively. Due to prior scientific investigations, the F1C fimbriae are able to bind to their specific receptors upon the whole zone of the urinary tract. There is a close homology between F1C and S fimbriae [7, 53, 55, 62, 66, 78] (**Table 3**).

4.2.4. S fimbriae

In addition to FIC, the S fimbriae organelles have also a close morphology to F9, P and Type 1 fimbriae and are detected in ≥22% of the UPEC pathotypes. The S fimbriae are encoded by *sfa* gene operon with nine genes. SfaA, SfaS and SfaH proteins contribute in S fimbrial adhesion. The SfaA protein is a dominant subunit, and the minor subunits are composed of SfaG, SfaH and SfaS. SfaS is located on the top of S fimbriae and adhere to alpha-sialyl-2,3-alpha-galactose residues upon the glycoproteins of urothelial tissues of the urinary bladder and kidneys. The presence or absence of S fimbriae is determined by environmental factors. The related regulations and phase variations are done by SfaB and SfaC [7, 22, 35, 50, 53, 55, 62, 66, 71, 77, 79] (**Table 3**).

4.2.5. P fimbriae

P fimbriae as considerable adhesins are encoded by 11 genes within a gene operon of *papA-K* in up to 70% of UPEC pathotypes. The predominant subunit in P fimbria is PapA fimbrin placed in the basis of the fimbrial stalk. PapG is known as the main adhesin which is linked to the stalk by PapE, PapF and PapK proteins. PapD and PapC have chaperone and usher roles, respectively. There are some isoclasses for PapG (PapGI, PapGII (major isoclass in UPEC strains) and PapGIII) in different UPEC pathotypes. The related receptor epitopes of P fimbriae are alpha-D-galactopyranosyl-(1-4)-beta-D-galactopyranoside which are located on the surface of entire urothelial cells covering the human urinary tract. P fimbriae are recognized as significant virulence factors in UPEC virulome [7, 22, 50, 53, 62, 66, 71, 77] (**Table 3**).

4.2.6. *Auf fimbriae*

Auf (acronym for another UPEC fimbria) fimbriae are detected in 67% of isolated UPEC pathotypes. The Auf fimbriae are encoded by the gene operon of *aufABCDEFG*. AufA protein is predominant subunit in Auf fimbria, whereas AufC is known as an usher protein. The Auf protein receptors are still unknown in human body cells [7, 22, 53, 62, 74] (**Table 3**).

4.2.7. *F9 fimbriae*

The F9 fimbriae encoded by *f9* gene operon including *c1931–c1936* are detectable in 78% of UPEC populations. The C1931 protein is the major subunit identified in F9 fimbriae. The genetic and structural characteristics of F9 fimbriae are very close to Type 1, F1C and S fimbriae. Gal-beta-(1-3)-Glc-NAc and lacto-N-tetraose glycans are recognized as the main F9 fimbriae receptors [22, 53, 59, 60] (**Table 3**).

5. Diagnostic methods for virulence genes of filamentous adhesins

Detection and identification of genes such as virulence genes of filamentous adhesins may be achieved by a vast range of molecular techniques. PCR tools from conventional and multiplex to real time are the commonest molecular diagnostic techniques which can be used for limited samples [80–86].

Furthermore there are advanced pangenomic techniques like microarray technology which can be applied for detection and identification of different types of genes, when there are huge numbers of specimens. Microarray technology is divided into three types of DNA, protein and RNA microarray tools. The outcome of microarray technology is reliable, sensitive, specific, flexible and rapid with high accuracy [4, 7, 8, 87–93].

6. Conclusion

UPEC strains are expanded pathogenic microorganisms which are able to carry a mass of virulence genes within their genomes. The environmental condition and the genomic abilities and capacity determine the expression of virulence genes and factors. The UPEC strains bear different types of virulence factors in different parts of their cellular structures. These properties make UPEC pathotypes interesting pathogenic microorganisms which can appear a vast range of UTIs: from acute to chronic, from light to severe, from complicated to uncomplicated, from lower to upper and from asymptomatic to symptomatic signs and syndromes. So, knowing the genotypic and phenotypic characteristics of UPEC strains in different regions of world helps us to recognize the probable UPEC strains with their local clinical demonstrations. This enables us to have an accurate diagnosis with a definite treatment to reduce the healthcare costs around the world. Moreover, equipped microbiology laboratories with normal molecular tools and techniques like PCR or advanced pangenomic technologies support us to have specific, sensitive and reliable outcome.

Adhesins	Type of adhesins	Genes	Role	Target structure	Type of UTIs
Curli	Afimbrial adhesin	*csgA, csgB,csgC, csgD, csgE,csgF,csgG*	Adhesion for colonization (biofilm formation) and invasion	Matrix Proteins like Fibronectin, Laminin and Plasminogen, Mucosal cells	Severe UTIs; Cystitis in particular
Dr	Fimbrial adhesin	*dra* gene family including: *draA, draB, draC, draD, draE, draP*	Adhesion for colonization, Preparing invasion	A vast range of cells with Dr blood group antigen on their surfaces like urothelia, Neutrophil cells, Connective tissues in upper part of human urinary tract	(Recurrent and/or chronic) Cystitis and pyelonephritis (mostly in pregnant women), Asymptomatic Bacteriuria (ABU) in few cases
AFA	Afimbrial adhesin	*afa* gene family including: *afaI, afaII, afaIII ,afaIV,nfaI ,drII*			
Type 1 fimbriae	Fimbrial adhesin (sensitive to mannose)	*fim* gene family including: *fimA, fimB, fimC, fimD, fimE, fimF, fimG, fimH, fimI*	Adhesion for colonization (biofilm formation), invasion	Red Blood Cells (RBCs), Mucosal membrane and Epithelium cells, Uroplakin receptors in urine bladder	UTIs
Type 3 fimbriae	Fimbrial adhesin	*mrk gene familyincluding: mrkA, mrkB, mrkC, mrkD, mrkE, mrkF*			UTIs in catheterized patients
F1C fimbriae	Fimbrial adhesin	*focA, focC, focD, focf, focG, focH, focI*	Adhesion for colonization (biofilm formation)	Glycolipids of endothelia, Mucosal membrane and Glomeruli	UTIs, Pyelonephritis in particular
S fimbriae	Fimbrial adhesin	*sfaA, sfaB, sfaC, sfaD, sfaE, sfaF, sfaG, sfaH, sfaS, sfaX, sfaY*	Adhesion and colonization	Sialic acid molecules on kidneys and glomeruli endothelial, epithelial and mucosal cells	Upper UTIs in most cases
P fimbriae	Fimbrial adhesin Resistance to mannose	*papa, papB, papC, papD, papE, papF, papG, papH, papI, papJ, papK*	Adhesion and colonization	vascular epithelia, urothelia and Mucosal cells	Acute forms of UTIs (particularly Pyelonephritis), ABU in few cases
F9 fimbriae	Fimbrial adhesin	*c1931, c1932, c1933, c1934, c1935, c1936*	Adhesion for colonization (biofilm formation) ?	Urothelial cells ?	UTIs ?
Auf fimbriae (Another UPEC Fimbriae)	Fimbrial adhesin	*aufA, aufB, aufC, aufD, aufE, aufF, aufG*	Adhesion for colonization (biofilm formation)	unknown	UTIs

Table 3. The UPEC fimbrial and afimbrial adhesins and their characteristics within human bodies [7, 22, 53, 55–64, 71].

Author details

Payam Behzadi

Address all correspondence to: behzadipayam@yahoo.com

Department of Microbiology, College of Basic Sciences, Shahr-e-Qods Branch, Islamic Azad University, Tehran, Iran

References

[1] Ciani O, Grassi D, Tarricone R. An economic perspective on urinary tract infection: The "costs of resignation". Clinical Drug Investigation. 2013;**33**:255-261. DOI: 10.1007/s40261-013-0069-x

[2] Kucheria R, Dasgupta P, Sacks S, Khan M, Sheerin N. Urinary tract infections: New insights into a common problem. Postgraduate Medical Journal. 2005;**81**:83-86. DOI: 10.1136/pgmj.2004.023036

[3] Behzadi P, Behzadi E. The microbial agents of urinary tract infections at central laboratory of Dr. Shariati hospital, Tehran, Iran. Turkiye Kliniklire Tip Bilim. 2008;**28**:445-449

[4] Behzadi P, Najafi A, Behzadi E, Ranjbar R. Microarray long oligo probe designing for *Escherichia coli*: An in-silico DNA marker extraction. Central European Journal of Urology. 2016;**69**:105-111. DOI: 10.5173/ceju.2016.654

[5] Behzadi E, Behzadi P. The role of toll-like receptors (TLRs) in urinary tract infections (UTIs). Central European Journal of Urology. 2016;**69**:404-410. DOI: 10.5173/ceju.2016.871

[6] Behzadi P, Behzadi E, Ranjbar R. Urinary tract infections and *Candida albicans*. Central European Journa of Urology. 2015;**68**:96-101. DOI: 10.5173/ceju.2015.01.474

[7] Jahandeh N, Ranjbar R, Behzadi P, Behzadi E. Uropathogenic *Escherichia coli* virulence genes: Invaluable approaches for designing DNA microarray probes. Central European Journal of Urology. 2015;**68**:452-458. DOI: 10.5173/ceju.2015.625

[8] Behzadi P, Behzadi E. Uropathogenic *Escherichia coli*: An Ideal Resource for DNA Microarray Probe Designing. In: Rojas I, Ortuño F, editors. Bioinformatics and Biomedical Engineering. 5th IWBBIO 2017. Lecture notes in computer science part II, vol 10209. Cham: Springer; 2017. pp. 12-19. DOI: 10.1007/978-3-319-56154-7_2

[9] Schwab S, Jobin K, Kurts C. Urinary tract infection: recent insight into the evolutionary arms race between uropathogenic *Escherichia coli* and our immune system. Nephrol Dial Transplant. 2017;**gfx022**:1-7. DOI: 10.1093/ndt/gfx022

[10] Johansen TB, Bonkat G, Cai T, Tandogdu Z, Wagenlehner F, Grabe M. Grey zones in the field of urinary tract infections. European Urology Focus. 2016;**2**:460-462. DOI: 10.1016/j.euf.2016.03.012

[11] Flores-Mireles AL, Walker JN, Caparon M, Hultgren SJ. Urinary tract infections: Epidemiology, mechanisms of infection and treatment options. Nature Reviews. Microbiology. 2015;**13**:269-284. DOI: 10.1038/nrmicro3432

[12] Kline KA, Lewis AL. Gram-positive uropathogens, polymicrobial urinary tract infection, and the emerging microbiota of the urinary tract. Microbiology spectrum. 2016;**4**(2). DOI: 10.1128/microbiolspec.UTI-0012-2012

[13] Behzadi P, Behzadi E, Yazdanbod H, Aghapour R, Cheshmeh MA, Omran DS. A survey on urinary tract infections associated with the three most common uropathogenic bacteria. Maedica. 2010;**5**:111-5

[14] Brubaker L, Wolfe AJ. The female urinary microbiota/microbiome: Clinical and research implications. Rambam Maimonides Medical Journal. 2017;**8**:e0015. DOI: 10.5041/RMMJ.10292

[15] Liu S, Jin D, Lan R, Wang Y, Meng Q, Dai H, et al. *Escherichia marmotae* sp. nov., isolated from faeces of Marmota Himalayana. International Journal of Systematic and Evolutionary Microbiology. 2015;**65**:2130-2134. DOI: 10.1099/ijs.0.000228

[16] Clermont O, Gordon DM, Brisse S, Walk ST, Denamur E. Characterization of the cryptic Escherichia lineages: Rapid identification and prevalence. Environmental Microbiology. 2011;**13**:2468-2477. DOI: 10.1111/j.1462-2920.2011.02519.x

[17] Ooka T, Ogura Y, Katsura K, Seto K, Kobayashi H, Kawano K, et al. Defining the genome features of *Escherichia albertii*, an emerging enteropathogen closely related to *Escherichia coli*. Genome Biology and Evolution. 2015;**7**:3170-3179. DOI: 10.1093/gbe/evv211

[18] NCBI > Genomes & Maps > Genome > *Escherichia* [Internet]. NCBI. Available from: https://www.ncbi.nlm.nih.gov/genome/?term=Escherichia [Accessed: 2017-08-23]

[19] Etymologia: *Escherichia coli*. Emerging Infectious Disease Journal. 2015;**21**:1310. DOI: 10.3201/eid2108.ET2108

[20] Schaechter M Editor. Desk Encyclopedia of Microbiology. 2nd ed. Academic press, Elsevier, UK; 2010

[21] Kaper JB, Nataro JP, Mobley HL. Pathogenic *Escherichia coli*. Nature Reviews. Microbiology. 2004;**2**:123-140. DOI: 10.1038/nrmicro818

[22] Donnenberg M. *Escherichia coli*: Pathotypes and principles of pathogenesis. 2nd ed. Academic press, Elsevier, UK; 2013

[23] Robins-Browne RM, Holt KE, Ingle DJ, Hocking DM, Yang J, Tauschek M. Are *Escherichia coli* Pathotypes still relevant in the era of whole-genome sequencing? Frontiers in Cellular and Infection Microbiology. 2016;**6**:141. DOI: 10.3389/fcimb.2016.00141

[24] Rossi E, Cimdins A, Lüthje P, Brauner A, Sjöling Å, Landini P, et al. "It's a gut feeling"–*Escherichia coli* biofilm formation in the gastrointestinal tract environment. Critical Reviews in Microbiology. 2017:1-30. DOI: 10.1080/1040841X.2017.1303660

[25] Leimbach A, Hacker J, Dobrindt U. *E. coli* as an all-rounder: The thin line between commensalism and pathogenicity. In: Dobrindt U, Hacker J, Svanborg C. (eds) Between Pathogenicity and Commensalism. Current Topics in Microbiology and Immunology, 1st ed. Springer, Berlin, Heidelberg; 2013;**358**:3-32. DOI: 10.1007/82_2012_30

[26] Croxen MA, Finlay BB. Molecular mechanisms of *Escherichia coli* pathogenicity. Nature Reviews. Microbiology. 2010;**8**:26-38. DOI: 10.1038/nrmicro2265

[27] Servin AL. Pathogenesis of human diffusely adhering *Escherichia coli* expressing Afa/Dr adhesins (Afa/Dr DAEC): Current insights and future challenges. Clinical Microbiology Reviews. 2014;**27**:823-869. DOI: 10.1128/CMR.00036-14

[28] da Silva LC, de Mello Santos AC, Silva RM. Uropathogenic *Escherichia coli* pathogenicity islands and other ExPEC virulence genes may contribute to the genome variability of enteroinvasive *E. coli*. BMC Microbiology. 2017;**17**:68. DOI: 10.1186/s12866-017-0979-5

[29] Nash JH, Villegas A, Kropinski AM, Aguilar-Valenzuela R, Konczy P, Mascarenhas M, et al. Genome sequence of adherent-invasive Escherichia coli and comparative genomic analysis with other *E. coli* pathotypes. BMC Genomics. 2010;**11**:667. DOI: 10.1186/1471-2164-11-667

[30] O'brien CL, Bringer M-A, Holt KE, Gordon DM, Dubois AL, Barnich N, et al. Comparative genomics of Crohn9s disease-associated adherent-invasive *Escherichia coli*. Gut 2016;**0**:1-8. DOI: 10.1136/gutjnl-2015-311059

[31] McInerney JO, McNally A, O'Connell MJ. Why prokaryotes have pangenomes. Natural Microbiology. 2017;**2**:17040. DOI: 10.1038/nmicrobiol.2017.40

[32] Snipen L-G, Ussery DW. A domain sequence approach to pangenomics: Applications to *Escherichia coli*. F1000Res. 2012;**1**:19. DOI: 10.12688/f1000research.1-19.v2

[33] Rouli L, Merhej V, Fournier P-E, Raoult D. The bacterial pangenome as a new tool for analysing pathogenic bacteria. NMNI. 2015;**7**:72-85. DOI: 10.1016/j.nmni.2015.06.005

[34] Marschall T, Marz M, Abeel T, Dijkstra L, Dutilh BE, Ghaffaari A, et al. Computational pan-genomics: Status, promises and challenges. BioRxiv. 2016;**043430**. DOI: 10.1101/043430

[35] Lo AW, Moriel DG, Phan M-D, Schulz BL, Kidd TJ, Beatson SA, et al. 'Omic'Approaches to study Uropathogenic *Escherichia coli* virulence. Trends in Microbiology. 2017;**25**:729-740. DOI: 10.1016/j.tim.2017.04.006

[36] Terlizzi ME, Gribaudo G, Maffei ME. UroPathogenic *Escherichia coli* (UPEC) infections: Virulence factors, bladder responses, antibiotic, and non-antibiotic antimicrobial strategies. Frontiers in Microbiology. 2017;**8**:1566. DOI: 10.3389/fmicb.2017.01566

[37] Karp P, Weaver D, Paley S, Fulcher C, Kubo A, Kothari A, et al. The EcoCyc Database. EcoSal Plus. 2014;**6**:10.1128/ecosalplus.ESP-0009-2013. DOI: 10.1128/ecosalplus.ESP-0009-2013

[38] Keseler IM, Collado-Vides J, Santos-Zavaleta A, Peralta-Gil M, Gama-Castro S, Muñiz-Rascado L, et al. EcoCyc: A comprehensive database of *Escherichia coli* biology. Nucleic Acids Research. 2010;**39**:D583-DD90. DOI: 10.1093/nar/gkq1143

[39] Zhou J, Rudd KE. EcoGene 3.0. Nucleic Acids Research. 2013;**41**:D613-D624. DOI: 10.1093/nar/gks1235

[40] Kanehisa M, Furumichi M, Tanabe M, Sato Y, Morishima K. KEGG: New perspectives on genomes, pathways, diseases and drugs. Nucleic Acids Research. 2017;**45**:D353-D361. DOI: 10.1093/nar/gkw1092

[41] Yamazaki Y, Niki H, Kato J. Profiling of *Escherichia coli* Chromosome Database. In: Osterman AL, Gerdes SY. (eds) Microbial Gene Essentiality: Protocols and Bioinformatics. Methods in Molecular Biology™. 1st ed. Humana Press, New Jersey, USA; 2008;**416**: 385-389. DOI: 10.1007/978-1-59745-321-9_26

[42] Finn RD, Coggill P, Eberhardt RY, Eddy SR, Mistry J, Mitchell AL, et al. The Pfam protein families database: Towards a more sustainable future. Nucleic Acids Research. 2016;**44**: D279-D285. DOI: 10.1093/nar/gkv1344

[43] Kersey PJ, Allen JE, Armean I, Boddu S, Bolt BJ, Carvalho-Silva D, et al. Ensembl genomes 2016: More genomes, more complexity. Nucleic Acids Research. 2015;**44**:D574-D580. DOI: 10.1093/nar/gkv1209

[44] Mashima J, Kodama Y, Fujisawa T, Katayama T, Okuda Y, Kaminuma E, et al. DNA data bank of Japan. Nucleic Acids Res. 2017;**45**:D25-D31. DOI: 10.1093/nar/gkw1001

[45] Benson DA, Cavanaugh M, Clark K, Karsch-Mizrachi I, Lipman DJ, Ostell J, et al. GenBank. Nucleic Acids Research. 2017;**45**:D37-D42. DOI: 10.1093/nar/gkw1070

[46] Gordienko EN, Kazanov MD, Gelfand MS. Evolution of pan-genomes of *Escherichia coli*, *Shigella* spp., and *Salmonella enterica*. Journal of Bacteriology. 2013;**195**:2786-2792. DOI: 10.1128/JB.02285-12

[47] Wiles TJ, Kulesus RR, Mulvey MA. Origins and virulence mechanisms of uropathogenic *Escherichia coli*. Experimental and Molecular Pathology. 2008;**85**:11-19. DOI: 10.1016/j.yexmp.2008.03.007

[48] Salvador E, Wagenlehner F, Köhler C-D, Mellmann A, Hacker J, Svanborg C, et al. Comparison of asymptomatic bacteriuria *Escherichia coli* isolates from healthy individuals versus those from hospital patients shows that long-term bladder colonization selects for attenuated virulence phenotypes. Infection and Immunity. 2012;**80**:668-678. DOI: 10.1128/IAI.06191-11

[49] Zdziarski J, Brzuszkiewicz E, Wullt B, Liesegang H, Biran D, Voigt B, et al. Host imprints on bacterial genomes—Rapid, divergent evolution in individual patients. PLoS pathogens. 2010;**6**(8):e1001078). DOI: 10.1371/journal.ppat.1001078

[50] Kot B. Virulence factors and innovative strategies for the treatment and control of uropathogenic *Escherichia coli*. In: Samie A. *Escherichia coli*-Recent Advances on Physiology, Pathogenesis and Biotechnological Applications. 1st ed. InTech, Rijeka, Croatia; 2017. DOI: 10.5772/67778

[51] Torres AG. *Escherichia coli* in the Americas. 1st ed. Springer, Switzerland; 2016. DOI: 10.1007/978-3-319-45092-6

[52] Subashchandrabose S, Mobley HLT. Virulence and fitness determinants of uropathogenic *Escherichia coli*. Microbiology spectrum. 2015;**3**:10.1128/microbiolspec.UTI-0015-2012. DOI: 10.1128/microbiolspec.UTI-0015-2012

[53] Klemm P, Hancock V, Schembri MA. Fimbrial adhesins from extraintestinal *Escherichia coli*. Environmental Microbiology Reports. 2010;**2**:628-640. DOI: 10.1111/j.1758-2229.2010.00166.x

[54] Quainoo S, Coolen JP, van Hijum SA, Huynen MA, Melchers WJ, van Schaik W, et al. Whole-genome sequencing of bacterial pathogens: The future of nosocomial outbreak analysis. Clinical Microbiology Reviews 2017;**30**:1015-1063. DOI: 10.1128/CMR.00016-17

[55] Virulence Factors of Pathogenic Bacteria: MOH Key Laboratory of Systems Biology of Pathogens, Institute of Pathogen Biology, CAMS&PUMC, Bejing, China; [Internet]. 2017. Available from: http://www.mgc.ac.cn/cgi-bin/VFs/genus.cgi?Genus=Escherichia [Accessed: 2017-08-23]

[56] Ong C-LY, Ulett GC, Mabbett AN, Beatson SA, Webb RI, Monaghan W, et al. Identification of type 3 fimbriae in uropathogenic *Escherichia coli* reveals a role in biofilm formation. Journal of Bacteriology. 2008;**190**:1054-1063. DOI: 10.1128/JB.01523-07

[57] Cordeiro MA, Werle CH, Milanez GP, Yano T. Curli fimbria: An *Escherichia coli* adhesin associated with human cystitis. Brazilian Journal of Microbiology. 2016;**47**:414-416. DOI: 10.1016/j.bjm.2016.01.024

[58] Klemm P, Schembri M. Type 1 fimbriae, Curli, and antigen 43: Adhesion, colonization, and biofilm formation. EcoSal Plus. 2004;**1**. DOI: 10.1128/ecosalplus.8.3.2.6

[59] Ulett GC, Mabbett AN, Fung KC, Webb RI, Schembri MA. The role of F9 fimbriae of uropathogenic *Escherichia coli* in biofilm formation. Microbiology. 2007;**153**:2321-2331. DOI: 10.1099/mic.0.2006/004648-0

[60] Wurpel DJ, Totsika M, Allsopp LP, Hartley-Tassell LE, Day CJ, Peters KM, et al. F9 fimbriae of uropathogenic *Escherichia coli* are expressed at low temperature and recognise Galβ1-3GlcNAc-containing glycans. PLoS One. 2014;**9**:e93177. DOI: 10.1371/journal.pone.0093177

[61] Emo L, Kerenyi M, Nagy G. Virulence factors of uropathogenic *Escherichia coli*. International Journal of Antimicrobial Agents. 2003;**22**:29-33. DOI: 10.1016/S0924-8579(03)00236-X

[62] Spurbeck RR, Stapleton AE, Johnson JR, Walk ST, Hooton TM, Mobley HL. Fimbrial profiles predict virulence of uropathogenic *Escherichia coli* strains: Contribution of ygi and yad fimbriae. Infection and immunity. 2011;**79**:4753-4763. DOI: 10.1128/IAI.05621-11

[63] Profiling of *Escherichia coli* chromosome (PEC) database; Japan: National Institute of Genetics. 1998-2016 ed. Availabl from: https://shigen.nig.ac.jp/ecoli/pec/ [Accessed: 2017-08-23]

[64] Fernández-Romero N, Romero-Gómez MP, Mora-Rillo M, Rodríguez-Baño J, López-Cerero L, Pascual Á, et al. Uncoupling between core genome and virulome in extraintestinal pathogenic *Escherichia coli*. Canadian Journal of Microbiology. 2015;**61**:647-652. DOI: 10.1139/cjm-2014-0835

[65] Behzadi P, Behzadi E. Environmental Microbiology. 1st ed. Tehran: Niktab Publisher; 2007

[66] Wurpel DJ, Beatson SA, Totsika M, Petty NK, Schembri MA. Chaperone-usher fimbriae of *Escherichia coli*. PLoS One. 2013;**8**:e52835. DOI: 10.1371/journal.pone.0052835

[67] Chapman MR, Robinson LS, Pinkner JS, Roth R, Heuser J, Hammar M, et al. Role of *Escherichia coli* curli operons in directing amyloid fiber formation. Science. 2002;**295**:851-855. DOI: 10.1126/science.1067484

[68] Van Houdt R, Michiels CW. Role of bacterial cell surface structures in *Escherichia coli* biofilm formation. Research in Microbiology. 2005;**156**:626-633. DOI: 10.1016/j.resmic.2005.02.005

[69] Barnhart MM, Chapman MR. Curli biogenesis and function. Annual Review of Microbiology. 2006;**60**:131-147. DOI: 10.1146/annurev.micro.60.080805.142106

[70] Van Loy CP, Sokurenko EV, Moseley SL. The major structural subunits of Dr and F1845 fimbriae are adhesins. Infection and Immunity. 2002;**70**:1694-1702. DOI: 10.1128/IAI.70.4.1694-1702.2002

[71] Baby S, Karnaker VK, Geetha R. Adhesins of Uropathogenic *Escherichia coli* (UPEC). Int J Med Microbiol Trop Dis. 2016;**2**:10-18

[72] Stubenrauch C, Belousoff MJ, Hay ID, Shen H-H, Lillington J, Tuck KL, et al. Effective assembly of fimbriae in *Escherichia coli* depends on the translocation assembly module nanomachine. Natural Microbiology. 2016;**1**:16064. DOI: 10.1038/nmicrobiol.2016.64

[73] Waksman G, Hultgren SJ. Structural biology of the chaperone–usher pathway of pilus biogenesis. Nature Reviews. Microbiology. 2009;**7**:765. DOI: 10.1038/nrmicro2220

[74] Nuccio S-P, Bäumler AJ. Evolution of the chaperone/usher assembly pathway: Fimbrial classification goes Greek. Microbiology and Molecular Biology Reviews. 2007;**71**: 551-575. DOI: 10.1128/MMBR.00014-07

[75] Busch A, Waksman G. Chaperone–usher pathways: Diversity and pilus assembly mechanism. Philosophical Transactions of Royal Society B. 2012;**367**:1112-1122. DOI: 10.1098/rstb.2011.0206

[76] Matuszewski MA, Tupikowski K, Dołowy Ł, Szymańska B, Dembowski J, Zdrojowy R. Uroplakins and their potential applications in urology. Central European Journal of Urology. 2016;**69**:252. DOI: 10.5173/ceju.2016.638

[77] Bien J, Sokolova O, Bozko P. Role of uropathogenic *Escherichia Coli* virulence factors in development of urinary tract infection and kidney damage. International Journla of Nephrology. 2012;**2012**:1-15. DOI: 10.1155/2012/681473

[78] Khan AS, Kniep B, Oelschlaeger TA, Van Die I, Korhonen T, Hacker J. Receptor structure for F1C fimbriae of uropathogenic *Escherichia coli*. Infection and Immunity. 2000;**68**:3541-3547. DOI: 10.1128/IAI.68.6.3541-3547.2000

[79] Ejrnæs K. Bacterial characteristics of importance for recurrent urinary tract infections caused by *Escherichia coli*. Dan Med Bull. 2011;**58**:B4187

[80] Ranjbar R, Bolandian M, Behzadi P. Virulotyping of *Shigella* spp. isolated from pediatric patients in Tehran, Iran. Acta Microbiologica et Immunologica Hungarica. 2017;**64**:71-80. DOI: 10.1556/030.64.2017.007

[81] Ranjbar R, Tabatabaee A, Behzadi P, Kheiri R. Enterobacterial repetitive intergenic consensus polymerase chain reaction (ERIC-PCR) genotyping of *Escherichia coli* strains isolated from different animal stool specimens. Iranian Journal of Pathology. 2017;**12**:25-34

[82] Behzadi E, Behzadi P, Sirmatel F. Identification of 30-kDa heat shock protein gene in *Trichophyton rubrum*. Mycoses. 2009;**52**:234-238. DOI: 10.1111/j.1439-0507.2008.01561.x

[83] Munkhdelger Y, Gunregjav N, Dorjpurev A, Juniichiro N, Sarantuya J. Detection of virulence genes, phylogenetic group and antibiotic resistance of uropathogenic *Escherichia coli* in Mongolia. Journal of Infection in Developing Countries. 2017;**11**:51-57. DOI: 10.3855/jidc.7903

[84] Ebadi M, Askari N, Jajarmi M, Ghanbarpour R. Detection of fimbrial genes, antibiotic resistance profile and phylogenetic background of uropathogenic *E. coli* isolated from clinical samples in Karaj City, Iranian Journal of Medical Bacteriology. 2017;**6**:15-20

[85] Paniagua-Contreras GL, Hernández-Jaimes T, Monroy-Pérez E, Vaca-Paniagua F, Díaz-Velásquez C, Uribe-García A, et al. Comprehensive expression analysis of pathogenicity genes in uropathogenic *Escherichia coli* strains. Microbial Pathogenesis. 2017;**103**:1-7. DOI: 10.1016/j.micpath.2016.12.008

[86] Yun KW, Kim HY, Park HK, Kim W, Lim IS. Virulence factors of uropathogenic *Escherichia coli* of urinary tract infections and asymptomatic bacteriuria in children. Journal of Microbiology, Immunology, and Infection. 2014;**47**:455-461. DOI: 10.1016/j.jmii.2013.07.010

[87] Behzadi P, Behzadi E, Ranjbar R. IL-12 family cytokines: General characteristics, pathogenic microorganisms, receptors, and signalling pathways. Acta Microbiologica et Immunologica Hungarica. 2016;**63**:1-25. DOI: 10.1556/030.63.2016.1.1

[88] Behzadi P, Behzadi E, Ranjbar R. Microarray probe set: Biology, bioinformatics and biophysics. Albanian Medical Journal. 2015;**2**:78-83

[89] Behzadi P, Ranjbar R. Microarray long oligo probe designing for Bacteria: An in silico pangenomic research. Albanian Medical Journal. 2016;**2**:5-11

[90] Ranjbar R, Behzadi P, Mammina C. Respiratory tularemia: *Francisella tularensis* and microarray probe designing. The Open Microbiology Journal. 2016;**10**:176-182. DOI: 10.2174/1874285801610010176

[91] Behzadi P, Ranjbar R, Alavian SM. Nucleic acid-based approaches for detection of viral hepatitis. Jundishapur Journal of Microbiol. 2015;**8**:e17449. DOI: 10.5812/jjm.17449

[92] Behzadi P, Behzadi E, Alavian SM. DNA microarray technology in HBV genotyping. Minerva Medica. 2017;**108**:473-476. DOI: 10.23736/S0026-4806.17.05059-5

[93] Ranjbar R, Behzadi P, Farshad S. Advances in diagnosis and treatment of *Helicobacter pylori* infection. Acta Microbiologica et Immunologica Hungarica. 2017;**64**:273-292. DOI: 10.1556/030.64.2017.008

10

Urinary Tract Infection in Renal Allograft Recipients

Lovelesh Kumar Nigam, Aruna V. Vanikar, Rashmi D. Patel, Kamal V. Kanodia and Kamlesh S. Suthar

Abstract

Renal replacement therapy in the form of renal transplantation (RT) is the treatment of choice in these patients. Various factors influence the graft survival, infections being most common. Infections account for 16% of patient deaths and 7.7% of death censored graft failure in renal transplant patients. Urinary tract infection (UTI) is the most common infectious complication accounting for 45–72% of all infections. According to few studies UTI may have a negative impact over the long term survival of renal allograft. There are multiple factors that predispose these patients to UTI. Elderly age group, female gender, increased duration of catheterization and anatomical abnormalities of the urinary tract are most common predisposing factors. E. coli is the most frequently isolated organisms from the urine of these patients. We would proceed further with two cases which presented as UTI in post-transplant period. The first patient transplanted (living donor related) for diabetes induced end stage renal disease had developed UTI 4 years post-transplant. The other patient underwent deceased donor renal transplant for adult polycystic disease related chronic kidney disease, presented 2 years post-transplant with UTI.

Keywords: renal transplantation, urinary tract infection, renal allograft, graft function, immunosuppression

1. Introduction

Clinical information (Case 1): A 53-year-old male patient, with a history of arterial hypertension, type 2 diabetes mellitus, and renal failure, caused by diabetic nephropathy diagnosed 5 years back and was on maintenance hemodialysis. The patient underwent live donor renal transplantation in June 2013. The intraoperative and post-operative period was unremarkable and he was put on Tacrolimus based immunosuppression thereafter consisting of Prednisone (20 mg/day), Mycophenolate sodium (360 mg/day), and Tacrolimus (1.5 mg/day level:4.6 ng/ml). He was on regular follow-up for routine urine examination, serum creatinine and serum electrolytes and hemogram. Nearly 4 years post-transplant he was admitted with complaints of low grade intermittent febrile episodes and painful micturition. There was slight rise in the serum creatinine levels to 2.4 mg/dL (baseline: 1.8 mg/dL). The urine output was however normal. Complete blood count performed revealed neutrophilic leukocytosis with total count of $14.2 \times 10^{6}/\mu l$, with predominance of neutrophils on differential, the absolute neutrophil count of $14 \times 10^{6}/\mu l$. Urine examination revealed urine albumin of +1 by dipstick method, pH of 5.0 and specific gravity of 1.020. **Clinical information (Case 2):** A 38-year-old female patient, underwent deceased donor renal transplantation for adult polycystic kidney disease induced chronic kidney disease. The intraoperative and post-operative period was unremarkable and she was on conventional Tacrolimus based immunosuppression thereafter consisting of Prednisone (20 mg/day), Mycophenolate sodium (360 mg/day), and Tacrolimus (1.5 mg/day; level:6.8 ng/dL). She was on regular monitoring for routine urine examination, renal function tests and complete blood counts. Nearly 2 years post-transplant she was admitted with complaints of intermittent high grade febrile episodes, pain in abdomen and nausea. The serum creatinine level at the time of presentation was found to be raised to 3.6 mg/dL (baseline: 1.2 mg/dL). The patient had normal urine output. Complete blood count performed revealed neutrophilic leukocytosis with total count of $18.6 \times 10^{6}/\mu l$, with predominance of neutrophils on differential, the absolute neutrophil count of $12 \times 10^{6}/\mu l$. Urine examination revealed urine albumin of +2 by dipstick method, pH of 4.6 and specific gravity of 1.040. **Summary**: So here we have two patients who underwent renal transplant for end stage renal disease and presented with signs and symptoms of urinary tract infection. Both the patients presented with rise in serum creatinine as well as pyuria on urine examination(not written in the text above)clinical suspicion of urinary tract infection. We would in further sections study how we proceeded with both the cases, investigations performed and management of both. In this brief review we would discuss the incidence of urinary tract infection in post-transplant patients, risk factors and how to manage a case with UTI.

1.1. Incidence of posttransplant urinary tract infections

Transplantation has become the gold standard treatment of end-stage disease in the present era. Of all the organs that are transplanted, kidneys remain the most frequently transplanted organ [1–5]. RT is regarded as an effective treatment for patients with advanced chronic renal disease [1–2]. Over the years various studies have been carried out globally to understand the factors that influence the graft function [1]. Multiple factors including technical expertise, donor-recipients related demographics, immunosuppressive regimens, infections, comorbid conditions have been implicated to influence the graft survival [1–3]. Infections are a common cause of morbidity and mortality after transplantation and it is widely known that RT patients have poor resistance to infection [4, 5]. Infections have been ranked second, as a cause of death in RT patients. According to the U.S. Renal Data System, the rate of first infection in the initial 3 years after kidney transplantation is reported to be 45.0 per 100 patient-years of follow-up. It has been postulated that in immunocompromised RT recipients, UTI is the most common infection that affects the graft function and is held responsible for longer hospital stay and increased health care cost [3, 6, 7]. Becerra et al. stated that the length of stay in patients who develop UTI is 74 and 76% higher in men and women renal transplant recipients respectively, when compared to those without UTI [8].

1.2. Burden of the disease

UTI is the most common type of hospital-acquired infection, accounting for nearly 40–50% of all infectious complications among RT patients followed by viral infections, pneumonia and surgical site infections [8, 9]. As per the data from Spanish Network for the Study of Infections in Transplantation (RESITRA) the incidence of cystitis per 100 recipient-years was 13.84 for renal, 3.09 for liver, 2.41 for heart and 1.36 for lung transplant recipients [10]. The incidence of pyelonephritis per 100 recipient-years was 3.66 for renal, 0.8 for liver, 0.3 for heart and 0.6 for lung transplant recipients. UTI-associated bacteremia was seen in 39% of renal, 3% of liver, 3% of heart and none of the lung transplant recipients [11, 12]. The prevalence of UTI in RT patients ranges from 13 to 80% according to various studies [1, 2, 6, 13–16]. Few authors have also reported an incidence as low as 4% to as high as 75% [17–20]. The vast difference could however be attributed largely due to lack of uniform diagnostic criteria to define UTI, implementation of prophylactic regimen and ill-defined period of follow-up. The incidence of UTI in the early post-transplant period (first 6 months) is higher as compared to late periods. However it is this early occurrence of UTI that has a profound effect over the allograft survival. Nearly 84% of symptomatic UTI cases are recorded in the first 6 months after transplant [21].

Recurrent UTI is also one of the major cause that poses threat to renal allograft and the prevalence ranges from 2.9 to 27% in renal transplant recipients. Mohammad et al. reported an incidence of recurrent UTI in nearly 51.7% patients who underwent renal transplantation [22].

1.3. Definition and diagnostic criteria for UTI

A urinary tract infection is an infection causing signs and symptoms of cystitis or pyelonephritis (including the presence of signs of systemic inflammation), which is documented to be caused by an infectious agent. The diagnostic criteria for UTI are similar to those that are used for general population, however all symptomatic UTI are considered as complicated UTI in RT patients [23–25].

Pain and tenderness over the renal allograft or costovertebral region indicates symptomatic infection of the upper urinary tract.

Asymptomatic bacteriuria in women is defined as two consecutive clean-catch voided urine specimens >24 hours apart with isolation of the same organism in quantitative counts of $\geq 10^5$ CFU/mL. However in males a single clean catch urine specimen with isolation of single organism in quantitative counts of $\geq 10^5$ CFU/mL is regarded as asymptomatic bacteriuria. In case of urethral catheterization bacteriuria is defined as isolation of a single organism in quantitative counts of $\geq 10^2$ CFU/mL in a single specimen.

2. Risk factors associated with development of UTI in renal transplant recipients

Post-transplant UTI in renal allograft recipients is of multifactorial origin and is determined by interaction between host factors, abnormalities associated with the anatomy of the uri nary tract and the virulence of the pathogenic organisms. A few common extensively studied factors are listed below. Few studies have found strong correlation of increased predilection to development of UTI, whereas other researchers have not been able to prove the association.

2.1. Gender

Most of the studies show that incidence of UTI is more common in females as compared to male patients who undergo renal transplantation [12]. The mean distance from the urethra to anus is less in females as compared to males, which leads to increased susceptibility for vaginal colonization with uropathogens [14, 26]. Menegueti et al. reported female sex as the only risk factor for post-transplant UTI [27]. Camargo et al. also reported a higher incidence of UTI in female patients [44.4%], despite higher prevalence of male patients in the study. However few studies do report a higher incidence of UTI in males. This could be due to the larger number of male patients receiving transplant in majority of the cohorts [8]. It is well documented that women with recurrent UTI have increased susceptibility to vaginal colonization with uropathogens. Sexual intercourse, using spermicidal products, maternal history of UTI and UTI at an early age predispose these patients to recurrent infections of the urogenital tract [1].

2.2. Catheterization and presence of ureteral stent

It has been observed that increased hospital stay and late removal of the catheter is an independent risk factor for developing UTI [1]. Ostaszewaska et al. reported a strong correlation between occurrence of UTI and length of hospital stay [28]. Stamm et al. reported that the risk of UTI in renal allograft recipients is more by approximately 5% with each day of bladder catheterization [29]. Dantass et al. also had similar observations [30]. Fayek et al. report a higher rate of UTI of 14.2% in transplant recipients with stents as compared to 7.9% without stent [31].

2.3. Anatomical abnormalities

Structural abnormalities of native or transplanted kidney predisposes to increased risk of developing UTI [1, 2]. The anatomical abnormalities could be vesicoureteral reflux, neurogenic bladder or presence of benign prostatic hyperplasia, are usually associated to increased risk for developing UTI [14, 28, 29].

2.4. Immunosuppressants

A wide variety of immunosuppressants are used in transplant medicine either as induction agents or for maintenance therapy. Recipients subjected to antimetabolite (azathioprine or mycophenolate mofetil) and induction therapy with cell depleting antibodies (antithymocyte globulin) are reported to have higher incidence of UTI [1, 32–34]. Prednisone dose of >20 mg/day and multiple rejection therapies are associated with increased risk [35].

2.5. Deceased versus living donor transplants

It has been documented by various studies that the incidence of UTI is more in patients who receive kidney from deceased donor as compared to living donor. Taminato et al., reported that there is a greater risk for the patients who receive organ from deceased donor as against recipients of living donor with an odds ratio of 2.65 [36]. Similar observations were reported by Ostaszewaska et al., R.Parasuraman et al., Camargo et al., Orhan Deniz Kara et al. and Abdulmalik MA et al. [2, 26, 28, 37, 38].

2.6. Human leucocyte antigen (HLA) match and rejection episodes

HLA compatibility and association with UTI was studied by Ostaszewaska et al. They observed that individuals with more than four HLA mismatches are more likely to develop UTI [28]. Patients who develop rejection episodes show increased incidence of UTI. These individuals are subjected to increased dosages of immunosuppression which may likely predispose these individuals to increased risk of developing UTI [9]. Moradi et al. evaluated the relationship between UTI and biopsy proven chronic rejection in a cohort of 100 patients over a period of 5 years. They concluded that patients with chronic rejection had more episodes of UTI as compared to those without rejection [39].

2.7. Other proposed factors

Apart from the important factors listed above, various other factors have been implicated in developing UTI. Older age has been related to an increased risk for UTI. The same study reported that an increase of 5 years in age at transplant increased the risk for UTI. Benign prostatic hyperplasia and menopause, was an additional risk factor for developing UTI [26, 37, 38]. Delayed graft function (DGF), usually associated with deceased donor organ transplant has been documented as a risk factor for development of UTI [9]. Study reported that occurrence of DGF strongly correlates with the incidence of UTI, with 61.8% patients with UTI developing delayed graft function [28]. Other factors that have been implicated are presence of comorbid conditions like hypertension and diabetes, prolonged cold ischemia time, serum creatinine levels of >2 mg/dL and chronic viral infections [6, 14, 26–28, 35, 37, 39].

3. Etiology of UTI in renal transplant patients

3.1. Etiological agents

The most common type of UTI is bacterial followed by fungi and rarely viruses are implicated in pathogenesis of UTI. Gram negative bacteria are the most common pathogens cultured from the urine of renal transplant patients with UTI, followed by candida and viruses.

3.2. Bacteria

E. coli is the most common, accounting for more than 70% of the cases. Enterobacteriaceae, *Enterococci*, *Pseudomonas* and coagulase-negative *staphylococci* are other common agents. Mycobacterium tuberculosis, Salmonella and Mycoplasma are encountered rarely [2, 6, 38, 41, 42]. A retrospective study by Espinar MJ et al., showed that renal allograft recipients are particularly susceptible to infection by Enterobacteriaceae-producing extended-spectrum β-lactamases (ESBLs). Diabetes mellitus, previous antibiotic prophylaxis or therapy, previous UTI, relapsing infection and patients with delayed graft function after transplant represented risk factors for infection by ESBL positive Enterobacteriaceae. It was also observed that these patients present early with UTI and exhibit higher resistance to fluoroquinolones, trimethoprim-sulfamethoxazole and gentamicin. Pourmand MR et al. and Tawab et al. studied renal transplant recipients who developed recurrent UTI. *E. coli* was the most common cultured organism from the urine of patients with recurrent UTI. Coagulase negative staphylococci and Bacillus were rare [2, 9, 22].

3.3. Fungus

Candida is the most common cause for UTI in renal transplant recipients and is usually asymptomatic. Serious complications can occur following ascending infections. Fungal balls can be formed that may cause obstruction at the ureterovesical junction [2, 3, 43].

3.4. Viruses

The most common viruses that cause viral UTI in a renal transplant patient are cytomegalovirus and type 1 human polyomavirus (BKV). Clinically they present with fever, acute graft rejection, tubulointerstitial nephropathy and renal vascular disease. BKV-associated nephropathy may be a frequent cause of recurrent post-transplant infections and these patients usually present as sterile pyuria, eosinophiluria and hematuria. Ureteral cell hyperplasia leading to ureteral obstruction has also been reported [2, 3, 40–43].

3.5. *Schistosoma haematobium*

Trematode involves the urinary tract and kidney, and the diagnosis is based on the visualization of parasite ova in urine specimens. The urine should be collected close to noon, when egg excretion is maximal. Reactivation of a prior infection due to immunosuppression has been described in solid organ transplant recipients. Any solid organ transplant recipient from an endemic at risk-area developing hematuria (with or without eosinophilia) should have urine examined to rule out the infection. *S. haematobium* should be treated with praziquantel both in the pre and post-transplant period, as chronic infection can lead to squamous cell carcinoma of the bladder [44].

3.5.1. Causative organisms and identification of the organisms in our cases

Case 1:*The microscopic examination of the urine sediment revealed plenty of pus cells with occasional red blood cells and bacilli. (***Figure 1***). Urine culture study was performed. On nutrient agar large, circular, low convex, grayish, white, moist, smooth and opaque colonies were observed. On MacConkey Agar media the colonies were circular, moist, smooth, and pink and found to be lactose fermenting. (***Figure 1a***) On Gram's stain, pink gram negative rods were identified. (***Figure 1b***) The sample was further subjected to VITEK 2 system for identification and culture sensitivity. Escherichia coli was identified as the causative organism with sensitivity to Piperacillin/ Tazobactum, Sulbactum, Imipenem, Meropenem, Amikacin, Colistin, Levofloxacin and Minocycline. However resistance to Trimetoprim/ Sulfamethoxazole, Gentamycin and Cefepime was observed.*

The patient was treated with intravenous administration of Cefoparazone-salbactam and Levofloxacin for 7 days. Urine routine and culture sensitivity studies were performed on sixth day. There was reduction in the total leucocyte count to 8.4 × $10^6/\mu l$, with normal differential count. The serum creatinine level dropped from 2.4 to 1.8 mg/dL on seventh day. Urine routine microscopic examination revealed

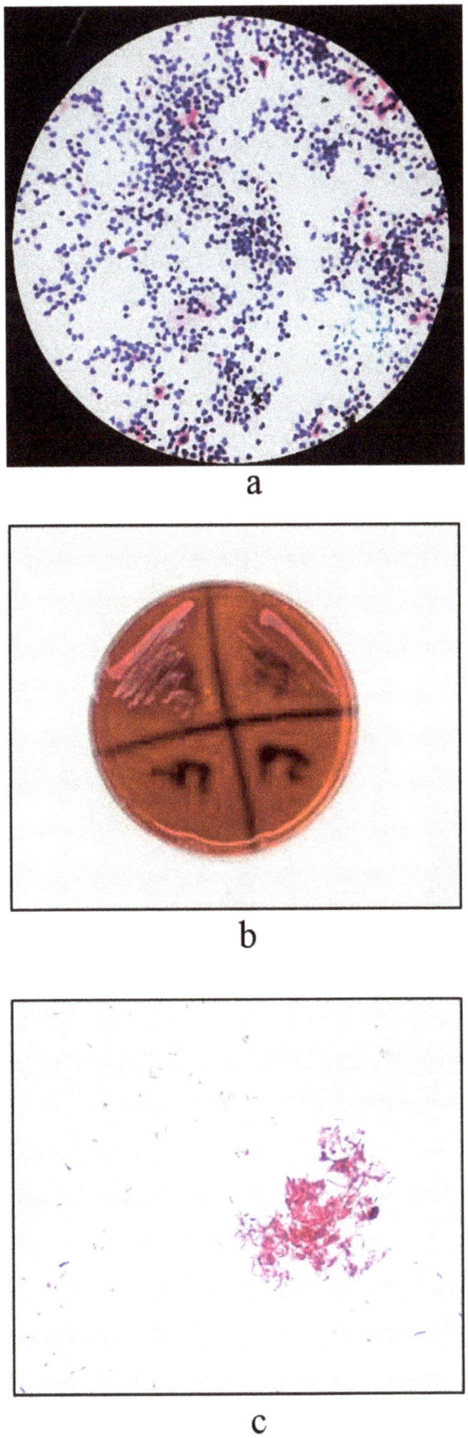

Figure 1. Urine microscopy stained with hematoxylin and eosin stain shows plenty of leucocytes and few bacilli. (Hematoxylin and eosin, x 400). (a) MacConkey agar media with circular, moist, smooth, and lactose fermenting pink colonies. The left upper quadrant is the patient sample and right upper quadrant depicts the positive control. (b) Gram's stain, these bacilli appeared to be as pink gram negative rods (Gram's stain, x 400).

scattered 15–20 WBC/ hpf. The patient was shifted to oral antibiotics for next 3 days. The immunosuppression regimen constituted of Tacrolimus, Prednisone and Mycophenolate sodium. No tapering of the drugs was done. Urine examination and culture studies were negative thereafter. The patient responded well to the treatment and is on regular follow-up. His present serum creatinine is 1.8 mg/dL, 4 months *after the episode of urinary tract infection.**Case 2:**The microscopic examination of the urine sediment revealed clusters of pus cells, scattered epithelial cells and fungal buds and pseudohyphae. (***Figure 2***) Urine culture study was performed on Sabouraud's dextrose agar. 65 g of the media was suspended in distilled water, mixed to form a uniform suspension, heated, boiled and then sterilized at 118–121°C for 15 min. The urine sample was streaked using inoculating loop and incubated in 37°C for 48 hours. The growth appeared in 48 hours as cream/white colored, smooth and pasty colonies. (***Figure 2a***). A drop of inoculated broth media was placed onto the slide and a drop of lactophenol cotton blue stain was added and examined under the microscope which revealed the presence of chlamydospores. (***Figure 2b***).*

The patient was treated with oral antifungal agent, fluconazole, 100 mg/day for 21 days along with conventional Tacrolimus-based immunosuppressive regimen. Urine routine and culture sensitivity studies were performed on tenth day. There was reduction in the total leucocyte count to 6.35 x 10 ^{6}/µl, with normal differential count. The serum creatinine level dropped to 1.6 mg/dL. Urine examination and culture studies were negative thereafter. The patient responded well to the treatment and is on regular follow-up. Her present serum creatinine is 1.76 mg/dL, 4 months after the episode of urinary tract infection.

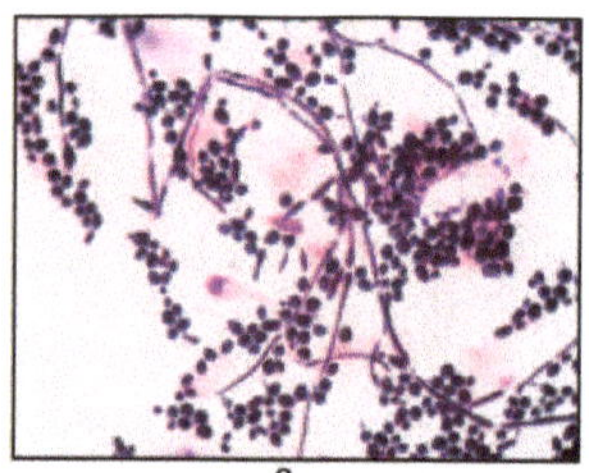

a

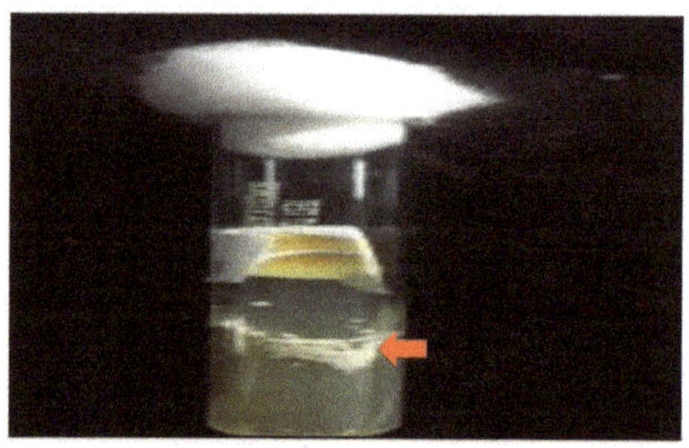

b

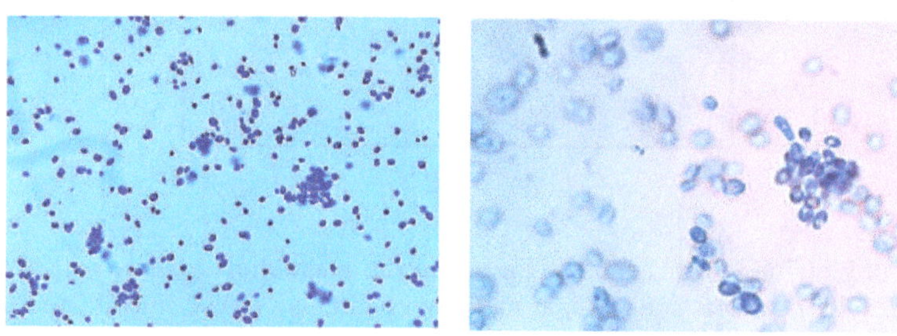

LCB, X 400 LCB, X 1000

c

Figure 2. Hematoxylin and eosin stained urine deposit reveals budding fungi along with pseudohyphae. (a) Creamy and smooth colonies of candida on Sabouraud's dextrose agar (red arrow). (b) Lactophenol cotton blue (wet preparation) reveals budding fungi (LCB, X 400)with chlamydospores (LCB, X 1000).

4. UTI and effect on renal allograft function

4.1. Negative impact of urinary tract infections in renal transplant recipients

It has been well documented that development of UTI in renal transplant recipients is associated with increased rates of health resource utilization, which includes length of stay as well as more economic burden. Longer hospital stay exposes these individuals to increased risk of development of nosocomial infection [2, 8].

4.2. Effect on graft function

Mohan et al., in their prospective study of 31 patients who underwent renal transplantation, found that infections in the immediate post-transplant period adversely affected the graft survival. Mortality rate in patients with UTI was reported as 12.9% [9].

Abbott and colleagues undertook a retrospective cohort study of 28,942 Medicare primary renal transplant recipients in the U.S. Renal Data System database from 1996 through 2000, assessing Medicare claims for UTI occurring later than 6 months after transplantation based on ICD-9 codes, and found that the cumulative incidence of UTI during the first 6 months after renal transplantation was 17% (equivalent for both men and women) and at 3 years was 60% for women and 47% for men ($P < 0.001$ in Cox regression analysis). Late UTI was significantly associated with an increased risk of subsequent death and graft loss [45].

In a study by Dhamidharka et al., who analyzed US Renal Data System database over the period of 1996 to 2000 (up to 36 months post-transplant). 265 (30.5%) pediatric patients had either inpatient or outpatient claims for UTI out of total 870 pediatric patients who qualified for the study. The authors found that early UTI (less than 6 months after transplant) was significantly [$P = 0.007$ upon multivariable Cox regression] associated with higher adjusted hazard ratio of graft loss, and late UTI was not associated with such an outcome. Risk for post-transplantation death was not increased significantly after either early UTI (AHR 1.23; 95% CI 0.37 to 4.08) or late UTI (relative risk 2.22; 95% CI 0.90 to 5.44) [46].

Pelle, et al. as well as Giral et al. reported that acute pyelonephritis of the graft is accompanied by renal failure and is an independent risk factor for impaired renal function as well as graft loss [47, 48]. Bodro et al. reported 1-year mortality rate of 3% in patients who developed worsening of graft function secondary to graft acute pyelonephritis. They further discovered that in patients with UTI due to a resistant strain of bacteria, the impairment of graft function is more frequent than in patients who develop UTI due to non-resistant strain bacteria [13]. Several hypotheses have been put forward to explain the negative impact of UTI on graft function. It has been postulated that bacterial infection activated the immune system, which can trigger the rejection cascades leading to acute or chronic rejections, causing deterioration of the graft function. Some authors propose that inflammation secondary to infection can cause scarring of the renal tissue, leading to loss of the functioning nephron mass causing impairment of renal function [49–51]. Reduction in the immunosuppressive agents following an episode of infection may accentuate the rejection process [13].

Various studies like the one by Ostaszewska et al., have found out no significant difference related to UTI and graft survival [28]. Fiorante et al. also in their study of 189 renal allograft recipients, over a follow-up of 36 months, did not find an association between asymptomatic and symptomatic bacteriuria with graft dysfunction. They also did not report statistically significant association between graft dysfunction and acute pyelonephritis of the graft [42]. Similarly, Ariza et al. and Lee et al. did not report any significant graft survival and UTI [52].

5. Management of UTI

Definitive diagnostic and treatment protocols for renal transplant patients are not well-defined. The current treatment protocols depend mainly on the severity of the infection, the local epidemiological data and the results of the culture reports. Complete urinalysis with microscopy along with culture studies is recommended. It has been proposed that bactericidal antibiotics should be preferred to bacteriostatic ones, which might be insufficient to cure the infection since the immune system cannot eradicate the dormant bacteria. Managing the predisposing factors is equally essential. The need for adequate immunosuppression and dose adjustment is also important. Various pharmacological interactions exist between antibiotics used to treat post-transplant UTI and immunosuppressant drugs. Ciprofloxacin and erythromycin are implicated in raising Calcineurin inhibitor (CNI) levels. Levofloxacin and ofloxacin usually do not interfere with CNI levels. Antifungal agents inhibit cytochrome P450 and increase CNI levels. Rifampin, imipenem and cephalosporin can reduce CNI levels. Nephrotoxic antibiotics (e.g., aminoglycosides, amphotericin) may have synergistic effects with CNIs, increasing renal damage.

UTI can co-exist with CMV, BKV and other viral and fungal diseases.

5.1. Management of asymptomatic bacteriuria

No definitive consensus or management is available for treatment of asymptomatic bacteriuria. However many of the researchers agree that there is no need to subject patients with asymptomatic bacteriuria to antibiotics as there are not enough studies that prove that asymptomatic bacteriuria heralds a negative outcome. Also studies have shown that treatment of this entity does not prevent occurrence of significant bacteriuria in the later post-transplant period [39]. Few studies have demonstrated that use of antimicrobials in patients with asymptomatic bacteriuria is usually unsuccessful in removing the offending agent; also it does not prevent the occurrence of subsequent UTI [53]. Study by Goya et al. proposed that considering asymptomatic bacteriuria as a precursor for symptomatic bacteriuria and subsequent development of pyelonephritis and high risk of developing symptomatic UTI in early transplant period that may affect the graft function it is recommended to keep patients with asymptomatic bacteriuria under screening schedules. Treatment with narrow-spectrum antibiotics of short duration of 5–7 days following culture report is recommended [54].

5.2. Symptomatic UTI

Symptomatic bacteriuria is classified further as mild, moderate and severe. Any predisposing conditions have to be treated. For mild cases empirical therapy with oral antibiotics, preferably ciprofloxacin with or without amoxicillin for a period of 5–7 days is recommended. For moderate infections, treatment with ciprofloxacin or ceftriaxone or ampicillin-salbactum is advised for 14 days after the culture sensitivity reports are obtained. For severe symptomatic UTI empirical treatment with pipercillin-tazobactum or cefepime is recommended over a period of 14–21 days following culture sensitivity report. Multi-drug resistant organisms need to be kept in mind before starting the empirical therapy. Carbapenem is the drug of choice for such cases. For recurrent UTI the treatment is extended to 6 weeks.

5.3. Candiduria

In patients with asymptomatic candiduria, there is no recommended treatment. In cases of symptomatic candiduria fluconazole, 200–400 mg, orally per day for 14 days is the treatment of choice. Fluconazole may have drug interactions with Calcineurin inhibitor, hence dose adjustment is recommended. Disseminated cases would require treatment by intravenous amphotericin B, 0.3–1 mg/kg/day for 1–7 days. Flucytosine [25 mg/kg every 6 h for 7–10 days] can also be used, but with caution, especially in cases of renal dysfunction. Monitoring for cytopenias, rash, gastrointestinal symptoms and hepatotoxicity is recommended [55, 56].

6. Prevention

Although the data from various studies does not provide a concrete evidence for post-transplant UTI to have a profound effect on graft dysfunction, but overall it is necessary to control infection related mortality. It is quite obvious from certain studies that UTI or any infection leads to increase in duration of stay at hospital as well as it adds to economic burden as discussed in this review. Infection of any sort can have a psychological effect on the transplant recipient too. With advent of wide range of antimicrobials available as well as vast advancement in the field of transplantation medicine, losing graft function to infections should not be acceptable. Hence it is important to identify the various risk factors and employ strategies to prevent the development of infections in these subset of patients. Individuals with high risk factors like those having structural anomalies of the urinary tract, old age patients, females, presence of comorbid conditions like diabetes, hypertension should be kept under proper surveillance. In case of living donors a thorough screening for infections before transplantation though serological tests, urine analysis and hematology is advisable to rule out possibility of any infections.

Certain studies have emphasized the role of antimicrobial prophylaxis with trimethoprim-sulfamethoxazole (TMP-SMZ) for prevention of UTI. TMP-SMZ is a broad spectrum

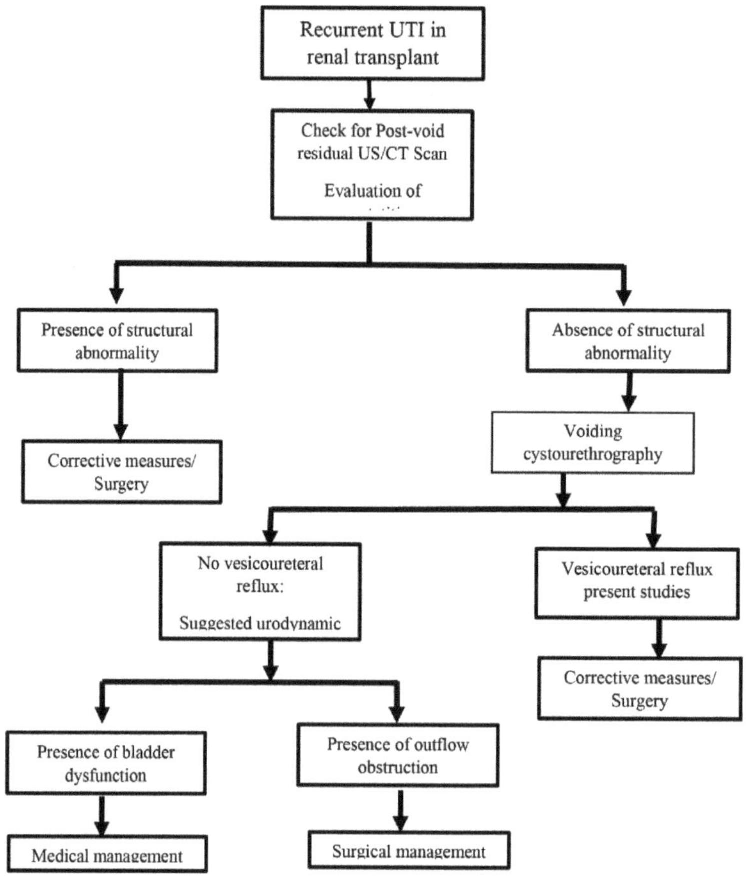

Figure 3. Scheme for evaluating a case of recurrent UTI.

antimicrobial agent, with relatively low cost and is mostly used for prevention of *Pneumocystis carinii* infection [2, 14, 51]. Ariza-Heredia et al. have reported the effect of TMP-SMZ prophylaxis offers great protection to prevent UTI in the first year. Four patients who were not offered this prophylaxis due to certain reasons developed UTI in first year of transplant as against those who received the prophylaxis [14].

In cases with recurrent UTI anatomical and functional abnormalities like vesicoureteral reflux and neurogenic bladder need to be addressed and managed accordingly. The patients should be educated for basic preventive measures like hydration and frequent voiding. Radiological studies should be implicated to rule out the anatomical defects, obstruction, calculi and retained foreign bodies. Prostatitis should be considered as an important differential diagnosis in men who present with recurrent post-transplant UTI. Mitra et al. have proposed a scheme for evaluating a case of recurrent UTI (**Figure 3**) [57].

7. Recommendations

As the risk of UTI is very high in the first week of transplantation, we recommend that every renal transplant recipient should undergo urine routine examination with microscopy for first 10 days in the post-operative period irrespective of the fact that the patient has any symptoms of UTI. This type of screening will be helpful in early diagnosis and treatment and preventing infection related mortality. Culture studies should be advised as and when required, and the treatment should be planned according to the organisms identified in the culture studies. Antibiotic prophylaxis should be given to patients who are at high risk for developing UTI. Urine examination should be advised during every follow-up. This practice will definitely help in early diagnosis of infection and help in preventing morbidity associated with UTI.

8. Conclusion

Urinary tract infections in the post-transplant period are quite common, more so during the early period of first 3 months. There are various risk factors attributed to development of UTI like female sex, delayed graft function, old age, anatomical anomalies and organs from the deceased donors being more common. Although few studies have identified UTI in post-transplant period as a negative predictor for graft function, further studies are still required to establish this relationship. The criteria to define asymptomatic bacteriuria and UTI are the same as that for general population. However in view of studies that show that post-transplant UTI has deleterious effect on graft function, it is necessary to design standard definitions, protocols for surveillance, prevention and management of UTI in renal transplant recipients.

However our protocol for renal transplant recipients involves regular follow-up by urine rou tine and microscopic examination and renal function tests, which helps in early detection of infections leading to prompt management. Thus, early intervention in both the patients led to restoration of the renal function with proper graft function.

Abbreviations

RT	renal transplant
UTI	urinary tract infection.
CFU	colony forming units.
DGF	delayed graft function.
CNI	calcineurin inhibitors.
TMP-SMZ	trimethoprim-sulfamethoxazole

Author details

Lovelesh Kumar Nigam*, Aruna V. Vanikar, Rashmi D. Patel, Kamal V. Kanodia and Kamlesh S. Suthar

*Address all correspondence to: drloveleshnigam@gmail.com

Department of Pathology, Lab Medicine, Transfusion Services and Immunohematology, Institute of Kidney Disease and Research Sciences, BJ Medical College Campus, Ahmedabad, Gujarat, India

References

[1] Tawab KA, Gheith O, Otaibi TA, Nampoory N, Mansour H, Halim AH, et al. Recurrent urinary tract infection among renal transplant recipients: Risk factors and long-term outcome. Experimental and Clinical Transplantation. 2017;**2**:157-163

[2] Parasuraman R, Julian K. Urinary tract infections in solid organ transplantation. American Journal of Transplantation. 2013;**13**:327-336

[3] Anastasopoulos NA, Duni A, Peschos D, Agnantis N, Dounousi E. The Spectrum of infectious diseases in kidney transplantation: A review of the classification, pathogens and clinical manifestations. Infectious Diseases in Kidney Transplantation. 2015;**29**:415-422

[4] Karuthu S, Blumberg EA. Common infections in kidney transplant recipients. Clinical Journal of the American Society of Nephrology. 2012;**7**:2058-2070

[5] Umesh L, Mahesh E, Kumar A, Punith K, Lalitha K, Suman G. Infections in renal transplant recipients. Journal, Indian Academy of Clinical Medicine. 2007;**8**(4):316-323

[6] Gondos AS, Al-Moyed KA, Al-Robasi ABA, Al-Shamahy HA, Alyousefi NA. Urinary tract infection among renal transplant recipients in Yemen. PLoS One. December 2015. DOI: 10.1371/journal.pone.0144266

[7] Espinar MJ, Miranda IM, Costa-de-Oliveira S, Rocha R, Rodrigues AG, Pina-Vaz C. Urinary tract infections in kidney transplant patients due to *Escherichia coli* and *Klebsiella pneumoniae*-producing extended-spectrum β-Lactamases: Risk factors and molecular epidemiology. PLoS One. 2015. DOI: 10.1371/journal.pone.0134737

[8] Becerra BJ, Becerra MB, Safdar N. A Nationwide assessment of the burden of urinary tract infection among renal transplant recipients. Journal of Transplantation. 2015 Article ID 854640, 8 pages:http://dx.doi.org/10.1155/2015/854640

[9] Mohan M, Neeraja M, Sudhaharan S, Raju SB, Gangadhar T, Lakshmi V. Risk factors for urinary tract infections in renal allograft recipients: Experience of a tertiary care center in Hyderabad, South India. Indian Journal of Nephrology. 2017;**27**:372-376. DOI: 10.4103/ijn.IJN_331_16

[10] Silva M, Marra AR, Pereira CA, Medina-Pestana JO, Camargo LF. Bloodstream infection after kidney transplantation: Epidemiology, microbiology, associated risk factors, and outcome. Transplantation 2010;**90**:581-587

[11] Vidal E, Torre-Cisneros J, Blanes M, et al. Bacterial urinary tract infection after solid organ transplantation in the RESITRA cohort. Transplant Infectious Disease. 2012;**14**:595-603

[12] Fontserè S, Chacón N, Cordero E. Review of bacterial urinary tract infection in kidney transplant recipients: Incidence, risk factors and impact on the graft survival. International Journal of Transplantation Research and Medicine 2017;**3**:026. doi.org/10.23937/2572-4045.1510026

[13] Bodro M, Sanclemente G, Lipperheide I, Allali M, Marco F, Bosch J, et al. Impact of urinary tract infections on short-term kidney graft outcome. Clinical Microbiology and Infection 2015;**21**:1104.e1-1101104.e8

[14] Ariza-Heredia EJ, Beam EN, Lesnick TG, Kremers WK, Cosio FG, Razonable RR. Urinary tract infections in kidney transplant recipients: Role of gender, urologic abnormalities, and antimicrobial prophylaxis. Annals of Transplantation. 2013;**18**:195-204. DOI: 10.12659/AOT.883901

[15] Brown PD. Urinary tract infections in renal transplant recipients. Current Infectious Disease Reports. 2002;**4**:525-528

[16] Elkehili IM, Kekli AB, Zaak AS, Salem EL. Urinary tract infections in renal transplant recipients. Arabian Journal of Nephrology and Transplantation. 2010;**3**(2):53-55

[17] Alangaden GJ, Thyagarajan R, Gruber SA, Morawski K, Gar nick J, et al. Infectious complications after kidney transplantation: Current epidemiology and associated risk factors. Clinical Transplantation. 2006;**20**:401-409

[18] Khosravi AD, Montazeri EA, Ghorbani A, Parhizgari N. Bacterial urinary tract infection in renal transplant recipients and their antibiotic resistance pattern: A four-year study. Iran Journal of Microbiology. 2014;**6**:74-78

[19] Origüen J, López-Medrano F, Fernández-Ruiz M, Polanco N, Gutiérrez E, et al. Should asymptomatic bacteriuria be systematically treated in kidney transplant recipients? Results from a randomized controlled trial. American Journal of Transplantation. 2016;**16**:2943-2953

[20] Papasotiriou M, Savvidaki E, Kalliakmani P, Papachristou E, Marangos M, et al. Predisposing factors to the development of urinary tract infections in renal transplant recipients and the impact on the long-term graft function. Renal Failure. 2011;**33**:405-410

[21] Albert X, Huertas I, Pereiro II, Sanfelix J, Gosalbes V, Perrota C. Antibiotics for preventing recurrent urinary tract infection in nonpregnant women. Cochrane Database Systematic Review. 2004 CD001209

[22] Pourmand MR, Keshtvarz M, Talebi M, Mashhadi R. Incidence of recurrent urinary tract infection after renal transplantation. Medical Bacteriology. 2012;**1**(2 [2013]):27-34

[23] Giessing M. Urinary tract infection in renal transplantation. Arab Journal of Urology. 2012;**10**:162-168

[24] Smelov V, Naber K, Johansen TEB. Improved classification of urinary tract infection: Future considerations. European Urology Supplements. 2016;**15**:71-80 http://dx.doi.org/10.1016/j.eursup.2016.04.002

[25] Hooton TM, Bradley SF, Cardenas DD, et al. Diagnosis, prevention, and treatment of catheter-associated urinary tract infection in adults: 2009 international clinical practice guidelines from the Infectious Diseases Society of America. Clinical Infectious Diseases. 2010;**50**:625-663

[26] Alkatheri AM. Urinary tract infections in Saudi renal transplant recipients. Journal of Infectious Diseases and Immunity. 2013;**5**(2):18-23. DOI: 10.5897/JIDI12.026

[27] Menegueti MG, Pereira MF, Bellissimo-Rodrigues F, Pisi Garcia TM, Saber LTS, Papini Nardim ME, et al. Study of the risk factors related to acquisition of urinary tract infections in patients submitted to renal transplant. Revista da Sociedade Brasileira de Medicina Tropical. 2015;**48**(3):285-290 http://dx.doi.org/10.1590/0037-8682-0098-2015

[28] Ostaszewska A, Wszoła M, Kuthan R, Domagała P, Góralski P, Diuwe P, et al. Urinary tract infection in patients after renal transplantation: Evaluation of risk factors. MEDtube Science. 2014;**2**:22-29

[29] Dantas SR, Kuboyama RH, Mazzali M, Moretti ML. Nosocomial infections in renal transplant patients: Risk factors and treatment implications associated with urinary tract and surgical site infections. The Journal of Hospital Infection. 2006;**63**(2):117-123

[30] Stamm WE. Catheter-associated urinary tract infections: Epidemiology, pathogenesis, and prevention. The American Journal of Medicine. 1991;**91**(3B):65S-71S

[31] Fayek SA, Keenan J, Haririan A, et al. Ureteral stents are associated with reduced risk of ureteral complications after kidney transplantation: A large single center experience. Transplantation. 2012;**93**:304-308

[32] Giral M, Pascuariello G, Karam G, et al. Acute graft pyelonephritis and long-term kidney allograft outcome. Kidney International. 2002;**61**:1880-1886

[33] Almond PS, Matas A, Gillingham K, et al. Risk factors for chronic rejection in renal allograft recipients. Transplantation. 1993;**55**(4):752-756 discussion 756-757

[34] Memikoglu KO, Keven K, Sengul S, Soypacaci Z, Erturk S, Erbay B. Urinary tract infections following renal transplantation: A single-center experience. Transplantation Proceedings. 2007;**39**:3131-3134

[35] Munoz P. Management of urinary tract infections and lymphocele in renal transplant recipients. Clinical Infectious Diseases. 2001;**33**(Suppl 1):S53-S57

[36] Taminato M, Fram D, Grothe C, Pereira RRF, Belasco A, Barbosa D. Prevalence of infection in kidney transplantation from living versus deceased donor: Systematic review and meta-analysis. Revista Da Escola De Enfermagem Da U S P. 2015;**49**(3):502-507

[37] Camargo LF, Esteves ABA, Ulisses LRS, Rivelli GG, Mazzali M. Urinary tract infection in renal transplant recipients: Incidence, risk factors, and impact on graft function. Transplantation Proceedings.**46**:1757e1759 http://dx.doi.org/10.1016/j.transproceed.2014.05.006

[38] Kara OD, Dincel N, Bulut IK, Ozdemir K, Yilmaz E, Gun ZH, et al. Infectious complications in pediatric renal transplant patients. World Journal of Nephrology and Urology. 2014;**3**(2):92-99

[39] Moradi M, Abbasi M, Moradi A, Boskabadi A, Jalali A. Effect of antibiotic therapy on asymptomatic bacteriuria in kidney transplant recipients. Urology Journal. 2005;**2**(1):32-35

[40] Satish R. Gokulnath. Intractable urinary tract infection in a renal transplant recipient. Saudi Journal of Kidney Disease Transplantation. 2009;**20**(3):458-461

[41] Korth J, Kukalla J, Rath PM, Dolff S, Krull M, Guberina H, et al. Increased resistance of gram-negative urinary pathogens after kidney transplantation. BMC Nephrology. 2017;**18**:164

[42] Fiorante S, Lopez-Medrano F, Lizasoain M, Lalueza A, Juan RS, et al. Systematic screening and treatment of asymptomatic bacteriuria in renal transplant recipients. Kidney International. 2010;**78**:774-781

[43] Lopez-Medrano F, Aguado JM. Urinary Tract Infection in a Renal Transplant Recipients. Monograph in Infectious Disease and Antimicrobial Agents

[44] Shams SF, Eidgahi ES, Lotfi Z, Khaledi A, Shakeri S, Sheikh M, et al. Urinary tract infection in a kidney transplant recipients 1st year after transplantation. Journal of Research in Medical Sciences;**2016**

[45] Abbott KC, Swanson SJ, Richter ER, et al. Late urinary tract infection after renal transplantation in the United States. *American Journal of Kidney Diseases*. 2004;**44**(2):353-362

[46] Dharnidharka VR, Agoda LY, Abbott KC. Effects of urinary tract infection on outcomes after transplantation in children. Clinical Journal of the American Society of Nephrology. 2007;**2**:100-106

[47] Pellé G, Vimont S, Levy PP, Hertig A, Ouali N, et al. Acute pyelonephritis represents a risk factor impairing longterm kidney graft function. American Journal of Transplantation. 2007;**7**:899-907

[48] Giral M, Pascuariello G, Karam G, Hourmant M, Cantarovich D, et al. Acute graft pyelonephritis and long-term kidney allograft outcome. Kidney International. 2000;**61**:1880-1886

[49] Audard V, Amor M, Desvaux D, Pastural M, Baron C, Philippe R, et al. Acute graft pyelonephritis: A potential cause of acute rejection in renal transplant. Transplantation. 2005;**80**:1128-1130

[50] Dupont PJ, Psimenou E, Lord R, Buscombe JR, Hilson AJ, Sweny P. Late recurrent urinary tract infections may produce renal allograft scarring even in the absence of symptoms or vesicoureteric reflux. Transplantation. 2007;**84**:351-355

[51] Lorenz EC, Cosio FG. The impact of urinary tract infection in a renal transplant recipients. Kidney International. 2010;**78**:719-721. DOI: 10.1038/ki.2010.219

[52] Chacon-Mora N, Diaz JP, Matia EC. Urinary tract infection in a renal transplant recipients. Enfermedades Infecciosas y Microbiología Clínica. 2017;**35**(4):255-259

[53] Green H, Rahamimov R, Goldberg E, et al. Consequences of treated versus untreated asymptomatic bacteriuria in the first year following kidney transplantation: Retrospective observational study. European Journal of Clinical Microbiology & Infectious Diseases. 2012

[54] Goya N, Takahashi K, Tanabe K, et al. Clinical studies of bacteriuria in renal transplantation recipients. Correlation with pyuria and symptomatic genitourinary tract infection. Nihon Hinyokika Gakkai Zasshi. 1991;**82**:947-954

[55] Pappas PG, Silveira FP. *Candida* in solid organ transplant recipients. American Journal of Transplantation. 2009;**9**(4):173-179

[56] Pappas PG, Rex JH, Sobel JD, et al. Guidelines for treatment of candidiasis. Clinical Infectious Diseases. 2004;**38**:161-189

[57] Mitra S, Alangaden GJ. Recurrent urinary tract infections in kidney transplant recipients. Current Infectious Disease Reports. 2011;**13**:579-587

11

Microbiology of Catheter Associated Urinary Tract Infection

Md. Mahabubul Islam Majumder, Tarek Ahmed,
Saleh Ahmed and Ashiqur Rahman Khan

Abstract

Urinary tract infection (UTI) is common ailment worldwide with female predominance. Catheter associated urinary tract infection (CAUTI) is the most common healthcare related infection commonly used in urinary obstruction and incontinence in critically ill patients with prolonged indwelling catheterization means more than 30 days, which is almost invariable in all patients within 14 days of catheterization which increases morbidity and mortality and treatment expenses. Approximately 80% of nosocomial UTI is CAUTI. CAUTI may be asymptomatic and symptomatic. 2–4% cases may develop bacteraemia. Organisms responsible for CAUTI is similar to UTI as *Escherichia coli* the commonest than proteus, Pseudomonas, Klebsiella, Enterobacter, Enterococci, Candida, Serratia and rarely with *Delftia tsuruhatensis, Achromobacter xylosoxidans* and few others. CAUTI can be multibacterial. In CAUTI infective organisms form biofilm and propagate from there. *E. coli* is the most common isolate of CAUTI but *Enterobacter cloacae* exhibit highest biofilm production. CAUTI organisms are more antibiotic resistance than UTI. Even due to extensive use of antibiotics now Extended Spectrum Beta Lactamase (ESBL) producing CAUTI organisms are isolated from catheter biofilm.

Keywords: UTI, catheterization, CAUTI, biofilm

1. General information about CAUTI

UTI affects approximately 150 million people worldwide, which is most common infection with female predominance [1]. Around 15–25% hospitalized patients receiving indwelling urinary catheter develops CAUTI with prolonged catheterization and in among 40% nosocomial UTI,

80% is due to CAUTI [2]. CAUTI causes about 20% of episodes of health-care acquired bacteraemia in intensive care facilities and over 50% in long term care facilities [3]. The microbiology of biofilm on an indwelling catheter is dynamic with continuing turnover of organisms in the biofilm. Patients continue to acquire new organisms at a rate of about 3–7%/day. In long term catheterization that is by the end of 30 days CAUTI develops in 100% patients usually with 2 or more symptoms or clinical sign of haematuria, fever, suprapubic or loin pain, visible biofilm in character or catheter tube and acute confusion all state [4]. In CAUTI the incidence of infection is *Escherichia coli* in 24%, Candida in 24%, Enterococcus in 14% Pseudomonas in 10%, Klebsiella in 10% and remaining part with other organisms [5]. Bacteraemia occurs in 2–4% of CAUTI patients where case fatality is three times higher than nonbacteremic patients [6]. Adhesions in bacteria initiate attachment by recognizing host cell receptors on surfaces of host cell or catheter. Adhesins initiate adherence by overcoming the electrostatic repulsion observed between bacterial cell membranes and surfaces to allow intimate interactions to occur [7]. A biofilm is an aggregate of micro-organisms in which cells adhere to each other on a surface embedded within a self-produced matrix of extracellular polymeric substance [8]. In biofilm micro-organisms growing in colonies within an extra-cellular mucopolysaccharide substance which they produce. Tamm-Horsfall protein and magnesium and calcium ions are incorporated into this material. Immediately after catheter insertion, biofilm starts to form and organisms adhere to a conditioning film of host proteins along the catheter surface. Both the inner and outer surfaces of catheter are involved. In CAUTI biofilms are initially formed by one organism but in prolonged Catheterization multiple bacteria's are present. In biofilm main mass is formed by extra cellular polymeric substance (EPS) within which organisms live. So there are three layers in biofilm, where deeper layer is abiotic, than environmental zone and on surface biotic zone [9]. Growth of bacteria in biofilms on the inner surface of catheters promotes encrustation and may protect bacteria from antimicrobial agents and the consequence is more drug resistance of biofilm organisms. When antibiotic treatment ends the biofilm can again shed bacteria, resulting recurrent acute infection. The patients may present as asymptomatic bacteriuria or symptomatic. In symptomatic bacteriuria patient present with fever, suprapubic or costovertebral angle tenderness, and systemic symptoms such as altered mentation, hypotension, or evidence of a systemic inflammatory response syndrome. In asymptomatic CAUTI diagnosis is made with presence of 10^5 cfu/mL of one bacterial species in a single catheter urine specimen [10]. In symptomatic CAUTI bacteriological criteria is present with clinical symptoms.

2. The collection of specimens

It is recommended that urine specimens be obtained through the catheter port using aseptic technique or, if a port is not present, puncturing the catheter tubing with a needle and syringe in patients with short term catheterization [11]. In long term indwelling catheterization, the ideal method of obtaining urine for culture is to replace the catheter and collect the specimen from the freshly placed catheter. In a symptomatic patient, this should be done immediately prior to initiating antimicrobial therapy. Culture specimens from the urine beg should not be obtained [10, 12]. Urine sample can be collected from suprapubic puncture also. Biofilm can be cultured from the catheter, for this swab is taken from inner side of catheter.

3. Microbiologic diagnosis of CAUTI

Catheter Associated Asymptomatic Bacteriuria (CA-ASB) is diagnosed when one or more organisms are present at quantitative counts ≥10^5 cfu/mL from an appropriately collected urine specimen in a patient with no symptoms [13]. Lower quantitative counts may be isolated from urine specimens prior to ≥10^5 cfu/mL being present, but these lower counts likely reflect the presence of organisms in biofilm forming along the catheter, rather than bladder bacteriuria [14]. Thus, it is recommended that the catheter be removed and a new catheter inserted, with specimen collection from the freshly placed catheter, before antimicrobial therapy is initiated for symptomatic infection [13]. In biofilm culture, most biofilm contains mixed bacterial communities meaning polymicrobial colonization.

Patients who remain catheterized without having antimicrobial therapy and who have colony counts ≥10^2 cfu/mL (or even lower colony counts), the level of bacteriuria or candiduria uniformly increases to >10^5 cfu/mL within 24–48 h [14]. Given that colony counts in bladder urine as low as 10^2 cfu/mL are associated with symptomatic UTI in non-catheterized patients [15], untreated catheterized patients and those who have colony counts ≥10^2 cfu/mL or even lower, the level of bacteriuria or candiduria uniformly increases to >10^5 cfu/mL within 24–48 h [10, 16]. Colony counts as low as 10^2 cfu/mL in bladder urine may be associated with symptomatic UTI in non-catheterized patients. Whereas low colony counts in catheter urine specimens are likely to be contaminated by periurethral flora, and the colony counts will increase rapidly if untreated. Low colony counts in catheter urine specimens are also reflective of significant bacteriuria in patients with intermittent catheterization [14].

4. Other laboratory tests

Pyuria is usually present in CA-UTI, as well as in CA-ASB. The sensitivity of pyuria for detecting infections due to enterococci or yeasts appears to be lower than that for gram-negative bacilli. Dipstick testing for nitrites and leukocyte esterase was also shown to be unhelpful in establishing a diagnosis in catheterized patients hospitalized in the ICU [17].

5. Microorganisms causing CAUTI

5.1. CAUTI with *E. coli*

5.1.1. Introduction

It is the most common cause of CAUTI in 24–60% patients [5, 18]. In CAUTI the source of this organism is usually patients own colonic flora. *E. coli* is large and diverse group of bacteria found in environment, foods and intestine of human and animal. Among many species of *E. coli* only a few causes disease in human being. It is beneficial in that it prevents the growth and proliferation of other harmful species of bacteria. Even it plays an important role in current biological engineering.

5.1.2. Structure and pathogenesis

E. coli was discovered in 1885 by Theodor Escherich, German bacteriologist, is gram negative rod, lactose fermenter, composed of one circular chromosome which is common facultative anaerobes in colon and farces of human. Distribution is diverse and most of them are harmless belonging to genus Escherichia. Harmful species causes infection of urinary tract, gastrointestinal tract, respiratory system and rarely bacteraemia and septicemia. Phylogenetic analysis of *E. coli* showed majority of the strains responsible for UTI belongs to the phylogenetic group B2 and D, while in smaller percentage belong to A and B1 [19].

It has three antigens O-cell was antigen, H- flagella antigen and k- Capsular antigen. It has pili—a capsule, fimbriae, endotoxins and exotoxins also. Uropathogenic *E. coli* use P fimbriae (pyelonephritis-associated pili) to bind urinary tract endothelial cells. Vast majority of catheter-colonizing cells (up to 88%) express type 1 fimbriae and around 73% in *E. coli* causing CAUTI [20]. In UPEC fimbrial genes are ygiL, yadN, yfcV, and c2395 [21]. Pathogenesis of CAUTI initiated with UPEC colonization in periurethral and vaginal areas. Then it ascends to bladder lumen and grows as planktonic cells in urine. Sequentially adherence to bladder epithelium, then biofilm formation and invasion with replication and kidney colonization and finally bacteremia [22] (**Figure 1**).

5.1.3. Laboratory diagnosis

Diagnosis of *E. coli* infection is simple, by isolation and laboratory identification of bacterium from urine or biofilm. Laboratory diagnosis by culture of specimen—urine or catheter biofilm in blood agar, MacConkey's agar or eosin-methylene blue agar (which reveal lactose fermentation). Immunomagnetic separation and specific ELISA, latex agglutination tests, colony immunoblot assays, and other immunological-based detection methods are other ways for diagnosis of *E. coli*.

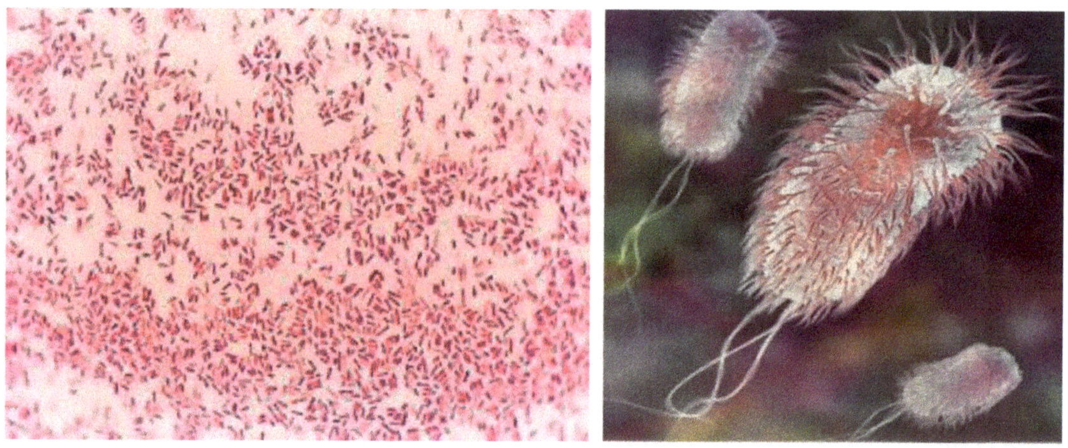

Figure 1. Gram stain picture and morphology of *E. coli*. Adapted from CCBC faculty web. BIOL 230 Lab Manual: gram stain of *E. coli* and infection landscapes: *Escherichia coli*. http://faculty.ccbcmd.edu/courses/bio141/labmanua/lab16/gramstain/gnrod.html.

5.2. Proteus in CAUTI

5.2.1. Introduction

Proteus species, member of the Enterobacteriaceae family of gram-negative bacilli are distinguishable from most other genera by their ability to swarm across an agar surface [23, 24]. Proteus species are most widely distributed in environment and as other enterobacteriaceae, this bacteria is part of intestinal flora of human being [25, 26]. Proteus also found in multiple environmental habitats, including long-term care facilities and hospitals. In hospital setting, it is not unusual for proteus species to colonize both the skin and mucosa of hospitalized patient and causing opportunistic nosocomial infections. It is one of the common causes of UTI in hospitalized patients undergoing urinary catheterization [26, 27].

UTIs are the most common manifestation of Proteus infection. Proteus infection accounts for 1–2% of UTIs in healthy women and 5% of hospital acquired UTIs. Catheters associated UTI have a prevalence of 20–45%. Proteus mirabilis causes 90% of proteus infection and proteus vulgaris and proteus penneri also isolated from long-term care facilities and hospital and from patients with underlying disease or specialized care. Most common age group is 20–50 years. More common in female group and the ratio between male female begins to decline after 50 years. UTI in men younger than 50 are usually caused by urologic abnormalities. Patients with recurrent infections, those with structural abnormalities of the urinary tract, those who have had urethral instrumentation or catheterization have an increase frequency of infection caused by proteus species [28].

5.2.2. Structure and pathogenesis

Proteus mirabilis produces an acidic capsular polysaccharide which was shown from glycose analysis, carboxyl reduction, methylation, periodate oxidation and the application high resolution nuclear magnetic resonance techniques. Proteus species possess an extra-cytoplasmic outer membrane, a common feature shared with other gram-negative bacteria. Infection depends upon the interacting organism and the host defense mechanism. Various component of the membrane interplay with the host to determine virulence. Virulence factors associated with adhesion, motility, biofilm formation, immunoavoidance, nutrient acquisition and as well as factors that cause damage to the host [29, 30] (**Figure 2**).

Certain virulence factors such as adhesin, motility and biofilm formation have been identified in Proteus species that has a positive correlation with risk of infection. After attachment of Proteus with urothelial cells, interleukin 6 and interleukin 8 secreted from the urothelial cells causes apoptosis and mucosal endothelial cell desquamation. Urease production of proteus also augments the risk of UTI. Urease production, together with the presence of bacterial motility and fimbriae or pili, as well as adhesins anchored directly within bacterial cell membrane may favor the upper urinary tract infection. Once firmly attached on the uroepithelium or catheter surface, bacteria begin to phenotypically change, producing exopolysaccharides that entrap and protect bacteria. These attached bacteria replicate and form microcolonies that eventually mature into biofilms [31, 32]. Once established, biofilms inherently protect uropathogens from antibiotic and the host immune response [33, 34]. Proteus mirabilis as with other uropathogens is capable of adapting to the urinary tract environment and acquiring nutrients. And this is accomplished by the production of degradative

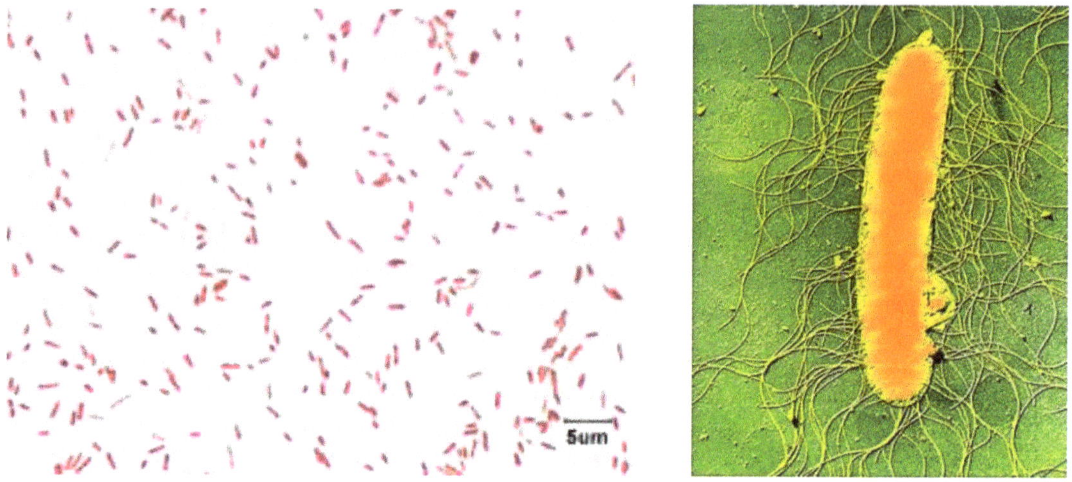

Figure 2. Gram stain picture and morphology of Proteus. Adapted from CCBC faculty web. BIOL 230 Lab Manual: gram stain of Proteus mirabilis and Proteus vulgaris bacteria (SEM) I Macro & Micro: Up Close and Personal I Pinterest I Microbiology, Bacteria shapes and Fungi. https://www.pinterest.com › pin.

enzymes such urease and proteases, toxins such as Haemolysin Hpm A and iron nutrient acquisition proteins.

5.2.3. Laboratory diagnosis

The infection with Proteus can be diagnosed by taking a urine sample for microscopy and culture which is sufficient in most of the cases except in few cases where advanced diagnostic tools are used. If the urine is alkaline, it is suggestive of infection with Proteus sp. The diagnosis of Proteus is made on swarming motility on media, unable to metabolized lactose and has a distinct fishy door. Ultrasound or CT scan to identify renal stone (Struvite stone) or to visualized kidneys or surrounding structures. It will allow to exclude other possible problems, mimicking symptoms of urinary tract infection [35, 36].

5.3. Pseudomonas in CAUTI

5.3.1. Introduction

Pseudomonas is a gram-negative bacteria belonging to the family Pseudomonadaceae and containing 191 validly described species [37]. Because of their widespread occurrence in water and plant seeds, the pseudomonas was observed in early history of microbiology. Pseudomonas is flagellated, motile, aerobic organism with Catalase and oxidase-positive. Pseudomonas may be the most common nuclear or of ice crystals in clouds, thereby being of utmost importance to the formation of snow and rain around the world [38]. All species of Pseudomonas are strict aerobes, and a significant number of organisms can produce exopolysaccharides associated with biofilm formation [39]. Pseudomonas is an opportunistic human pathogen that is especially adept at forming surface associated biofilms. Pseudomonas causes catheter associated urinary tract infection(CAUTIs) through biofilm formation on the surface of indwelling catheters, and biofilm mediated infection including ventilator associated pneumonia, infections related to mechanical heart valves, stents, grafts, sutures, and contract lens associated corneal infection [40].

Pseudomonas is third ranking causes nosocomial UTI about 12%, where *E. coli* remain on the top [41]. CAUTI is directly associated with duration of catheterization. Within 2–4 days of catheterization 15–25% patients develop bacteriuria [42].

5.3.2. Structure and pathogenesis

Pseudomonas aeruginosa is a gram-negative, rod shaped, asporogenous and monoflagellated, noncapsular bacterium but many strains have a mucoid slime layer. Pseudomonas has an incredible nutritional versatility. Pseudomonas can catabolize a wide range of organic molecule including organic compounds such as benzoate. This, then make Pseudomonas a very ubiquitous microorganism and Pseudomonas is the most abundant organism on earth [43] (**Figure 3**).

Pseudomonas is widely distributed in nature and is commonly present in moist environment of hospitals. It is pathogenic only when introduce into areas devoid of normal defense such as disruption of mucous membrane and skin, usage of intravenous or urinary catheters and neutropenia due to cancer or in cancer therapy. Its pathogenic activity depends on its antigenic structure, enzymes and toxins [44]. Among the enzymes Catalase, Pyocyanin, Proteases, elastase, haemolysin, Phospholipase C, exoenzyme S and T and endotoxin and endotoxin A play role in disease process and as well as immunosuppression. Pseudomonas can infect almost any organ or external site. Pseudomonas in invasive and toxigenic. It attached to and colonized the mucous membrane of skin. Pseudomonas can invade locally to produce systemic disease and septicemia. Pseudomonal UTs are usually hospital acquired and are associated with catheterization, instrumentation and surgery. These infections can involve the urinary tract through an ascending infection or through bacteriuria spread. These UTIs may be a source of bacteraemia or septicemia [45].

5.3.3. Laboratory diagnosis

Identification of bacterium with microscopy is simple method of identification of pseudomonas. Culture and antibiotic sensitivity pattern can be done in most laboratory media commonly on blood agar or eosin-methylthionine blue agar. Pseudomonas has inability to ferment lactose and has a positive oxidase reaction. Fluorescence under UV light is helpful in

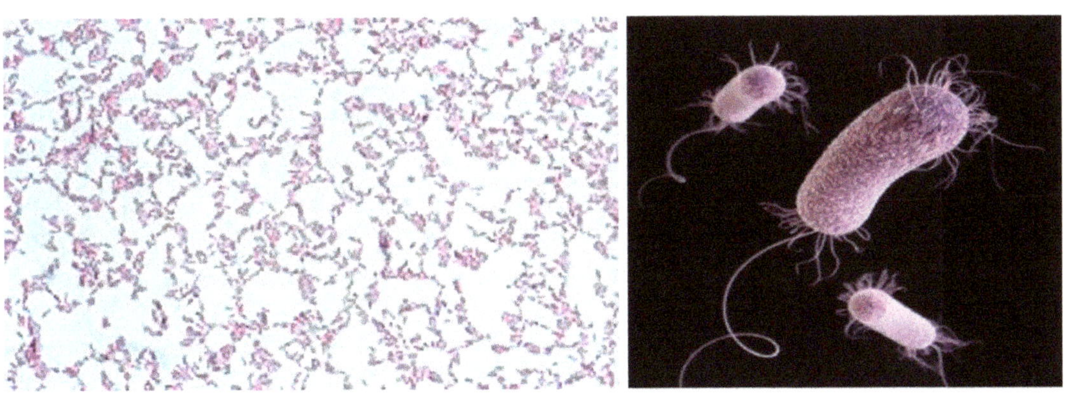

Figure 3. Gram stain picture and morphology of Pseudomonas aeroginosa. Adapted from Science News. A new antibiotic uses sneaky tactics to kill drug-resistant Pseudomonas aeruginosa illustration and Pseudomonas Aeruginosa Stock Photos & Pseudomonas Aeruginosa Stock Images—Alams. https://www.alamy.com › stock-photo.

early identification of colonies. Fluorescence is also used to suggest the presence of pseudomonas in wounds [46].

5.4. CAUTI with Klebsiella

5.4.1. Introduction

Urinary catheters are standard medical devices utilized in both hospital and nursing home settings are associated with a high frequency of catheter-associated urinary tract infections (CAUTI). The contribution of Klebsiella spp. in CAUTI is near about 7.7% [47].

5.4.2. Structure and pathogenesis

Klebsiella pneumoniae is a gram-negative pathogenic bacterium, is part of the Enterobacteriaceae family. It has got polysaccharide capsule attached to the bacterial outer membrane, and it ferments lactose. Klebsiella species are found ubiquitously in nature, including in plants, animals, and humans. They are the causative agent of several types of infections in humans. It has a large accessory genome of plasmids and chromosomal gene loci. This accessory genome divides *K. pneumoniae* strains into opportunistic, hyper virulent, and multidrug-resistant groups [48] (**Figure 4**).

The source of Klebsiella causing CAUTI can be endogenous typically via meatal, rectal, or vaginal colonization or exogenous, such as via equipment or contaminated hands of healthcare personnel. They typically migrate along the outer surface of the indwelling urethral catheter, until they enter the urethra.

Migration of the Klebsiella along the inner surface of the indwelling urethral catheter occurs much less frequently, compared with along the outer surface Internal (intraluminal) bacterial ascension occurs by Klebsiella tend to be introduced when opening the otherwise closed urinary drainage system, ascend from the urine collection bag into the bladder via reflux, biofilm formation occurs.

A critical step in progression to CAUTI by Klebsiella is to adhere to host surfaces, which is frequently achieved using pili (fimbriae) [49]. Pili are filamentous structures extending from

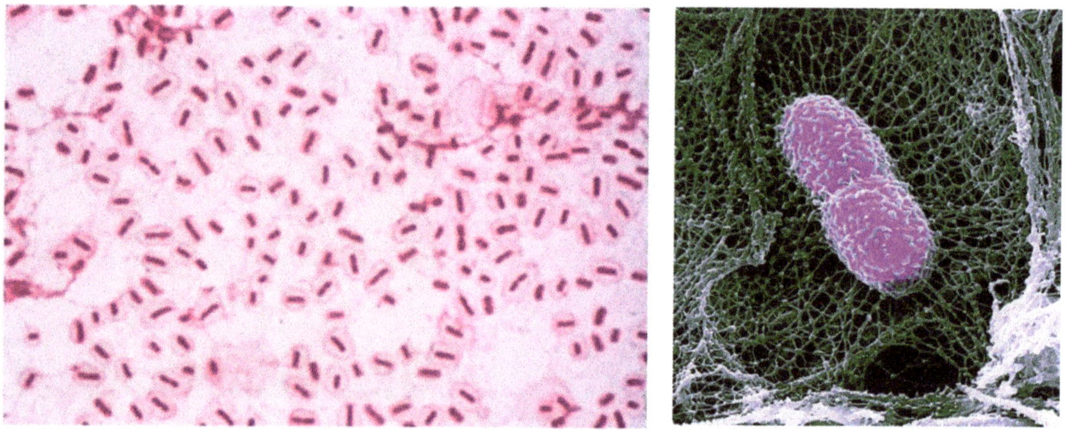

Figure 4. Gram stain picture and morphology of Klebsiella pneumonie. Adapted from studyblue.com. Microbio Lab Practical I—Microbiology 101 with Johnson at University of Vermont—StudyBlue. Study 368 Microbio Lab Practical I flashcards from Tess H. on StudyBlue and Klebsiella Pneumoniae Stock Photos and Pictures. Getty Images https://www.gettyimages.com › photos.

the surface of Klebsiella. They can be as long as 10 μm and between 1 and 11 nm in diameter. Among the two types of pili—type 1 (fim) pili and type 3 (mrk) pili, type 1 aids virulence by their ability to adhere with mucosal surfaces and type 3 pili strongly associated with biofilm production [50]. Both fim and mrk pili are considered part of the core genome [51]. It is thought that both types of pili play a role in colonization of urinary catheters, leading to CAUTI [52]. In addition to fim and mrk pili, a number of additional usher-type pili have been identified in Klebsiella with an average of ~8 pili clusters per strain. Based on varying gene frequencies, some of these appear to be part of the accessory genome. Immediately after catheterization Klebsiella starts biofilm production on the inner as well as outer surface of the catheter and on urothelium. Biofilm augments migration of Klebsiella into urethra and urinary bladder. Biofilm formation on the catheter surface by *Klebsiella pneumoniae* causes severe problem. Type 1 and type 3 fimbriae expressed by *K. pneumoniae* enhance biofilm formation on urinary catheters in a catheterized bladder model that mirrors the physicochemical conditions present in catheterized patients. These two fimbrial types does not is expressed when cells are grown planktonically. Interestingly, during biofilm formation on catheters, both fimbrial types are expressed, suggesting that they are both important in promoting biofilm formation on catheters [53]. The biofilm life cycle illustrated in three steps: initial attachment events with inert surfaces type 1 and type 3 fimbriae encoded by the mrk ABCDF gene cluster within *K. pneumoniae* promotes biofilm formation [54, 55]. Detachment events by clumps of Klebsiella or by a 'swarming' phenomenon within the interior of bacterial clusters, resulting in so-called 'seeding dispersal'.

Modifiable risk factor are prolonged catheterization, lack of adherence to aseptic catheter care, insertion of the indwelling urethral catheter in a location other than an operating room, presence of a urethral stent, feecal incontinence. Non-modifiable risk factor—renal disease (i.e., serum creatinine >2 mg/dL), diabetes mellitus, older age (i.e., age > 50 years old), female sex, malnutrition and severe underlying illness [53]. For infection several virulence factors such as surface factors (fimbriae, adhesins, and P and type 1 pili) and extracellular factors toxins, siderophores, enzymes, and polysaccharide coatings are necessary for initial adhesion with colonization of host mucosal surfaces for tissue invasion overcoming the host defense mechanisms, and causing chronic infections [55].

5.4.3. Laboratory diagnosis

Diagnosis of klebsiella infection is by isolation and laboratory identification of bacterium from urine or biofilm. Laboratory diagnosis can be done by culture of specimen—urine or catheter biofilm in blood agar, MacConkey's agar. Specific ELISA, latex agglutination tests, PCR and other immunological-based detection methods are sophisticated alternatives for diagnosis of klebsiella. Determination of a gene on capsule of Klebsiella is rapid and simple method for the determination of the K types of most *K. pneumoniae* clinical isolates [56].

5.5. CAUTI with Enterobacter

5.5.1. Introduction

Enterobacter species, particularly Enterobacter cloacae and *Enterobacter aerogenes*, are important nosocomial pathogens responsible for about 1.9–9% CAUTI, rarely causes bacteremia [57, 58]. *Enterobacter cloacae* exhibited the highest biofilm production (87.5%) among isolated pathogens [53].

5.5.2. *Structure and pathogenesis*

Enterobacter bacteria are motile, rod-shaped cells, facultative anaerobic, non-spore-forming, some of which are encapsulated belonging to the family Enterobacteriaceae. They are important opportunistic and multi-resistant bacterial pathogens. As facultative anaerobes, some Enterobacter bacteria ferment both glucose and lactose as a carbon source, presence of ornithine decarboxylase (ODC) activity and the lack of urease activity. In biofilms they secrete various cytotoxins (enterotoxins, hemolysins, pore-forming toxins. Though it is microflora in the intestine of humans, it is pathogens in plants and insects. Amp C β-lactamase production by *E. cloacae* is responsible for cephalosporin resistance. They possess peritrichous, amphitrichous, lophotrichous, polar flagella. *E. aerogenes* flagellar genes and its assembly system have been acquired in bloc from the Serratia genus [59] (**Figure 5**).

5.5.3. *Laboratory diagnosis*

The most important test to document Enterobacter infections is culture. Direct gram staining of the specimen is also useful. In the laboratory, growth of Enterobacter isolates is occurs in 24 h or less; Enterobacter species grow rapidly on selective (i.e., MacConkey) and nonselective (i.e., sheep blood) agars.

5.6. CAUTI with Enterococcus

5.6.1. *Introduction*

Enterococci are gram-positive facultative anaerobic cocci, two species are common commensal organisms in the intestines of humans: Enterococcus faecalis (90–95%) and Enterococcus faecium (5–10%) [60]. Though normally a gut commensal, these organisms are commonly responsible for nosocomial infection of urinary tract, biliary tract and blood, particularly in intensive care units (ICU) [61]. *E. coli* is usually the most frequent species isolated from

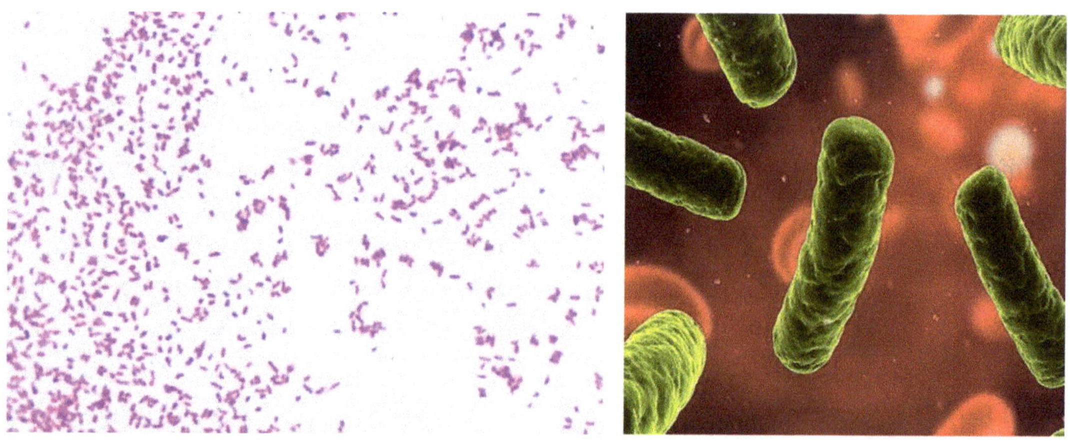

Figure 5. Gram stain picture and morphology of Enterobacter species. Adapted from Gram Stain Kit | Microorganism Stain | abcam.comAdwww.abcam.com/ and Science Prof Online. Gram-negative Bacteria Images: photos of *Escherichia coli*, Salmonella & Enterobacter and Enterobacter aerogenes | Gram-negative microorganism—HPV Decontamination | Hydrogen Peroxide Vapour—Bioquellhealthcare.bioquell.com › microbiology.

bacteremic catheter associated urinary tract infections (CAUTI). However, Enterococcus spp. (28.4%) and Candida spp. (19.7%) were also reported to be most common [62]. In another study, *E. coli* was found the commonest (36%) followed by Enterococcus spp. (25%), Klebsiella species (20%) and Pseudomonas spp. (5%) [63].

5.6.2. Structure and pathogenesis

The most important cause of bacteriuria is the formation of biofilm along the catheter surface [64]. Enterococcus is gram positive bacteria often found in pairs or short chains. Broadly, Enterococcus is in two groups—faecalis and non-faecalis (*E. gallinarum* and *E. casseliflavus*). Enterococcus faecalis formerly classified as part of the group D Streptococcus is a gram-positive, commensal bacterium inhabiting the gastrointestinal tracts of humans and other mammals, survive harsh environmental conditions including drying, high temperatures, and exposure to some antiseptics [65]. *E. faecalis* has the important characteristics of complex set of biochemical reactions, including fermentation of carbohydrates, hydrolysis of arginine, tolerance to tellurite, and motility and pigmentation. Presence of the catheter itself is essential for *E. faecalis* persistence in the bladder, *E. faecalis* depends on the catheter implant for persistence via an unknown mechanism that more than likely involves its ability to produce biofilms on the silicone tubing and immune-suppression [66].

E. faecalis produce a heteropolymeric extracellular hair-like fimbrial structure called the endocarditis- and biofilm-associated pilus-Ebp, having three components the organelle (EbpC), a minor subunit that forms the base of the structure (EbpB) and a tip-located adhesin (EbpA) [67]. EbpA is responsible for adhesion in urothelial and catheter surface for biofilm production (**Figure 6**).

5.6.3. Laboratory diagnosis

Urine sample and biofilm microscopy can identify this gram positive organism. Culture yields the growth of *E. faecalis* in appropriate media. Advanced diagnostic methods like immunological-based detection methods and PCR are rarely needed for diagnosis.

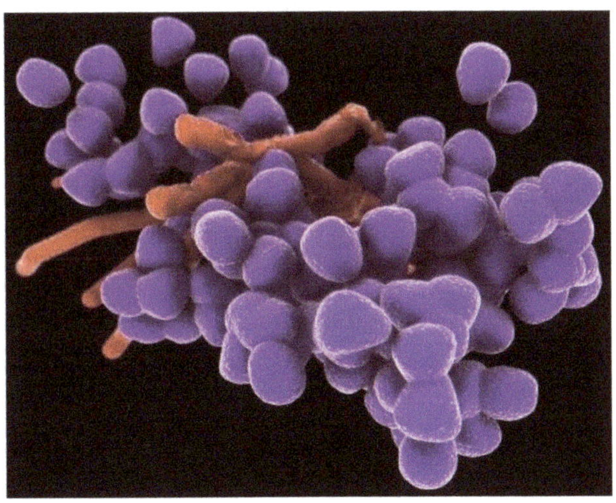

Figure 6. Morphology of Enterococcus. Adapted from Science Photo Library/Alamy Stock Photo Image ID: F6YBC3.

5.7. CAUTI with Candida

5.7.1. Introduction

One of the common causes of catheter associated urinary tract infection is fungal infection. Bacterial infections are accounted for 70.9% of catheter associated urinary infection. *E. coli* is the most commonly isolated organism (41.6%) whereas fungal infections are accounted for 16.6% and mixed fungal and bacterial infections accounted for 12.5% [68]. The National nosocomial infections surveillance (NNIS) data indicated that *C. albicans* caused 21% of catheter-associated urinary tract infections, in contrast to 13% of non-catheter-associated infections [69]. In one study 24% of the cases showing fungal yeast growth. Candida spp. was the commonest. Non-albicans Candida (86%) isolated more commonly than *Candida albicans* (14%) [70]. Candida are commensals, and to be pathogenic, interruption of normal host defenses is crucial which is facilitated in conditions like immunocompromised states as AIDS, diabetes mellitus, prolonged broad spectrum antibiotic use, indwelling devices, intravenous drug use and hyperalimentation fluids [71]. Diabetes mellitus has been reported as the most common risk factor for fungal infection [72, 73]. The duration of catheterization is also an important risk factor as the duration increases the incidence of fungal infection is increased [74].

5.7.2. Structure and pathogenesis

Candida albicans is an oval, budding yeast, which is a member of the normal flora of mucocutaneous membrane. Twenty species of Candida yeasts can cause in human infection but most common is *Candida albicans*. Sometimes it can gain predominance and can produce disease. Other candida species that can cause disease occasionally are *Candida parapsilosis, Candida tropicalis* and *Candida krusei* [75]. Although *Candida albicans* are common isolates in CAUTI, *Candida tropicalis* is increasingly reported in CAUTI [76]. The majority of *Candida albicans* infections are associated with biofilm formation on host or abiotic surfaces such as indwelling medical devices, which carry high morbidity and mortality [63, 77]. Several factors and activities contribute to the pathogenesis of this fungus which mediate adhesion to and invasion into host cells, which are in sequences are the secretion of hydrolases, the yeast-to-hypha transition, contact sensing and thigmotropism, biofilm formation, phenotypic switching and a range of fitness attributes [78] (**Figure 7**).

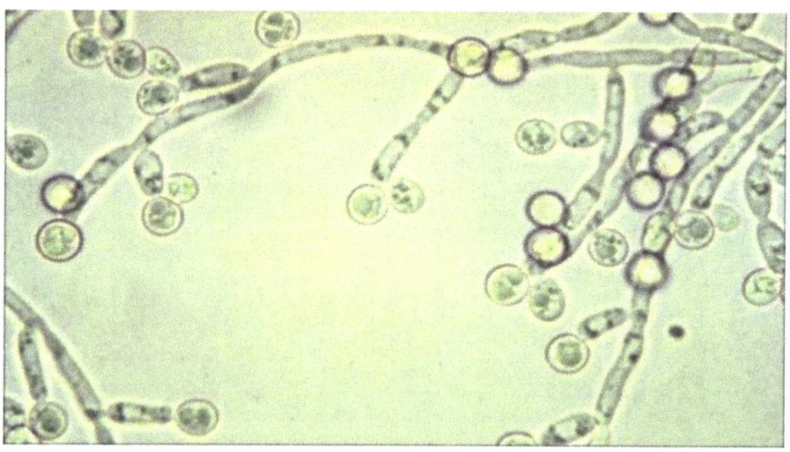

Figure 7. Morphology of Candida albicans. Adapted from biomedik8888, Aug 24, 2011. http://www.BioMedik.com.au3.

5.7.3. Laboratory diagnosis

Urine and materials removed from catheter are needed. Microscopic examinations of gram-stained specimen showed pseudohyphae and budding cells. Culture on Sabouraud's agar at room temperature and at 37°C showed typical colonies and budding pseudomycelia [79].

5.8. CAUTI with *Serratia marcescens*

It is facultative anaerobic bacilli gram-negative rod of Enterobacteriaceae family considered opportunistic human pathogen but not a component of human facial flora. It is capable of producing a pigment called prodigiosin, which ranges in color from dark red to pale pink. It is ubiquitously spent in nature and has preference for damp conditions. Though previously known as nonpathogenic, but since 1970s it is associated with multi drug resistant infection due to presence of R factor—a plasmid. A study in Japan showed 6.8% incidence of UTI with this organism [80]. It also causes bacteraemia rarely. Diagnosis is confirmed by culture of the urine specimen or catheter biofilm. Automated bacterial identification systems and Matrix-Assisted Laser Desorption Ionization-Time of Flight Mass Spectrometry (MALDI-TOF MS) is the other modality for diagnosis of serratia as well as other enterobacteriaceae [81].

5.9. CAUTI with *Delftia tsuruhatensis*

This non-fermentative gram-negative rod discovered as plant growth-promoting bacterium and potential biocontrol agent against plant pathogens. Infection with this uncommon organism in CAUTI occurs in combination with commonest bacteria *E. coli*, *Klebsiella pneumoniae* and *Pseudomonas aeruginosa*. *D. tsuruhatensis* and *E. coli* coexist and tend to co-aggregate over time and also cooperate synergistically [82]. *D. tsuruhatensis* metabolized citric acid more rapidly leaving more uric acid available in the medium to be used by *E. coli* for dynamic growth of both organisms. Identification of this organism is not confirmatory with culture, so molecular methods are more reliable [83].

5.10. CAUTI with *Achromobacter xylosoxidans*

Achromobacter denitrificans is gram negative bacterium formerly known as *Alcaligenes denitrificans*. Infection with this organism predominantly observed in elderly patients with predisposing factors as urological abnormalities, malignancies and immune-suppression. Rarely it causes bacteraemia. This bacterium has high level of antibiotic resistance [84].

In polymicrobial biofilm, *Achromobacter xylosoxidans* cohabits with common organisms *E. coli*, *Pseudomonas aeruginosa* and *Klebsiella pneumoniae*. Diagnosis is by bacterial culture and molecular methods.

5.11. CAUTI with Staphylococci

Staphylococci (methicillin-sensitive *Staphylococcus aureus* [MSSA] and methicillin-resistant *S. aureus* [MRSA], *Staphylococcus saprophyticus*. These are the common gram positive bacteria usually responsible for skin and soft tissue infections but rarely cause CAUTI and bacteraemia [85].

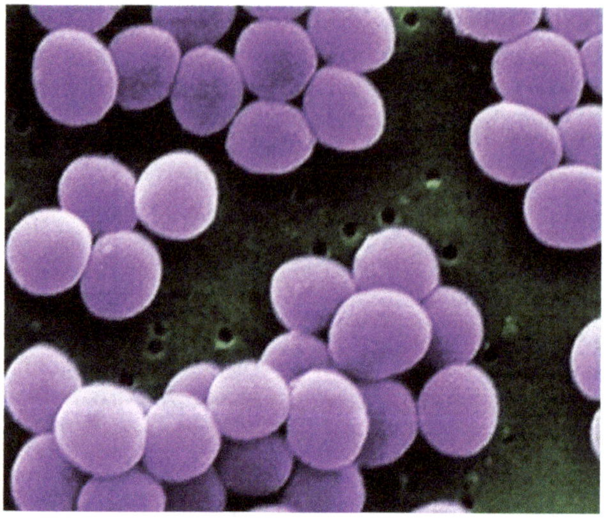

Figure 8. Morphology of Staphylococcus aureus. Adapted from abcam.comAdwww.abcam.com/ pharmacist-driven intervention improves care of patients with S aureus Bacteremia/Staph aureus. Nebraska Medicine https://asap.nebraskamed.com.

The incidence of Staphylococcal UTI as well as CAUTI is increasing and the organisms carry wide variety of multidrug-resistant genes on plasmids, which augment spread of resistance among other species [86].

Diagnosis is easy, gram stain of the sample, culture is sufficient. Advanced techniques rarely needed (**Figure 8**).

6. Conclusion

CAUTI is one of the most nosocomial Infection worldwide resulting from rational as well as sometimes irrational use of indwelling urinary catheter. Cause of CAUTI is formation of pathogenic biofilm commonly due to UPEC, Proteus, Klebsiella, Pseudomonas, Enterobacter rarely Candida and other uncommon opportunistic organisms. CAUTI has got high impact on morbidity and mortality as biofilm producing organisms are more antibiotic resistant. Antibiotic resistance is a global problem. Early detection of CAUTI is simple by examination of urine and catheter biofilm with microscopy as well as culture with antibiogram. It is easy and cost effective with early diagnosis and treatment for good clinical outcome. Advanced and sophisticated methods like Immunomagnetic separation, specific ELISA, colony immunoblot assays and PCR for diagnosis of CAUTI is seldom necessary.

Author details

Md. Mahabubul Islam Majumder*, Tarek Ahmed, Saleh Ahmed and Ashiqur Rahman Khan

*Address all correspondence to: mahabubmazumder@yahoo.com; m.i.majumder@gmail.com

Department of Medicine, Comilla Medical College, Comilla, Bangladesh

References

[1] Florece-Mireles AL, Waslker JN, Caparon M, Hultgren SJ. Urinary tract infections: Epidemiology, mechanisms of infection and treatment options. Nature Reviews Microbiology. 2015;**13**(5):269-264. DOI: 10.1038/nrmicro3432

[2] Esposito S, Noviello S, Leone S. Catheter-associated urinary tract infections: Epidemiology and prevention. Le Infezioni in Medicina. 2008;**16**(3):130-143

[3] Nicolle LE. Catheter associated urinary tract infections. Antimicrobial Resistance and Infection Control. 2014;**3**:23. DOI: 10.1186/2047-2994-3-23

[4] Parida S, Mishra SK. Urinary tract infections in the critical care unit: A brief review. Indian Journal of Critical Care Medicine. 2013;**17**(6):370-374. DOI: 10.4103/0972-5229.123451

[5] Weiner LM, Webb AK, Limbago B, et al. Antimicrobial-resistant pathogens associated with healthcare-associated infections: Summary of data reported to the national healthcare safety network at the centers for disease control and prevention, 2011-2014. Infection Control and Hospital Epidemiology. 2016;**37**(11):1288

[6] Walter E, Stamm MD. Catheter-associated urinary tract infections: Epidemiology, pathogenesis, and prevention. The American journal of Medicine. 1991;**91**(3, Supplement 2.19):S65-S71

[7] Jacobsen SM, Stickler DJ, Mobley HLT, Shirtliff ME. Complicated catheter associated urinary tract infections due to *Escherichia coli* and *Proteus mirabilis*. Clinical Microbiology Reviews. 2008;**21**(1):26-59. DOI: 10.1128/CMR.00019-07

[8] Tomar R, Paviaya R, Ghosh S, Murthy R, Pradhan S, Agrawal E. Biofilm production by uropathogens causing catheter associated urinary tract infection. International Journal of Medical Research and Review. 2017;**5**(07):710 Available online at: www.ijmrr.in

[9] Buhmann MT, Stiefel P, Maniura-Weber K, Ren Q. In vitro biofilm models for device-related infections. Trends in Biotechnology. 2016;**34**(12):945-948. DOI: 10.1016/j.tibtech.2016.05.016

[10] Hooton TM, Bradley SF, Cardenas DD, Colgan R, Geerlings SE, Rice JC, et al. Diagnosis, prevention and treatment of catheter-associated urinary tract infection in adults 2009 international clinical practice guidelines from the Infectious Diseases Society of America. Clinical Infectious Diseases. 2010;**50**:625-663

[11] Bergqvist D, Bronnestam R, Hedelin H, et al. The relevance of urinary sampling methods in patients with indwelling Foley catheters. British Journal of Urology. 1980;**52**:92-95

[12] Grahn D, Norman DC, White ML, et al. Validity of urinary catheter specimen for diagnosis of urinary tract infection in the elderly. Archives of Internal Medicine. 1985;**145**:1858-1860

[13] Stark RP, Maki DG. Bacteriuria in the catheterized patient. What quantitative level of bacteriuria is relevant? The New England Journal of Medicine. 1984;**311**:560-564

[14] Nicolle LE. Catheter-related urinary tract infection. Drugs & Aging. 2005;**22**:627-639

[15] Tambyah PA, Maki DG. The relationship between pyuria and infection in patients with indwelling urinary catheters: A prospective study of 761 patients. Archives of Internal Medicine. 2000;**160**:673-677

[16] Nicolle LE, Bradley S, Colgan R, et al. Infectious Diseases Society of America guidelines for the diagnosis and treatment of asymptomatic bacteriuria in adults. Clinical Infectious Diseases. 2005;**40**:643-654

[17] Schwartz DS, Barone JE. Correlation of urinalysis and dipstick results with catheter-associated urinary tract infections in surgical ICU patients. Intensive Care Medicine. 2006;**32**:1797-1801

[18] Majumder MI, Ahmed T, Hossain D, et al. Bacteriology and antibiotic sensitivity patterns of urine and biofilm in patients with indwelling urinary catheter in a tertiary hospital in Bangladesh. Journal of Bacteriology and Parasitology. 2014;**5**:3. DOI: 10.4172/2155-9597.1000191

[19] Lee JH, Subhadra B, Son YJ, et al. Phylogenetic group distributions, virulence factors and antimicrobial resistance properties of uropathogenic *Escherichia coli* strains isolated from patients with urinary tract infections in South Korea. Letters in Applied Microbiology. 2016;**62**(1):84-90. DOI: 10.1111/lam.12517 Epub 2015 Dec 9

[20] Reisner A, Maierl M, Jörger M, et al. Type 1 fimbriae contribute to catheter-associated urinary tract infections caused by *Escherichia coli*. Journal of Bacteriology. 2014;**196**(5): 931-939. DOI: 10.1128/JB.00985-13

[21] Spurbeck RR, Stapleton AE, Johnson JR, Walk ST, Hooton TM, Mobley HL. Fimbrial profiles predict virulence of uropathogenic *Escherichia coli* strains: Contribution of ygi and yad fimbriae. Infection and Immunity. 2011;**79**(12):4753-4763

[22] Terlizzi ME, Gribaudo G, Maffei ME. UroPathogenic Escherichia coli (UPEC) infections: Virulence factors, bladder responses, antibiotic, and non-antibiotic antimicrobial strategies. Frontiers in Microbiology. 15 Aug, 2017;**8**:1566. DOI: 10.3389/fmicb.2017.01566. eCollection 2017

[23] Penner JL. Genus XI Proteus. In: Krieg NR, Holt JG, editors. Bergey's Annual of Systemic Bacteriology. Vol. 1. Baltimore, M.D: Williams & Wilkins Co; 1984. pp. 491-494

[24] Penner JL, Hennessy J. Clinical isolates of *Proteus mirabilis* and *Proteus vulgaris*. Journal of Clinical Microbiology. 1980;**12**:304-309

[25] Luzzaro F, Brigante G, D'Andrea MM, Pini B, Giani T, Mantengoli E, et al. Spread of multidrug-resistant *Proteus mirabilis* isolates producing AmpC-type beta-lactamase: Epidemiology and clinical management. International Journal of Antimicrobial Agents. 2009;**33**(4):328-333

[26] Chow AW, Taylor PR, Yoshikawa TT, et al. A nosochomial outbreak of infections due to multiply resistant *Proteus mirabilis*: Role of intestinal colonization as a major reservoir. The Journal of Infectious Diseases; Jun 1979;**139**(6):621-627

[27] Wang JT, Chen PC, Chang SC, Shiau YR, Wang HY, Lai JF, et al. Antimicrobial susceptibilities of *Proteus mirabilis*: A longitudinal nationwide study from the Taiwan Surveillance of antimicrobial resistance (TSAR) program. BMC Infectious Diseases. 2014;**14**:486

[28] Lipsky BA. Urinary tract infection in men. Epidemiology, pathophysiology, diagnosis and treatment. Annals of Internal Medicine. 1989;**110**(2):138-150

[29] Beynon LM, Dumanski AJ, MacLean RJ, et al. Capsule structure of *Proteus mirabilis*. Journal of Bacteriology. 1992;**174**(7):2172-2177

[30] Jacobsen SM, Stickler DJ, Mobley THL, Shirtliff EM. Complicated cather-associated urinary tract infection due to *E. coli* and *Proteus mirabilis*. Clinical Microbiology Reviews. 2008;**21**(1):26-59

[31] Costerton JW, Lewandowski DE, Caldwell DR. Korberetal microbial bioflims. Annual Review of Microbiology. 1995;**49**:711-745

[32] Williams GJ, Stickler DJ. Effect of triclosan on the formation of crystalline biofilms by mixed communities of Urinary tract pathogens on urinary catheters. Journal of Medical Microbiology. 2008;**57**:1135-1140

[33] Kucheria R, Dasgupt P, Sacks SH, Khan MS, Sheerin NS. Urinary tract infection: New insight into a common problem. Postgraduate Medical Journal. 2005;**81**:83-86

[34] Kunin CM. Can we built a better urinary catheter? The New England Journal of Medicine. 1988;**319**:365-366

[35] Mobley HL, Belas R. S warming and pathogenicity of *Proteus mirabilis* in the urinary tract. Trends in Microbiology. 1995;**3**:280-284

[36] Mobley HL, Island MD, Hausinger RP. Molecular biology of microbial urease. Microbiological Reviews. 1995;**59**:451-480

[37] Madigan MT, Bender KS, Buckley DH, Sattkey WM, Stahl DA, editors. Brock Biology of Microbiology. 15th ed. London: Pearson; 2017

[38] Biello D. Do Microbes Makev Sniw? Scientific American. 2008;**2**:45-61

[39] Ryan KJ, Ray CG. Sherris Medical Microbiology. 6th ed. New York: McGRaw Hill; 2014

[40] Costerton JW, Stewart PS, Greenberg EP, et al. Bacterial biofilms: A common cause of persistent infection. Science; 21 May, 1999;**284**(5418):1318-1322

[41] Kunin CM. Infection of the urinary tract due to pseudomonas. In: Baltch AL, Smith RP, editors. Pseudomonas Infections and Treatment. New York: Marcel Dekker; 1994

[42] Warren JW. Catheter-associated urinary tract infections. International Journal of Antimicrobial Agents. 2001;**17**:299-303

[43] Costerton JW, Anwar H. *Pseudomonas aeruginosa*: The microbe and Pathogen. In: *Pseudomonas aeruginosa* Infections and Treatment. 1994. pp. 2-17

[44] Stewart PS, Costerton JW. Antibiotic resistance of bacteria on biofilms. Lancet; Jul 14, 2001;**358**(9276):135-138

[45] Flux CA, Costerton JW, Stewart PS, Stoodley P. Survival strategies of infectious biofilms. Trends in Microbiology. 2005;**13**:34-40

[46] Cole SJ, Angela R, Mona W, et al. Catheter-associated urinary tract infection by *Pseudomonas aeruginosa* is mediated by exopolysaccharide-dependent biofilms. Infection and Immunity. 2014;**82**(5):2048-2058

[47] Gould C, Umscheid C, Agarwal R, et al. Healthcare Infections Control Practices Advisory Committee (HICPAC). In: Guideline for Prevention of Catheter-associated Urinary Tract Infections. 2009 Available at: www.cdc.gov/hicpac/pdf/CAUTI/CAUTIguideline2009final.pdf

[48] Podschun and Ullmann. Klebsiella spp. as Nosocomial Pathogens: Epidemiology, Taxonomy, Typing Methods, and Pathogenicity Factors. 1998;**11**(4):589-603

[49] Ofek I, Doyle RJ. Bacterial Adhesion to Cells and Tissues. 1st edition. Principles of Bacterial Adhesion. US: Springer; 1994; Chapter-1. Pages 1-15. ISBN: 978-1-4684-6437-5. Online ISBN: 978-1-4684-6435-1. DOI: https://doi.org/10.1007/978-1-4684-6435-1

[50] Schroll et al. Role of type 1 and type 3 fimbriae in *Klebsiella pneumoniae* biofilm formation. BMC Microbiology. 2010;**10**:179

[51] Andrade BGN, de Veiga Ramos N, Marin MFA, Fonseca EL, Vicente ACP. The genome of a clinical *Klebsiella variicola* strain reveals virulence-associated traits and a pl9-like plasmid. FEMS Microbiology Letters. 2014;**360**:13-16. DOI: 10.1111/1574-6968.12583

[52] Murphy CN, Mortensen MS, Krogfelt KA, Clegg S. Role of *Klebsiella pneumoniae* type 1 and type 3 fimbriae in colonizing silicone tubes implanted into the bladders of mice as a model of catheter-associated urinary tract infections. Infection and Immunity. 2013; **81**:3009-3017. DOI: 10.1128/IAI.00348-13

[53] Clarke K. Catheter-Associated Urinary Tract Infections (CAUTIs). Austin Journal of Clinical Medicine. 2015;**2**(1):1022.1-1022.3

[54] Stahlhut SG, Struve C, Krogfelt KA, Reisner A. Biofilm formation of *Klebsiella pneumoniae* on urethral catheters requires either type 1 or type 3 fimbriae. Fems Immunology and Medical Microbiology. 2012;**65**(2):350-359. DOI: 10.1111/j.1574-695X.2012.00965.x

[55] Delcaru C, Alexandru I, Podgoreanu P, et al. Microbial biofilms in urinary tract infec tions and prostatitis: Etiology, pathogenicity, and combating strategies. Young LS, ed. Pathogens. 2016;**5**(4):65. DOI: 10.3390/pathogens5040065

[56] Brisse S, Passet V, Haugaard AB, et al. wzi gene sequencing, a rapid method for deter mination of capsular type for Klebsiella strains. Journal of Clinical Microbiology. 2013;**51**(12):4073-4078. DOI: 10.1128/JCM.01924-13

[57] Afzal S, Ashraf M, Bukhsh A, et al. Efficacy of anti-microbial agents with ascorbic acid in catheter associated urinary tract infection. Journal of Infectious Diseases & Preventive Medicine. 2017;**5**:3. ISSN: 2329-8731. DOI: 10.4172/2329-8731.100016

[58] Sabir N, Ikram A, Zaman G, et al. Bacterial biofilm-based catheter-associated urinary tract infections: Causative pathogens and antibiotic resistance. American Journal of Infection Control. 2017;**45**(10):1101-1105. DOI: 10.1016/j.ajic.2017.05.009 Epub 2017 Jun 16

[59] Bhani D, Bachhiwal R, Sharma R, Maheshwari RK. Microbial profile and antimicrobial susceptibility pattern of uropathogens isolated from Catheter Associated Urinary Tract Infection (CAUTI). International Journal of Current Microbiology and Applied Sciences. 2017;**6**(8):2446-2453 ISSN: 2319-7706

[60] Abdallah NMA, Elsayed SB, Yassin MM, et al. Biofilm forming bacteria isolated from urinary tract infection, relation to catheterization and susceptibility to antibiotics. International Journal for Biotechnology and Molecular Biology Research. 2011;**2**(10):172-178 Available online at: http://www.academicjournals.org/IJBMBR

[61] Davin-Regli A, Pagès JM. *Enterobacter aerogenes* and *Enterobacter cloacae*; versatile bacterial pathogens confronting antibiotic treatment. Frontiers in Microbiology. 18 May, 2015;**6**:392. DOI: 10.3389/fmicb.2015.00392. eCollection 2015

[62] Gilmore MS et al., editors. The Enterococci: Pathogenesis, Molecular Biology, and Antibiotic Resistance. Washington, D.C.: ASM Press; 2002

[63] Brooks GF, Carroll KC, Butel JS, Morse SA. Mietzner TA, editors. Jawetz, Melnick & Adelburg's Medical Microbiology. 26th ed. NewYork, London: Mc-Graw Hill; 2013

[64] Chang R, Greene MT, Chenoweth CE, Kuhn L, Shuman E, Rogers NAM, Saint S. Epidemiology of hospital-acquired urinary-tract related blood stream infection at a university hospital. Infection Control and Hospital Epidemiology. 2011;**32**:1127-1129

[65] Murray BE. The life and times of the Enterococcus. Clinical Microbiology Reviews. 1990;**3**(1):46

[66] Guiton PS, Hannan TJ, Ford B, Caparon MG, Hultgren SJ. *Enterococcus faecalis* overcomes foreign body-mediated inflammation to establish urinary tract infections. Morrison RP, ed. Infection and Immunity. 2013;**81**(1):329-339. DOI: 10.1128/IAI.00856-12

[67] Schembri MA, Lo AW, Ulett GC. Blocking the "MIDAS" touch of *Enterococcus faecalis*. Annals of Translational Medicine. 2015;**3**(Suppl 1):S3. DOI: 10.3978/j.issn.2305-5839. 2015.03.32

[68] Warren JW. The catheter and urinary tract infection. The Medical Clinics of North America. 1991;**75**:481-493

[69] Warren JW, Tenney JH, Hoopes JM, Muncie HL, Anthony WC. A prospective microbiologic study of bacteriuria in patients with chronic indwelling urethral catheters. The Journal of Infectious Diseases. 1982;**146**:719-723

[70] Mohammad EJ. Catheter associated fungal urinary tract infection. The Iraqi Post Graduate Medical Journal. 2012;**11**(3):11

[71] Kojic EM, Darouiche RO. Candida infections of medical devices. Clinical Microbiology Reviews. 2004;**17**:255-267

[72] Sangamithra V, Sneka, Praveen S, Manonmoney. Incidence of catheter associated urinary tract infection in medical ICU in a tertiary care hospital. International Journal of Current Microbiology and Applied Sciences. 2017;**6**(4):662-669

[73] Kremery V, Barnes AJ. Non-albicans Candida spp. causing fungaemia: pathogenicity and antifungal resistance. The Journal of Hospital Infection. 2002;**50**:243-260

[74] Kauffman CA, Vazquez JD, Sobei HA, Gallis DSMK, Karchmer AW, Sugar AM, et al. Prospective multicenter surveillance study of funguria in hospitalized patients and the National Institute for Allergy and Infectious Diseases (NIAID) Mycoses Study Group. Clinical Infectious Diseases. 2000;**30**:14-18

[75] Wey SB, Mori M, Pfaller MA, Woolson RF, Wenzel RP. Risk factors for hospital-acquired candidemia. A matched case-control study. Archives of Internal Medicine. 1989;**149**: 2349-2353

[76] Hamory BH, Wenzel RP. Hospital associated candiduria: Predisposing factors and review of the literature. The Journal of Urology. 1978;**120**:444-448

[77] Mayer FL, Wilson D, Hube B. Candida albicans pathogenicity mechanisms. Virulence. 2013;**4**(2):119-128

[78] Deorukhkar SC, Saini S, Raytekar NA, Sebastian MD. Catheter associated urinary tract candida infections in intensive care unit patients. Journal of Clinical Microbiology and Biochemical Technology. 2016;**2**(1):015-017

[79] Tsui C, Kong EF, Jabra-Rizk MA. Pathogenesis of *Candida albicans* biofilm. Pathogens and Disease. 2016;**74**(4):ftw018. DOI: 10.1093/femspd/ftw018

[80] Ishikawa K, Matsumoto T, Yasuda M, Uehara S, Muratani T, et al. The nationwide study of bacterial pathogens associated with urinary tract infections conducted by the Japanese Society of Chemotherapy. Journal of Infection and Chemotherapy. 2011;**17**(1):126-138 Epub 2010 Dec 21

[81] Rodriguesa NMB, Bronzatoa GF, Santiago GS, et al. The Matrix-Assisted Laser Desorption Ionization-Time of Flight Mass Spectrometry (MALDI-TOF MS) identification versus biochemical tests: A study with enterobacteria from a dairy cattle environment Braz. Journal of Microbiology. 2017;**48**(1). DOI: 10.1016/j.bjm.2016.07.025

[82] Preiswerk B, Ullrich S, Speich R, Bloemberg GV, Hombach M. Human infection with Delftia tsuruhatensis isolated from a central venous catheter. Journal of Medical Microbiology. 2011;**60**:246-248. DOI: 10.1099/jmm.0.021238-0

[83] Azevedo AS, Almeida C, Gomes LC, Ferreira C, Mergulhão FJ, Melo LF, Azevedo NF. An in vitro model of catheter-associated urinary tract infections to investigate the role of uncommon bacteria on the *Escherichia coli* microbial consortium. Biochemical Engineering Journal. 2017;**118**:64-69

[84] Tena D, Praetorius AG, Balsalobre MP, Bisquert J. Urinary tract infection due to *Achromobacter xylosoxidans*. Report of 9 cases. Infectious Diseases. 2008;**40**(2):84-87. DOI: 10.1080/00365540701558714

[85] Romero-Vivas J, Rubio M, Fernandez C, Picazo JJ. Mortality associated with nosocomial bacteremia due to methicillin-resistant *Staphylococcus aureus*. Clinical Infectious Diseases. 1995;**21**(6):1417-1423. DOI: 10.1093/clinids/21.6.1417

[86] Looney AT, Redmond EJ, Davey NM, et al. Methicillin-resistant *Staphylococcus aureus* as a uropathogen in an Irish setting. Medicine (Baltimore). 2017;**96**(14):e4635. DOI: 10.1097/MD.0000000000004635

12

Urinary Tract Infections in Neuro-Patients

Charalampos Konstantinidis and
Achilleas Karafotias

Abstract

The majority of neurological diseases may have an impact on lower urinary tract function. High intravesical pressure, post-void residual and incontinence are the main consequences of this dysfunction. All the mentioned conditions are inductive factors for urinary tract infections (UTIs). In addition, the potential complications of neurogenic urinary disorders (reflux, stone formation, incomplete emptying of the bladder), and the methods of urine drainage (intermittent or indwelling catheters, urinary diversion) contribute even more to UTIs. In neuro-patients, all UTIs are considered as complicated ones and there is a different microbiology as compared to the general population. In this chapter, inductive factors for UTIs in neuro-patients will be analyzed and the potential solutions will be exposed. There is a special mention in asymptomatic bacteriuria, which is correlated to neurogenic urinary dysfunction and it is clinically total different from UTI. Asymptomatic bacteriuria should not be treated as the treatment has a negative final outcome for the patient.

Keywords: neurogenic low urinary tract dysfunction, UTIs

1. Introduction

The normal functioning of the urinary system is closely related to the functional integrity of the central nervous system (CNS). Neuro-urological symptoms may be caused by a variety of diseases and events affecting the nervous system controlling the lower urinary tract (LUT). The resulting neuro-urological symptoms depend predominantly on the location and the extent of the neurological lesion. There are no exact figures on the overall prevalence of neuro-urological disorders in the general population, but data are available on the prevalence of the underlying conditions and the relative risk of these for the development of neuro-urological symptoms. The majority of the data show a very wide range of prevalence/incidence. This reflects the variability in the cohort (e.g. early or late stage disease) and the frequently small sample sizes, resulting in a low level of evidence in most published data. Spinal cord injury patients may be the most studied group among neurogenic patients.

Spinal cord injury (SCI) is a damage to the spinal cord from traumatic or nontraumatic etiology, as defined by the International Spinal Cord Society (ISCoS) [1]. It is difficult to accurately calculate the worldwide prevalence and incidence of SCI due to the lack of standardized methods of assessment across regions and limited information in the data collected. The incidence varies from 12 to more than 65 cases/million per year. Data from Olmsted County, Minnesota, United States, from 1975 to 1981, showed an age- and sex-adjusted incidence rate of 71 spinal cord injuries/million [2]. The annual incidence of SCI reported for the year 1991 was around 30.0–32.1 persons/million population in the United States, meaning 7500 and 8000 new cases per year at that time [3]. In 2016, the estimated annual incidence of SCI was approximately 54 cases/million population or 17,000 new SCI cases each year [4]. The annual incidence varies widely by country. From 27 per million persons in Japan, 8–13.4 in Switzerland, 12.7 in France, and 16.7 in South Africa [5]. A systematic review in 2010 by Van den Berg et al. showed up to threefold variation in incidence rates between developed countries. The highest rates reported in Canada and Portugal. Most traumatic SCI studies show a bimodal age distribution. The first peak was found in young men between 15 and 29 years of age and the second peak in older adults (mostly ≥65 years old and women) [6]. The National Spinal Cord Injury Statistical Center at the University of Alabama at Birmingham reported approximately 12,000 new cases each year, with 4:1 male-to-female ratio. The average age at injury was 40 years. The most common injury was incomplete tetraplegia at 30%, followed by 25.6% for complete paraplegia, 20.4% for complete tetraplegia, and 18.5% for incomplete paraplegia. In the past, the leading cause of death among SCI patients was the renal failure while nowadays, is pneumonia, pulmonary emboli, and septicemia supersede renal failure. SCI patients seem to have a higher prevalence of several comorbidities than the general population. It is reported high blood pressure (49% vs. 26%, respectively), high cholesterol (47% vs. 30%), and diabetes (19% vs. 7%). Obesity is also a significant problem for individuals with SCI (25%).

Spinal cord injury (SCI) patients clinically face urinary incontinence during the bladder filling phase and incomplete emptying during the micturition phase. The main aggravating factors are the increased intravesical pressure and the residual urine. These may result in vesicoureteral reflux, bladder diverticula, and urinary stones formation. These conditions also lead to an increased risk of urinary tract infection (UTI) [7, 8]. Despite improved treatment methods, UTI is considered the second leading cause of death in SCI patients [9]. It is known that UTIs are the most common hospital infections with known repercussions for the patient and the national economy. Approximately 5–10% of patients admitted to hospital are infected during their hospitalization and UTIs account for the highest (40–50%) [10, 11]. In addition, SCI patients usually have asymptomatic bacteriuria. In this way, positive urine culture is not the foundation stone for the diagnosis of urinary tract infection. The clinical signs and symptoms of urinary tract infection are differentiated in these individuals as the neural sensation is affected or absent. The review of the following literature aims to highlight the specificities of urinary tract infections in people with SCI or other neurogenic conditions in order to prevent and treat the infections and recognize asymptomatic bacteriuria without treatment necessity.

The physiological function of the lower urinary tract is characterized by the central control of the urinary reflexes (inhibition or removal of reflex inhibition) from the upper cortical centers of the cortex. Urine concentration within the bladder results in an increase in intravesical pressure that causes stimulation of the thoracic-lymphatic sympathetic center (T10-L2) via transient and adductor nerve fibers. Adjacent nerve fibers transfer the stimulus to the breech centers of urination and from there to the upper centers of the cerebral cortex. Then, if there is no central depression, the urinary reflex is manifested through the contraction of the detrusor resulting in the sympathetic nerves. However, if urination is undesirable, this reflex is inhibited as cationic signals inhibit sympathetic stimulation at the level of the thoracic-lumbar sympathetic center and increase the muscular tone of the external sphincter by suture from the pelvic neural mesh formed by the S2–S4 level. From the above, it is clear that any damage at any level of SC results in disorders of lower urinary function. These disorders vary according to level [11, 12], the degree (complete or incomplete) [13] and the extent of the damage.

2. Associated risk factors

2.1. Increased intravesical pressures

Neurogenic urinary tract dysfunction characterized by increased intravesical pressures and/or urine residual [14]. These patients have decreased microorganism removal capacity [15]. Both incomplete emptying of the bladder [16] and high intravesical pressure [17, 18] are accompanied by an increased risk of UTI. Patients who have been using Credé maneuver for a long time to empty their bladder have had severe complications in the upper urinary tract (82% pyuria, 60% ureter dilation, 35% hydronephrosis, and 16% renal failure). Men appeared more susceptible to upper urinary tract damage than to women [19]. According to Esclarin De Ruz et al [20] in patients with SCI with detrusor overactivity, the coexistence of detrusor-sphincter dyssynergia duplicates the risk of urinary tract infections.

2.2. Vesicoureteral reflux

Under normal circumstances, the ureterovesical junction allows urine to enter the bladder but prevents urine from regurgitating into the ureter and the kidney. This results in the kidney being protected from high pressure in the bladder and from contamination by vesical bacteria. In this way, vesicoureteral reflux is considered to be an important factor in urinary tract infection [20]. It occurs in 10% of patients over 4 years of SCI [21]. Although the reflux is the result of high intravesical pressure, it must be controlled by another neurological mechanism since patients with a T10-L2 lesion exhibit more regressive effects than patients who have a level of damage above or below this level [22]. The damage at this level is probably related to the ureteral peristaltic mechanisms.

2.3. Intermittent catheterization

Intermittent catheterization (IC) during the recovery period appears to reduce the rate of urinary tract infections and substantially eliminate many of the complications associated with the use of an indwelling catheter [23, 24]. However, IC may also present certain complications, such as traumatic urethral injury (immediate) or urethral restenosis and recurrent epididymitis (late). In one study, SCI patients, using pure intermittent catheterization for more than 5 years, showed urine stasis at 19% and epididymitis at 28.5% [23]. The appearance of the above complications appears to be increased according to the number of years of pure IC performed [23]. Research supports the use of sterile IC technique in the acute phase of the neurogenic bladder [25] and agrees with a study in which few cases of bacteriuria and urinary tract infection were observed using sterile intermittent catheterization as compared to using a non-sterile procedure [26]. On the other hand, Shekelle et al. reported contradictory results in the value of sterile techniques or techniques without direct catheter contact compared to pure intermittent catheterization, as there is insufficient evidence of risk associated with psychological, behavioral and hygienic factors [27]. Hydrophilic catheters for clean intermittent catheterization are associated with lower rates of long-term complications (urethral stenosis) and may cause a lower degree of bacteriuria [28]. Another type of catheter, with an insertion sheath, which bypasses the first 1.5 cm of the urethra, appears to reduce the incidence of urinary tract infections in hospitalized men with SC damage [29].

2.4. Permanent indwelling catheters

Permanent indwelling catheters are the greatest risk factor for complicated UTIs [30]. They are responsible for most in-hospital UTIs, 3–10% per day and with 100% bacteriuria in their long-term use [31]. Silver-coated catheters are more effective in preventing urinary tract infections in patients who require short-term catheterization and reduce the incidence of symptomatic urinary tract infection and bacteriemia compared to simple catheters [32, 33]. For short-term catheters not exceeding 2–3 weeks, the use of nitrofurazone, minocycline, and rifampin-impeded catheters reduce the risk of urinary tract infection [34, 35] due to antibiotic overlap.

2.5. Suprapubic catheters

The use of a permanent suprapubic catheter is an effective way of draining the bladder in SCI patients with a low rate of urinary tract infection [36, 37]. Suprapubic catheterization may be an alternative drainage method for female patients who cannot perform self-IC [38]. The disadvantage is the continuous presence of the catheter (foreign material) within the bladder associated with the formation of urinary lithiasis as compared to intermittent catheterization at rates of 9 and 4%, respectively, over a period of more than 9 years [39]. On the other hand, this chronic irritation from the catheter is accompanied by an increased incidence of bladder cancer as compared to intermittent catheterization [40]. Nomura et al. [41] reported that 25% of patients with long-term use of suprapubic catheter showed bladder stone formation, which was accompanied by a 7.24 urine pH. Suprapubic drainage in patients with neurogenic urinary disorders is preferred (against urethral catheterization) as it appears to reduce the risk of urethritis, orchiepididymitis, testicular abscess and urethral erosion as compared to permanent catheterization [42].

2.6. Condom catheter drainage

Condom catheters are used in male patients to manage incontinence but not bladder emptying. Their application is accompanied by the same degree of urinary tract infection as in the use of intermittent catheterization. However, condom catheters do not ensure complete bladder drainage and can (in cases of poor application) be considered a cause of occlusion [43]. It is recommended that the condom catheter is applied daily, although no increase in infections has been reported in non-daily applications [44]. In addition, although condom catheters are external, they appear to be related to colonization of the urethra by pathogenic microbes. They are accompanied by Pseudomonas [45] and Klebsiella [46] infections due to the colonization of the regions of the urethra, perineum, penis, and rectum by the above microorganisms. In addition, the urine trap is a very good reservoir of microorganisms. In male patients using condom catheter, urine culture was 73% positive for Pseudomonas, although the degree of bacteriuria was much lower [47, 48]. Also, the colonization of the urethra with Pseudomonas is combined with the presence of the condom catheter [49]. From the above, it can be seen that the chronic use of a condom catheter drainage and urine collector predisposes to the colonization of the patient and the upward introduction of microorganisms into the anterior urethra.

2.7. Biofilm (biomembranes)

According to their initial description, microorganisms are referred to as non-adherent "planktonic" cells [50] based on their developmental characteristics in enriched liquids and solids. Today, it is now known that bacteria in their natural environment are typically attached to some biological or non-surface area. It is also known that adhering microorganisms under suitable conditions form complex structures, biofilms (bio-membranes). These structures are formed as the microorganisms are surrounded by an extracellular exopolysaccharide (EPS) layer which themselves produce [50, 51]. Bacteria are the best-studied microorganisms regarding surface colonization and subsequent biofilm formation.

Fungi, protozoa, viruses, and algae have also been isolated from corresponding extracellular material in direct contact with organic or inorganic surfaces [52]. Stable microbial attachment to the underlying surfaces and the formation of biofilms creates significant and often insoluble problems both in the medical community and in the industry [53]. *Staphylococcus aureus, Staphylococcus epidermidis, Enterococcus faecalis* and *Pseudomonas aeruginosa* often colonize implanted medical devices [54] (such as pacemakers, intravenous catheters, urinary catheters, prosthetic implants, and heart valves) as well as pathological tissue structures (such as respiratory epithelium in patients with cystic fibrosis or cystic fibrosis mucosal in patients with neurogenic bladder) and create biofilms, thus causing chronic and often resistant to treatment infections.

Bacterial biomembranes are observed in 73% [55] patients with SCI using IC, and no relationship has been found between the presence of bio-membrane and symptoms [56]. However, the presence of at least 20 bacterial adherence in each bladder cell appears to be related to the symptomatology of the infection [57]. Bacterial cells are detached individually or in groups from the upper layers of the biofilm circulating in the fluid medium, urine in this case, and attempting to adhere to a new substrate which is more conducive to their growth. These detachable bacteria can cause systemic infection [53, 58].

3. Clinical symptoms

The specificity of individuals with SCI is that asymptomatic bacteriuria is usually present and the sensory disorder results in the lack of a clear symptom of urinary tract infection. The clinician should carefully evaluate the patient to decide whether a positive urine culture reveals infection or is an asymptomatic bacteriuria. Additionally, fever should not be attributed to urinary tract infection if the only positive point is bacteriuria unless other possible causes of fever are excluded. Approximately 45% of feverish conditions in these patients are thought to be due to urinary tract infections [59]. Other causes are respiratory infections as well as thromboembolic events. The septic condition in quadriplegic patients may also occur as hypothermia [60]. Approximately 10% of febrile episodes may be the result of a temperature control malfunction and not an infection [61]. The coexistence of elevated CRP and routine serum test values should be considered. UTI is accompanied by a specimen of urine blisters with microbes above 10^5 CFU/ml, and symptoms such as fever, back pain in the lumbar region of the kidney, upper urinary tract infection, and if the patient has a sensation at this level, urinary urgency and increased spasticity. A characteristic symptom is the reduction of cystic functional capacity and the aggravation of overactive bladder syndrome, in the case of a neurogenic overactive detrusor, or the discontinuation of response to previously well-regulated treatment for increased extravasation activity. The incidence of urinary tract infections in SCI patients is 2.5 episodes per patient per year. Bacteremia and sepsis occur in 1% of SCI patients [62]. The urinary system is considered to be the most common source of bacteremia [62, 63]. Bacteremia in SCI patients is accompanied by 90% fever, 17% hypotension, and death rate of about 15%. [62, 63]. Approximately 20–25% of episodes are characterized by polymicrobial infections. Bacteriemia is more common in quadriplegic patients and in patients with complete SCI [64]. Urogenital tube manipulations are considered as risk factors for bacteremia [65].

4. Microbiology—urine culture

Urinary tract colonization often follows colonization of the urogenital tract, perineum or urethra with enteropathogenic microorganisms [66, 67]. In a study of 15 adult men with SCI and other neurogenic urinary dysfunctions, the normal flora of the perineum, penis and urethra regions was compared with the flora of 10 control men without neurogenic urinary disorders [68]. The predominant microorganisms with respect to the control group were Gram-positive granules and diphtheroids. In the individuals with the neurogenic urinary disorder, the microorganisms isolated from the skin flora include species such as Enterobacteriaceae, Pseudomonas, Acinetobacter, and Enterococcus [68]. In addition, other studies of individuals with SCI as compared to non-injured patients, the presence of *E.coli* microorganisms and Klebsiella spp. are less, and have a higher frequency of infections than Pseudomonas, Proteus, and Serratia. Esclarin De Ruz et al. [20] reported that *E. coli,* 36% enterobacteria, 15% *Pseudomonas aeruginosa,* 15% *Acinetobacter* spp., 12% Enterococcus, 6% other microorganisms, and 26% multiple strains were isolated in 45%. In another study in 43 of 50 individuals with SCI, the same types of microorganisms as those from various areas of the skin, including perineal, peripubic, and perinatal regions, were isolated in urine [69]. In 50% of the cases, the same microorganism was isolated from the anterior urethra and from the bladder [70]. Also, the catheter insertion mode is also considered to be significant, which appears to cause an increase of approximately 10 times the number of bladder colonies [70]. The above results demonstrate the important role of bacterial colonization of the skin and urethra as a source of vaccination, through the catheters, of the bladder with microorganisms.

When a UTI is suspected, it is important that the urine specimen is obtained in an appropriate manner in order to prevent contamination and a potential false-positive result. For patients with indwelling catheters (either the urethral catheter or suprapubic), the indwelling catheter should be changed to a new catheter, and the specimen should be obtained from the new catheter after capping the catheter for a few minutes to allow a small amount of urine to collect in the bladder. The urine specimen should then be collected by uncapping the catheter. For patients with external catheters or those who perform IC, the specimen should be collected by catheterization with a new sterile catheter.

5. Pyuria

The significance of pyuria in neurogenic patients in combination with the use of intermittent catheterization or permanent catheter is often difficult to assess. Changing the Foley catheter in symptomatic patients causes an increase in the leucocytes without affecting the microbial strain or the number of colonies [71]. Positive urine culture (10^5 CFU/ml colonies), with the presence of >50 leucocytes per field of vision, is associated with an increased risk of fever. In addition, Gram-positive microorganisms such as *Staphylococcus epidermidis* and *Streptococcus faecalis* are accompanied by a small number of leukocytes despite the occurrence of a large number of colonies, while Gram-negative microorganisms are accompanied by significant pyuria [72]. According to the above significant pyuria is associated with the presence of catheters, infection with Gram-negative microorganisms, as well as bacterial tissue filtration.

6. Bacteriuria

Comparative studies are difficult to perform in these patient groups due to different definitions of bacteriuria and urinary tract infection, different urinary tract drainage methods, as well as the severity of acute, subacute, chronic, or total and partial lesions. In 1992, according to the National Institute on Disability Rehabilitation Research, severe bacteriuria is defined as the number of colony counts of 10^2 CFU uropathogenic micro granules per ml of urine in samples taken by catheterization, 10^4 CFU/ml urine samples under pure micturition and any detectable uropathogenic concentration in samples from permanent catheter or supraventricular puncture. Other researchers continue to regard the concentration of 10^5 CFU/ml in urine as a criterion for significant bacteriuria even in samples after catheterization [73]. Waites et al. reported that patients with 10 CFU/ml in urine have a 10% risk of a febrile episode, while the presence of pyuria is more associated with fever and shivering [73]. In patients receiving 40% IC, the source of bacteriuria was the upper urinary tract, while in 60%, the source was the lower urinary tract [74]. Pyuria was much higher in patients with upper urinary tract infection [75].

7. Asymptomatic bacteriuria

Asymptomatic bacteriuria is defined as the presence of a significant number of urine microbes (10^5 CFU/ml) in patients without clinical symptoms or signs of infection. The incidence varies depending on the age of the patients, the sex and the presence or absence of functional or anatomical urinary tract abnormalities. Bladder catheterization is the most important predisposing factor for asymptomatic microbial growth. In hospitalized catheterized patients with an open urine collection system, the incidence of the asymptomatic microbial disease is 100% of the patients within 3–4 days.

Microorganisms most commonly isolated in bladder catheterized patients are *Escherichia coli*, Klebsiella, Proteus, Enterococcus, Enterobacter, Pseudomonas, Serratia, and Candida. Most are part of the microbial flora of the bowel colonizing the anterior part of the urethra. In patients with a bladder catheter for a short or long period of time, urine specimen collection should be taken by catheter puncture after meticulous antisepsis of the puncture site and not through the catheter's mouth. The presence of leucocytes with or without hematuria is taken into account but does not necessarily require the diagnosis of active infection. Asymptomatic bacteriuria in individuals with SCI requires treatment only in cases where symptomatic urinary tract infection develops [76, 77].

8. Skin colonization

As mentioned, bacterial colonization of the skin and the urethra is an important source of bladder infection using catheters. Differences in microbial species and their presence in normal skin flora of SCI patients and other neurogenic urinary disorders in relation to individuals without neurogenic disorders may result from the use of antibiotic therapy, use of condom catheters, pH and skin temperature in the area, personal hygiene, or fecal contamination. Pseudomonas colonizes the perineum, in addition to the high pH of the skin of the area appears to contribute positively to the high risk of colonization [78, 79]. The meticulous soap wash of the perineum area only has temporary effects in reducing its colonization by Gram-negative microorganisms, whereas the use of antiseptics, such as chlorhexidine and povidone-iodine, has no effect [80, 81].

9. Bladder catheterization

Efforts to eliminate bacteriuria due to the use of permanent or intermittent catheterization have no effect. Intensive or continuous catheterization is a frequent but not documented method of treatment to prevent sedimentation, bacteriuria, urinary tract infection and/or bacteremia. Intravenous administration with neomycin/polymyxin has no effect. Spinal hygiene, perineal wash, and frequent catheter changes have found ineffective methods in reducing urinary tract infection due to catheterization [82]. In addition, it is important for both coating and catheter composition. Prevention of *P. aeruginosa* biofilm formation is observed using silver-coated catheters [83].

10. Biofilm management

As mentioned above, a general feature of the microorganisms that form the bio-membranes is their resistance to various antimicrobial substances, as opposed to free-flowing cells. The main objective should prevent biofilm formation by the prophylactic administration of antibiotics and strict adherence to antisepsis rules when attaching any prosthetic material and in this case a catheter. It is also proposed to incorporate antimicrobial agents into the material to be implanted and to modify the physical or chemical properties of the material so as not to favor biofilm formation.

To achieve satisfactory penetration of antimicrobial drugs into the bio-membrane, experimentally liposomal forms of drugs have been tested with encouraging results. Reid et al. claimed that the daily use of cranberry helmet juice drastically reduced the formation of biofilm and reduced the adhesion of Gram-negative and -positive microorganisms to bladder cells [84]. Respectively, in more recent studies and post-analysis, the clinical benefit of using cranberry juice to reduce urinary tract infections appears to be limited to recurrent urothelial infections in women without neurogenic urinary disorders of young and middle age [85, 86].

The use of antimicrobial drugs for the prevention of UTIs in people who have intermittent catheterization or carry an indwelling bladder catheter has some positive results. In some studies, prophylactic antibiotics are reported to be effective. The use of methenamine orally and intake of acidic substances contributes to the reduction of urinary tract infection in the case of intermittent catheterization [87]. A low dose of ciprofloxacin appears to be more effective than placebo in preventing urinary tract infection [88]. In a study, administration of the 500 mg twice daily dose for 10 days reduced the incidence of Gram-negative organisms in the perineum and urethra but ciprofloxacin-susceptible microorganisms were replaced by resistant microorganisms such as staphylococci, including methicillin-resistant *S. aureus*, Enterococci and Acinetobacter spp. [89]. In contrast to the above, comparative studies of prophylactic administration of ascorbic acid, TMP-SMX, nalidixic acid, methenamine hippurate, or nitrofurantoin microcrystals to prevent urinary tract infection in patients with SCI did not provide statistically significant results. In a daily use of TMP-SMX study compared to placebo as a prophylaxis for urinary tract infections in SCI patients, the use of TMP-SMX did not reduce the incidence of symptomatic bacteremia while there was an increase in TMP-SMX resistance in asymptomatic patients [90].

11. External sphincterotomy

The efficacy of the sphincterotomy has been well documented since Emmett JL and Dunn JH described the trans-urethral resection of the bladder neck and prostate in SCI patients with outlet obstruction. Ross JC introduced the resection of the external urinary sphincter. Large series have shown that sphincterotomy is successful in the treatment of vesical outlet obstruction in certain male patients with quadriplegia, in order to reduce detrusor leak point pressure, followed by condom catheter drainage. Patients who develop UTIs after sphincterotomy are should undergo assessment of PVR to ensure adequate bladder emptying. Urodynamic testing should also be considered to assess the efficacy of the sphincterotomy. If there is evidence of urethral obstruction, repeat sphincterotomy may be indicated. Sphincterotomy can also be indicated when patients use Credé or Valsalva to empty their bladder, but first, surgeons must have assessed that the lower urinary tract is urodynamically safe and that the upper urinary tract is not damaged [91].

12. Bladder augmentation

The aim of bladder augmentation is to reduce detrusor overactivity (DO), improve bladder compliance and reduce the pressure effect of DO [92, 93]. Complications associated with these procedures are recurrent infection, stone formation, perforation or diverticula, possible malignant changes, metabolic abnormality, mucus production and impaired bowel function [94–96]. Special attention should be paid to patients with preoperative renal scars since metabolic acidosis can develop [97]. Several different techniques have been published [98–106]. Bladder substitution, even by performing a supratrigonal cystectomy [93], is also indicated in patients with a severely fibrotic bladder wall. IC may become necessary after this procedure.

13. Urinary diversion

Following supravesical urinary diversion, pyelonephritis may occur, usually accompanied by fever, chills, leukocytosis, nausea and vomiting. Upper tract imaging should be performed, due to possible urinary obstruction. If there is an obstruction, the system should be drained via percutaneous nephrostomy. In this case, urine culture should be obtained from the nephrostomy tube.

13.1. Continent diversion

It is the first choice for urinary diversion. The continent urinary reservoir is indicated when the native bladder and urethra are severely devastated functionally or anatomically, as well as bladder neck closure and ureteral re-implantation are not avoidable. All of the different techniques have complications such as leakage or stenosis. The short-term continence rates are >80% and good protection of the UUT is achieved [107–119].

13.2. Incontinent diversion

If catheterization is impossible, incontinent diversion is indicated. The ileal conduit is the most common form of incontinent urinary diversion used. It could be considered in patients who show intractable and untreatable incontinence, in patients with LUT dysfunction, when the upper urinary tract is severely compromised and in patients who refuse other therapy [119]. An ileal segment is used for the deviation in most cases [120–124] and patients gain better functional status and quality of life [125]. Incontinent diversion has also an acceptable rate of complications. Especially in children, there are concerns about long-term effects on renal function, and while conduit diversion may be considered in this population, alternative methods may be preferable.

13.3. Undiversion

Long-standing diversions may be successfully undiverted or an incontinent diversion changed to a continent one with the cause of better techniques for control of detrusor pressure and incontinence [120]. The patient must be carefully counseled and must comply with the instructions [120]. Only then successful undiversion can be performed [126].

14. Continent catheterizable channel

Some patients with spinal cord injury have difficulty or are unable to perform IC through a native urethra. In such cases, the creation of an abdominal stoma using a continent catheterizable channel (CCC) should be considered. A CCC is particularly helpful in women because their ability to access their urethra is more difficult than in men [127–129]. A concomitant bladder neck closure with a CCC becomes an option when urethral dysfunction or destruction does not result in acceptable continence over anti-incontinence surgeries.

The majority of patients with bladder augmentation or continent urinary diversion will have mucus production that can act as an incubation material for infection. Irrigation of the bladder or pouch at regular intervals with normal saline decrease the incidence of symptomatic urinary tract infection.

15. Treatment

Generally, asymptomatic bacteriuria does not require treatment because the microorganism cannot be eliminated or will recur after the treatment is complete. In addition, antimicrobial therapy will lead to resistant strains of microorganisms [130, 131]. Therefore, there is no indication that treatment reduces virulence or mortality. Systemic antimicrobial therapy for asymptomatic bacteriuria is recommended only in special cases such as:

- patients who undergo urological surgery or prosthetic graft
- treatment may be a part of the control of a hospital infection due to a particular prevalent virulent microorganism

- patients belonging to high-risk groups (immunosuppressed)
- strains of microorganisms suspected of bacteremia such as Serratia marcescens [132–135].

Symptomatic UTI in the neurogenic patient is defined as a urinary culture with $\geq 10^2$ CFU bacteria/mL and symptoms including, but not limited, to LUTS, urinary incontinence, increased spasticity, autonomic dysreflexia, pelvic discomfort, fever, and decreased energy level. Moreover, it has not been shown that the type of microbe isolated in urine culture of an asymptomatic patient is the cause of infection when a symptomatic episode occurs. In 30–50% of cases, urinary catheter removal is accompanied by urinary tract purification by the microorganism [40, 134]. People with symptomatic bacteriuria—UTI should be treated with the most specific antibiotic treatment for the shortest but sufficient period. Since the urinary catheter surface, due to biofilm formation becomes a source of bacterial growth, it is justified and important to remove it and replace it with a new one before treatment of symptomatic infection [40, 136–139]. The guidelines for choosing the right antimicrobial treatment are the same as those of the general population. They include the identification of the microorganism, antimicrobial susceptibility, the location of the infection, its complexity, and the risk factors.

Although there are insufficient clinical studies on the duration of treatment for urinary tract infections in neurogenic patients, the duration of treatment varies from 3 to 21 days depending on the microorganism, the accompanying factors of infection and the condition of the patient [138, 140, 141]. When oral treatment is sufficient, it is usually given for a period of 5–7 days, and when intravenous treatment is required, it remains from 7 to 14 days depending on the clinical and laboratory findings [142]. In the appearance of fungi in urethral cultures, treatment is unnecessary. In this case, either local (intravesical) or systemic antifungal treatment [143, 144] is not recommended, and it is recommended to replace the catheter with a new one. If the infection is accompanied by symptoms of the urinary tract or the presence of fungus is a symptom of systemic infection, then antifungal treatment is necessary [145].

16. Conclusion

Urinary tract infections are a grade issue for medical doctors and patients. It is even more difficult to diagnose and treat neurogenic patients rather than general population. The higher frequency of recurrent infections in these patients and resistant microorganisms remain the main problems as for this specific population. In summary, based on the criteria of evidence-based medicine, there is currently no preventive measure for recurrent urinary tract infections in neurogenic patients that can be recommended without limitations. Individualized concepts, including immunostimulation, phytotherapy, and complementary medicine, should be taken into consideration [146]. Prophylaxis is important to pursue, but there are no data favoring one approach over another. In this case, prophylaxis is essentially a trial and error approach. Nowadays, the quality of life of the neurogenic patients is the primary concern. Antibiotics, catheterization techniques and urinary diversions are the main features of treatment applied. The medical community contributes in this direction with the proper diagnosis of the diseases in this group of patients. Personalized physician and patient collaboration and the timely recognition of symptoms by the patient remain the cutting edge of early symptoms relief. The proper and efficient control of the "neurogenic bladder" is essential for the prevention and the management of the UTIs. The controlled bladder pressure and its complete periodical evacuation under a low-pressure environment can ensure that the UTIs will be less frequent and less severe.

Author details

Charalampos Konstantinidis[1]* and Achilleas Karafotias[2]

*Address all correspondence to: konstantinidischaralampos@yahoo.com

1 Urology and Neuro-Urology Unit, National Rehabilitation Center, Athens, Greece

2 Urology Department, General Hospital "Asklepieio Voulas", Athens, Greece

References

[1] New PW, Sundararajan V. Incidence of non-traumatic spinal cord injury in Victoria, Australia: A population-based study and literature review. Spinal Cord. 2008;**46**(6):406-411

[2] Griffin MR, Opitz JL, Kurland LT, et al. Traumatic spinal cord injury in Olmsted County, Minnesota, 1935-1981. American Journal of Epidemiology. 1985;**121**(6):884-895

[3] National Spinal Cord Injury Statistical Center (NSCISC). Spinal cord injury facts and figures at a glance. The Journal of Spinal Cord Medicine. 2010;**33**(4):439-440

[4] National Spinal Cord Injury Statistical Center (NSCISC). Spinal Cord Injury (SCI) Facts and Figures at a Glance. 2016. Available from: https://www.nscisc.uab.edu/Public/Facts%202016.pdf [Accessed: May 1, 2016]

[5] Key AG, Retief PJ. Spinal cord injuries. An analysis of 300 new lesions. Paraplegia. 1970;**7**(4):243-249

[6] van den Berg MEL, Castellote JM, Mahillo-Fernandez I, de Pedro-Cuesta J. Incidence of spinal cord injury worldwide: A systematic review. Neuroepidemiology. 2010;**34**(3):184-192

[7] The prevention and management of urinary tract infections among people with spinal cord injuries. National Institute on Disability and Rehabilitation Research consensus statement. The Journal of the American Paraplegia Society. 1992;**15**(3):194-204

[8] Carderas DD, Hooton TM. Urinary tract infection in persons with spinal cord injury. Archives of Physical Medicine and Rehabilitation. 1995;**76**:272-280

[9] Frankel HL, Coll JR, Charlifue SW, Whiteneck GG, Gardner BP, Jamous MA, Krishnan KR, Nuseibeh I, Savic G, Sett P. Long-term survival in spinal cord injury: A fifty-year investigation. Spinal Cord. 1998;**36**:266-274

[10] Noreau L, Proulx P, Gagnon L, Drolet M, Laramee MT. Secondary impairments after spinal cord injury: A population-based study. American Journal of Physical Medicine & Rehabilitation. 2000;**79**:526-535

[11] Siroky MB, Krane RJ. Neurologic aspects of detrusor-sphincter dyssynergia, with reference to the guarding reflex. The Journal of Urology. 1982;**127**:953-957

[12] Weld KJ, Dmochowski RR. Association of level of injury and bladder behavior in patients with post-traumatic spinal cord injury. Urology. 2000;**55**:490-494

[13] Pikov V, Wrathall JR. Coordination of the bladder detrusor and the external urethral sphincter in a rat model of spinal cord injury: Effect of injury severity. The Journal of Neuroscience. 2001;**21**:559-569

[14] Hansson S, Hjalmas K, Jodal U, Sixt R. Lower urinary tract dysfunction in girls with untreated asymptomatic or covert bacteriuria. The Journal of Urology. 1990;**143**:333-335

[15] Merritt JL. Residual urine volume: Correlate of urinary tract infection in patients with spinal cord injury. Archives of Physical Medicine and Rehabilitation. 1981;**62**:558-561

[16] MacMillan RD. Complicated urinary tract infections in patients with voiding dysfunction. The Canadian Journal of Urology. 2001;**8**(Suppl 1):13-17

[17] Ruutu M. Cystometrographic patterns in predicting bladder function after spinal cord injury. Paraplegia. 1985;**23**:243-252

[18] Chang SM, Hou CL, Dong DQ, Zhang H. Urologic status of 74 spinal cord injury patients from the 1976 Tangshan earthquake, and managed for over 20 years using the Credé maneuver. Spinal Cord. 2000;**38**:552-554

[19] Foley SJ, McFarlane JP, Shah PJ. Vesicoureteric reflux in adult patients with spinal injury. British Journal of Urology. 1997;**79**:888-891

[20] Esclarin de Ruz A, Garcia Leoni E, Herruzo Cabrera R. Epidemiology and risk factors for urinary tract infection in patients with spinal cord injury. The Journal of Urology. 2000;**164**:1285-1289

[21] Lamid S. Long-term follow-up of spinal cord injury patients with vesicoureteral reflux. Paraplegia. 1988;**26**:27-34

[22] Suzuki T, Ushiyama T. Vesicoureteral reflux in the early stage of spinal cord injury: A retrospective study. Spinal Cord. 2001;**39**:23-25

[23] Firlit CF, Canning JR, Lloyd FA, Cross RR, Brewer R Jr. Experience with intermittent catheterization in chronic spinal cord injury patients. The Journal of Urology. 1975;**114**:234-236

[24] Perrouin-Verbe B, Labat JJ, Richard I, Mauduyt de la Greve I, Buzelin JM, Mathe JF. Clean intermittent catheterisation from the acute period in spinal cord injury patients. Long-term evaluation of urethral and genital tolerance. Paraplegia. 1995;**33**:619-624

[25] Matsumoto T, Takahashi K, Manabe N, Iwatsubo E, Kawakami Y. Urinary tract infection in neurogenic bladder. International Journal of Antimicrobial Agents. 2001;**17**:293-297

[26] Prieto-Fingerhut T, Banovac K, Lynne CM. A study comparing sterile and nonsterile urethral catheterization in patients with spinal cord injury. Rehabilitation Nursing. 1997;**22**:299-302

[27] Shekelle PG, Morton SC, Clark KA, Pathak M, Vickrey BG. Systematic review of risk factors for urinary tract infection in adults with spinal cord dysfunction. The Journal of Spinal Cord Medicine. 1999;**22**:258-272

[28] Hedlund H, Hjelmas K, Jonsson O, Klarskov P, Talja Ml. Hydrophilic versus non-coated catheters for intermittent catheterization. Scandinavian Journal of Urology and Nephrology. 2001;**35**:45-53

[29] Bennett CJ, Young MN, Razi SS, Adkins R, Diaz F, McCrary A. The effect of urethral introducer tip catheters on the incidence of urinary tract infection outcomes in spinal cord injured patients. The Journal of Urology. 1997;**158**:519-521

[30] Biering-S¢rensen F, Bagi P, H¢iby N. Urinary tract infections in patients with spinal cord lesions: Treatment and prevention. Review of aetiology, bladder management, treatment and prevention related to UTI in SCL individuals. Drugs. 2001;**61**:1275-1287

[31] Nicolle LE. A practical guide to antimicrobial management of complicated urinary tract infection. Drugs Ageing. 2001;**18**:243-254

[32] Saint S, Elmore JG, Sullivan SD, Emerson SS, Koepsell TD. The efficacy of silver alloy-coated urinary catheters in preventing urinary tract infection: A meta-analysis. The American Journal of Medicine. 1998;**105**:236-241

[33] Saint S, Veenstra DL, Sullivan SD, Chenoweth C, Fendrick AM. The potential clinical and economic benefits of silver alloy urinary catheters in preventing urinary tract infection. Archives of Internal Medicine. 2000;**160**:2670-2675

[34] Guay DR. An update on the role of nitrofurans in the management of urinary tract infections. Drugs. 2001;**61**:353-364

[35] Maki DG, Tambyah PA. Engineering out the risk for infection with urinary catheters. Emerging Infectious Diseases. 2001;**7**:342-347

[36] MacDiarmid SA, Arnold EP, Palmer NB, Anthony A. Management of spinal cord injured patients by indwelling suprapubic catheterization. The Journal of Urology. 1995;**154**:492-494

[37] Sheriff MK, Foley S, McFarlane J, Nauth-Misir R, Craggs M, Shah PJ. Long-term suprapubic catheterisation: Clinical outcome and satisfaction survey. Spinal Cord. 1998;**36**:171-176

[38] Grundy DJ, Fellows GJ, Gillett AP, Nuseibeh I, Silver JR. A comparison of fine-bore suprapubic and an intermittent urethral catheterisation regimen after spinal cord injury. Paraplegia. 1983;**21**:227-232

[39] Mitsui T, Minami K, Furuno T, Morita H, Koyanagi T. Is suprapubic cystostomy an optimal urinary management in high quadriplegics? A comparative study of suprapubic cystostomy and clean intermittent catheterization. European Urology. 2000;**38**:434-438

[40] West DA, Cummings JM, Longo WE, Virgo KS, Johnson FE, Parra RO. Role of chronic catheterization in the development of bladder cancer in patients with spinal cord injury. Urology. 1999;**53**(2):292-297

[41] Nomura S, Ishido T, Teranishi J, Makiyama K. Long-term analysis of suprapubic cystostomy drainage in patients with neurogenic bladder. Urologia Internationalis. 2000;**65**:185-189

[42] Konstantinidis C, Kalokerinou K, Siatelis A, Kartsaklis P, Nikolia A, Karyotis I, Gekas A, Delakas D. Urethral erosion after long-term urethral catheterization. Urology. 2007;**70**(Suppl 3A):287

[43] Pidde TJ, Little JW. Hydronephrosis due to improper condom catheter use. The Journal of the American Paraplegia Society. 1994;**17**:168-170

[44] Stelling JD, Hale AM. Protocol for changing condom catheters n males with spinal cord injury. SCI Nursing. 1996;**13**:28-34

[45] Montgomerie JZ, Morrow JW. Long-term pseudomonas colonization in spinal cord injury patients. American Journal of Epidemiology. 1980;**112**:508-517

[46] Montgomerie JZ, Gilmore DS, Graham IE, Schick DG, Ashley MA, Morrow JW, Bruce SK. Klebsiella pneumoniae colonization in patients with spinal cord injury. Diagnostic Microbiology and Infectious Disease. 1987;**7**:229-235

[47] Gilmore DS, Schick DG, Young MN, Montgomerie JZ. Effect of external urinary collection system on colonization and urinary tract infections with Pseudomonas and Klebsiella in men with spinal cord injury. The Journal of the American Paraplegia Society. 1992;**15**:155-157

[48] Gilmore DS, Bruce SK, Jimenez EM, Schick DG, Morrow JW, Montgomerie JZ. Pseudomonas aeruginosa colonization in patients with spinal cord injuries. Journal of Clinical Microbiology. 1982;**16**:856-860

[49] Montgomerie JZ, Morrow JW. Pseudomonas colonization in patients with spinal cord injury. American Journal of Epidemiology. 1978;**108**:328-336

[50] Donlan RM. Biofilms: Microbial life on surfaces. Emerging Infectious Diseases. 2002;**8**: 881-890

[51] Donlan RM, Costerton JW. Biofilms: Survival mechanisms of clinically relevant microorganisms. Clinical Microbiology Reviews. 2002;**15**:167-193

[52] Lindsay D, von Holy A. Bacterial biofilms within the clinical setting: What healthcare professionals should know. The Journal of Hospital Infection. 2006;**64**:313-325

[53] Kierek-Pearson K, Karatan E. Biofilm development in bacteria. Advances in Applied Microbiology. 2005;**57**:79-111

[54] Davey ME, O' Toole GA. Microbial biofilms: From ecology to molecular genetics. Microbiology and Molecular Biology Reviews. Dec 2000;**64**:847-867

[55] Reid G, Charbonneau-Smith R, Lam D, Kang YS, Lacerte M, Hayes KC. Bacterial biofilm formation in the urinary bladder of spinal cord injured patients. Paraplegia. 1992;**30**:711-717

[56] Reid G, Kang YS, Lacerte M, Tieszer C, Hayes KC. Bacterial biofilm formation on the bladder epithelium of spinal cord injured patients. II. Toxic outcome on cell viability. Paraplegia. 1993;**31**:494-499

[57] Reid G, Dafoe L, Delaney G, Lacerte M, Valvano M, Hayes KC. Use of adhesion counts to help predict symptomatic infection and the ability of fluoroquinolones to penetrate bacterial biofilms on the bladder cells of spinal cord injured patients. Paraplegia. 1994;**32**:468-472

[58] Jain A, Gupta Y, Agrawal R, Khare P, Jain SK. Biofilms—A microbial life perspective: A critical review. Critical Reviews in Therapeutic Drug Carrier Systems. 2007;**24**(5):393-443

[59] Montgomerie JZ, Guerra DA, Schick DG, Gilmore DS, Tabatabai MF, Morrow JW. Pseudomonas urinary tract infection in patients with spinal cord injury. The Journal of the American Paraplegia Society. 1989;**12**:8-10

[60] Ohry A, Heim M, Rozin R. Peculiar septic responses in traumatic tetraplegic patients. Paraplegia. 1983;**21**:318-321

[61] Colachis SC III, Otis SM. Occurrence of fever associated with thermoregulatory dysfunction after acute traumatic spinal cord injury. American Journal of Physical Medicine & Rehabilitation. 1995;**74**:114-119

[62] Bhatt K, Cid E, Maiman D. Bacteremia in the spinal cord injury population. The Journal of the American Paraplegia Society. 1987;**10**:11-14

[63] Montgomerie JZ, Chan E, Gilmore DS, Canawati HN, Sapico FL. Low mortality among patients with spinal cord injury and bacteremia. Reviews of Infectious Diseases. 1991;**13**:867-871

[64] Waites KB, Canupp KC, Chen Y, DeVivo MJ, Moser SA. Bacteremia after spinal cord injury in initial versus subsequent hospitalizations. The Journal of Spinal Cord Medicine. 2001;**24**:96-100

[65] Faarvang KL, Muller P, Lomberg B, Biering-S¢rensen F. Screening for bacteriuria in patients with spinal cord lesion: Dipstick test, microscopic examination and urine culture. Spinal Cord. 2000;**38**:106-108

[66] Moloney PJ, Doyle AA, Robinson BL, Fenster H, McLoughlin MG. Pathogenesis of urinary infection in patients with acute spinal cord injury on intermittent catheterization. The Journal of Urology. 1981;**125**:672-673

[67] Montgomerie JZ, McCary A, Bennett CJ, Young M, Matias B, Diaz F, Adkins R, Anderson J. Urethral cultures in female patients with a spinal cord injury. Spinal Cord. 1997;**35**:282-285

[68] Taylor TA, Waites KB. A quantitative study of genital skin flora in male spinal cord-injured outpatients. American Journal of Physical Medicine & Rehabilitation. 1993;**72**:117-121

[69] Hamamci N, Dursun E, Akbas E, Aktepe OC, Cakc A. A quantitative study of genital skin flora and urinary colonization in spinal cord injured patients. Spinal Cord. 1998;**36**:617-620

[70] Barnes DG, Timoney AG, Moulas G, Shaw PJ, Sanderson PJ. Correlation of bacteriological flora of the urethra, glans and perineum with organisms causing urinary tract infection in the spinal injured male patient. Paraplegia. 1992;**30**:851-854

[71] Ho CH, Kirshblum S, Linsenmeyer TA, Millis SR. Effects of the routine change of chronic indwelling Foley catheters in persons with spinal cord injury. The Journal of Spinal Cord Medicine. 2001;**24**:101-104

[72] Anderson RU, Hsieh-Ma ST. Association of bacteriuria and pyuria during intermittent catheterization after spinal cord injury. The Journal of Urology. 1983;**130**:299-301

[73] Waites KB, Canupp KC, DeVivo MJ. Epidemiology and risk factors for urinary tract infection following spinal cord injury. Archives of Physical Medicine and Rehabilitation. 1993;**74**:691-695

[74] Hooton TM, O'Shaughnessy EJ, Clowers D, Mack L, Cardenas DD, Stamm WE. Localization of urinary tract infection in patients with spinal cord injury. The Journal of Infectious Diseases. 1984;**150**:85-91

[75] Newman E, Price M. Bacteriuria in patients with spinal cord lesions: Its relationship to urinary drainage appliances. Archives of Physical Medicine and Rehabilitation. 1977;**58**:427-430

[76] Nicolle LE, Bradley S, Colgan R, Rice J, Schaeffer A, Hooton TM. Infections Diseases Society of America Guidelines for the diagnosis and treatment of asymptomatic bacteriuria in adults. Clinical Infectious Diseases. 2005;**40**:643-654

[77] Zhanel GG, Harding GK, Guay DR. Asymptomatic bacteriuria. Which patients should be treated? Archives of Internal Medicine. 1990;**150**:1389-1396

[78] Montgomerie JZ, Gilmore DS, Ashley MA, Schick DG, Jimenez EM. Long-term colonization of spinal cord injury patients with Klebsiella pneumoniae. Journal of Clinical Microbiology. 1989;**27**:1613-1616

[79] Montgomerie JZ, Schick DG, Gilmore DS, Graham IE. pH and water content of Pseudomonas aeruginosa- and Klebsiella pneumoniae-colonized perineal skin of men with spinal cord injuries. Journal of Clinical Microbiology. 1983;**18**:844-848

[80] Gilmore DS, Aeilts GD, Alldis BA, Bruce SK, Jimenez EM, Schick DG, Morrow JW, Montgomerie JZ. Effects of bathing on Pseudomonas and Klebsiella colonization in patients with spinal cord injuries. Journal of Clinical Microbiology. 1981;**14**:404-407

[81] Gilmore DS, Montgomerie JZ, Graham IE, Schick DG, Jimenez EM. Effect of antiseptic agents on skin flora of the perineum of men with spinal cord injury. Infection Control. 1984;**5**:431-434

[82] Muncie HL Jr, Hoopes JM, Damron DJ, Tenney JH, Warren JW. Once-daily irrigation of long-term urethral catheters with normal saline. Lack of benefit. Archives of Internal Medicine. 1989;**149**:441-443

[83] Liedberg H, Ekman P, Lundeberg T. Pseudomonas aeruginosa: Adherence to and growth on different urinary catheter coatings. International Urology and Nephrology. 1990;**22**:487-492

[84] Reid G, Hsiehl J, Potter P, Mighton J, Lam D, Warren D, Stephenson J. Cranberry juice consumption may reduce biofilms on uroepithelial cells: Pilot study in spinal cord injured patients. Spinal Cord. 2001;**39**:26-30

[85] Guay DR. Cranberry and urinary tract infections. Drugs. 2009;**69**(7):775-807

[86] Jepson RG, Craig JC. Cranberries for preventing urinary tract infections. Cochrane Database of Systematic Reviews. 2008;**1**:CD001321

[87] Krebs M, Halvorsen RB, Fishman IJ, Santos-Mendoza N. Prevention of urinary tract infection during intermittent catheterization. The Journal of Urology. 1984;**131**:82-85

[88] Biering-Sorensen F, Hoiby N, Nordenbo A, Ravnborg M, Bruun B, Rahm V. Ciprofloxacin as prophylaxis for urinary tract infection: Prospective, randomized, cross-over, placebo-controlled study in patients with spinal cord lesion. The Journal of Urology. 1994;**151**:105-108

[89] Waites KB, Canupp KC, Brookings ES, DeVivo MJ. Effect of oral ciprofloxacin on bacterial flora of perineum, urethra, and lower urinary tract in men with spinal cord injury. The Journal of Spinal Cord Medicine. 1999;**22**:192-198

[90] Sandock DS, Gothe BG, Bodner DR. Trimethoprim-sulfamethoxazole prophylaxis against urinary tract infection in the chronic spinal cord injury patient. Paraplegia. 1995;**33**:156-160

[91] Reynard JM, Vass J, Sullivan ME, Mamas M. Sphincterotomy and the treatment of detrusor-sphincter dyssynergia: Current status, future prospects. Spinal Cord. 2003;**41**(1):1-11

[92] Vainrib M et al. Differences in urodynamic study variables in adult patients with neurogenic bladder and myelomeningocele before and after augmentation enterocystoplasty. Neurourology and Urodynamics. 2013;**32**:250. Available from: https://www.ncbi.nlm.nih.gov/pubmed/22965686

[93] Krebs J, Bartel P, Pannek J. Functional outcome of supratrigonal cystectomy and augmentation ileocystoplasty in adult patients with refractory neurogenic lower urinary tract dysfunction. Neurourol Urodyn. 2016 Feb;**35**(2):260-266. DOI: 10.1002/nau.22709. (Epub 2014 Dec 18)

[94] Gough DC. Enterocystoplasty. BJU International. 2001;**88**:739. Available from: https://www.ncbi.nlm.nih.gov/pubmed/11890246

[95] Greenwell TJ et al. Augmentation cystoplasty. BJU International. 2001;**88**:511. Available from: https://www.ncbi.nlm.nih.gov/pubmed/11678743

[96] Vajda P et al. Histological findings after colocystoplasty and gastrocystoplasty. The Journal of Urology. 2002;**168**:698. Available from: https://www.ncbi.nlm.nih.gov/pubmed/12131353

[97] Mitsui T et al. Preoperative renal scar as a risk factor of postoperative metabolic acidosis following ileocystoplasty in patients with neurogenic bladder. Spinal Cord. 2014;**52**:292. Available from: https://www.ncbi.nlm.nih.gov/pubmed/24469144

[98] Chapple CR et al. Surgery for detrusor overactivity. World Journal of Urology. 1998;**16**:268. Available from: https://www.ncbi.nlm.nih.gov/pubmed/9775426

[99] Comer MT et al. Reconstruction of the urinary bladder by auto-augmentation, enterocystoplasty, and composite enterocystoplasty. Advances in Experimental Medicine and Biology. 1999;**462**:43. Available from: https://www.ncbi.nlm.nih.gov/pubmed/10599412

[100] Cranidis A, Nestoridis G. Bladder augmentation. International Urogynecology Journal and Pelvic Floor Dysfunction. 2000;**11**(1):33-40. Available from: https://www.ncbi.nlm.nih.gov/pubmed/10738932

[101] Leng WW, Blalock HJ, Fredriksson WH, English SF, McGuire EJ. Enterocystoplasty or detrusor myectomy? Comparison of indications and outcomes for bladder augmentation. The Journal of Urology. 1999;**161**(3):758-763. Available from: https://www.ncbi.nlm.nih.gov/pubmed/10022679

[102] Niknejad KG, Atala A. Bladder augmentation techniques in women. International Urogynecology Journal and Pelvic Floor Dysfunction. 2000;**11**(3):156-169. Available from: https://www.ncbi.nlm.nih.gov/pubmed/11484743

[103] Oge O, Tekgul S, Ergen A, Kendi S. Urothelium-preserving augmentation cystoplasty covered with a peritoneal flap. BJU International. 2000;**85**:802. Available from: https://www.ncbi.nlm.nih.gov/pubmed/10792156

[104] Siracusano S, Trombetta C, Liguori G, De Giorgi G, d'Aloia G, Di Benedetto P, et al. Laparoscopic bladder auto-augmentation in an incomplete traumatic spinal cord injury. Spinal Cord. 2000;**38**:59. Available from: https://www.ncbi.nlm.nih.gov/pubmed/10762200

[105] Westney OL, McGuire EJ. Surgical procedures for the treatment of urge incontinence. Techniques in Urology. 2001;**7**:126-132. Available from: https://www.ncbi.nlm.nih.gov/pubmed/11383990

[106] Zhang F, Liao L. Sigmoidocolocystoplasty with ureteral reimplantation for treatment of neurogenic bladder. Urology. 2012;**80**:440-445. Available from: https://www.ncbi.nlm.nih.gov/pubmed/22857763

[107] Khavari R, Fletcher SG, Liu J, Boone TB. A modification to augmentation cystoplasty with catheterizable stoma for neurogenic patients: Technique and long-term results. Urology. 2012;**80**:460-464. Available from: https://www.ncbi.nlm.nih.gov/pubmed/22704181

[108] Hadley D, Anderson K, Knopick CR, Shah K, Flynn BJ. Creation of a continent urinary channel in adults with neurogenic bladder: Long-term results with the Monti and Casale (Spiral Monti) procedures. Urology. 2014;**83**:1176. Available from: https://www.ncbi.nlm.nih.gov/pubmed/24612618

[109] Leslie B, Lorenzo AJ, Moore K, Farhat WA, Bägli DJ, Pippi Salle JL. Long-term follow up and time to event outcome analysis of continent catheterizable channels. The Journal of Urology. 2011;**185**:2298-2302. Available from: https://www.ncbi.nlm.nih.gov/pubmed/21511280

[110] Duckett JW, Lotfi AH. Appendicovesicostomy (and variations) in bladder reconstruction. The Journal of Urology. 1993;**149**:567-569. Available from: https://www.ncbi.nlm.nih.gov/pubmed/8437267

[111] Kajbafzadeh AM, Chubak N. Simultaneous Malone antegrade continent enema and Mitrofanoff principle using the divided appendix: Report of a new technique for prevention of stoma complications. The Journal of Urology. 2001;**165**:2404-2409. Available from: https://www.ncbi.nlm.nih.gov/pubmed/11371987

[112] Kawai K, Hattori K, Akaza H. Tissue-engineered artificial urothelium. World Journal of Surgery. 2000;**24**:1160-1162. Available from: https://www.ncbi.nlm.nih.gov/pubmed/11071451

[113] Liard A, Séguier-Lipszyc E, Mathiot A, Mitrofanoff P. The Mitrofanoff procedure: 20 years later. The Journal of Urology. 2001;**165**:2394-2398. Available from: https://www.ncbi.nlm.nih.gov/pubmed/11371985

[114] Moreno JG, Chancellor MB, Karasick S, King S, Abdill CK, Rivas DA. Improved quality of life and sexuality with continent urinary diversion in quadriplegic women with umbilical stoma. Archives of Physical Medicine and Rehabilitation. 1995;**76**:758-762. Available from: https://www.ncbi.nlm.nih.gov/pubmed/7632132

[115] Sekar P, Wallace DD, Waites KB, DeVivo MJ, Lloyd LK, Stover SL, et al. Comparison of long-term renal function after spinal cord injury using different urinary management methods. Archives of Physical Medicine and Rehabilitation. 1997;**78**:992-997. Available from: https://www.ncbi.nlm.nih.gov/pubmed/9305274

[116] Stein R, Fisch M, Ermert A, Schwarz M, Black P, Filipas D, et al. Urinary diversion and orthotopic bladder substitution in children and young adults with neurogenic bladder: A safe option for treatment? The Journal of Urology. 2000;**163**:568-573. Available from: https://www.ncbi.nlm.nih.gov/pubmed/10647686

[117] Sylora JA, Gonzalez R, Vaughn M, Reinberg Y. Intermittent self-catheterization by quadriplegic patients via a catheterizable Mitrofanoff channel. The Journal of Urology. 1997;**157**:48-50. Available from: https://www.ncbi.nlm.nih.gov/pubmed/8976213

[118] Van Savage JG, Yepuri JN. Transverse retubularized sigmoidovesicostomy continent urinary diversion to the umbilicus. The Journal of Urology. 2001;**166**:644-647. Available from: https://www.ncbi.nlm.nih.gov/pubmed/11458110

[119] Karsenty G, Chartier-Kastler E, Mozer P, Even-Schneider A, Denys P, Richard F. A novel technique to achieve cutaneous continent urinary diversion in spinal cord-injured patients unable to catheterize through native urethra. Spinal Cord. 2008;**46**(4):305-310. Epub Aug 14, 2007

[120] Drake M et al. Conservative management in neuropathic urinary incontinence. In: Abrams P, Cardozo L, Khoury S, Wein A, editors. Incontinence. Plymouth: Health Publication; 2013. pp. 827-1000

[121] Atan A, Konety BR, Nangia A, Chancellor MB. Advantages and risks of ileovesicostomy for the management of neuropathic bladder. Urology. 1999;**54**:636-640. Available from: https://www.ncbi.nlm.nih.gov/pubmed/10510920

[122] Cass AS, Luxenberg M, Gleich P, Johnson CF. A 22-year follow up of ileal conduits in children with a neurogenic bladder. The Journal of Urology. 1984;**132**:529-531. Available from: https://www.ncbi.nlm.nih.gov/pubmed/6471190

[123] Hald T, Hebjøorn S. Vesicostomy—An alternative urine diversion operation. Long term results. Scandinavian Journal of Urology and Nephrology. 1978;**12**:227-231. Available from: https://www.ncbi.nlm.nih.gov/pubmed/725543

[124] Schwartz SL, Kennelly MJ, McGuire EJ, Faerber GJ. Incontinent ileo-vesicostomy urinary diversion in the treatment of lower urinary tract dysfunction. The Journal of Urology. 1994;**152**:99-102. Available from: https://www.ncbi.nlm.nih.gov/pubmed/8201699

[125] Sakhri R, Seigle-Murandi F, Jacqmin D, Lang H, Saussine C. Laparoscopic cystectomy and ileal conduit urinary diversion for neurogenic bladders and related conditions. Morbidity and better quality of life. Progrès en Urologie. 2015;**25**:342-347. Available from: https://www.ncbi.nlm.nih.gov/pubmed/25726693

[126] Herschorn S, Rangaswamy S, Radomski SB. Urinary undiversion in adults with myelodysplasia: Long-term follow up. The Journal of Urology. 1994;**152**:329-333

[127] Herschorn S, Thijssen AJ, Radomski SB. Experience with the hemi-Kock ileocystoplasty with a continent abdominal stoma. The Journal of Urology. 1993;**149**(5):998-1001

[128] Hakenberg OW, Ebermayer J, Manseck A, Wirth MP. Application of the Mitrofanoff principle for intermittent self-catheterization in quadriplegic patients. Urology. 2001;**58**(1):38-42

[129] Perrouin-Verbe MA, Chartier-Kastler E, Even A, Denys P, Roupret M, Phé V. Long-term complications of continent cutaneous urinary diversion in adult spinal cord injured patients. Neurourology and Urodynamics. 2016;**35**(8):1046-1050

[130] Darouiche RO, Hull RA. Bacterial interference for prevention of urinary tract infection: An overview. The Journal of Spinal Cord Medicine. 2000;**23**:136-141

[131] Stover SL, Lloyd LK, Waites KB, Jackson AB. Neurogenic urinary tract infection. Neurologic Clinics. 1991;**9**:741-755

[132] Rutala WA, Kennedy VA, Loflin HB, Sarubbi FA Jr. Serratia marcescens nosocomial infections of the urinary tract associated with urine measuring containers and urinometers. The American Journal of Medicine. 1981;**70**:659-663

[133] Maki DG, Hennekens CG, Phillips CW, Shaw WV, Bennett JV. Nosocomial urinary tract infection with Serratia marcescens: An epidemiologic study. The Journal of Infectious Diseases. 1973;**128**:579-587

[134] Schaberg DR, Weinstein RA, Stamm WE. Epidemics of nosocomial urinary tract infection caused by multiply resistant gram-negative bacilli: Epidemiology and control. The Journal of Infectious Diseases. 1976;**133**:363-366

[135] Kumon H. Management of biofilm infection in the urinary tract. World Journal of Surgery. 2000;**24**:1193-1196

[136] Raz R, Schiller D, Nicolle LE. Replacement of catheter improves the outcome of patients with permanent urinary catheter and asymptomatic bacteriuria. In: Abstracts of the 38th Interscience Conference on Antimicrobial Agents and Chemotherapy (ICAAC). American Society for Microbiology; 1998. pp. 532-537

[137] Zimakoff JD, Pontoppidan B, Larsen SO, Poulsen KB, Stickler DJ. The management of urinary catheters: Compliance of practice in Danish hospitals, nursing homes and home care, to national guidelines. Scandinavian Journal of Urology and Nephrology. 1995;**29**:299-309

[138] Nicolle LE. The chronic indwelling catheter and urinary infection in long-term-care facility residents. Infection Control and Hospital Epidemiology. 2001;**22**:316-321

[139] Harding GK, Nicolle LE, Ronald AR, Preiksaitis JK, Forward KR, Low DE, Cheang M. How long should catheter-acquired urinary tract infection in women be treated? A randomized controlled study. Annals of Internal Medicine. 1991;**114**:713-719

[140] Nicolle LE. Catheter-related urinary tract infection. Drugs & Aging. 2005;**22**:627-639

[141] Everaert K, Lumen N, Kerckhaert W, Willaert P, van Driel M. Urinary tract infections in spinal cord injury: Prevention and treatment guidelines. Acta Clinica Belgica. 2009;**64**(4):335-340

[142] Sobel JD, Kauffman CA, McKinsey D, Zervos M, Vazquez JA, Karchmer AW, et al. Candiduria: A randomized, double-blind study of treatment with fluconazole and placebo. The National Institute of Allergy and Infectious Diseases (NIAID) Mycoses Study Group. Clinical Infectious Diseases. 2000;**30**:19-24

[143] Jacobs LG, Sidmore EA, Freeman K, Lipschultz D, Fox N. Oral fluconazole compared with bladder irrigation with amphotericin B for treatment of fungal urinary tract infections in elderly patients. Clinical Infectious Diseases. 1996;**22**:30-35

[144] Sobel JD, Lundstrom T. Management of candiduria. Current Urology Reports. 2001;**2**:321-325

[145] Hamory BH, Wenzel RP. Hospital-associated candiduria: Predisposing factors and review of the literature. The Journal of Urology. 1978;**120**:444-448

[146] Pannek J et al. Usefulness of classical homoeopathy for the prevention of urinary tract infections in patients with neurogenic bladder dysfunction: A case series. Indian Journal of Research in Homoeopathy. 2014;**8**:31

Permissions

All chapters in this book were first published in UTITRSPWH, by InTech Open; hereby published with permission under the Creative Commons Attribution License or equivalent. Every chapter published in this book has been scrutinized by our experts. Their significance has been extensively debated. The topics covered herein carry significant findings which will fuel the growth of the discipline. They may even be implemented as practical applications or may be referred to as a beginning point for another development.

The contributors of this book come from diverse backgrounds, making this book a truly international effort. This book will bring forth new frontiers with its revolutionizing research information and detailed analysis of the nascent developments around the world.

We would like to thank all the contributing authors for lending their expertise to make the book truly unique. They have played a crucial role in the development of this book. Without their invaluable contributions this book wouldn't have been possible. They have made vital efforts to compile up to date information on the varied aspects of this subject to make this book a valuable addition to the collection of many professionals and students.

This book was conceptualized with the vision of imparting up-to-date information and advanced data in this field. To ensure the same, a matchless editorial board was set up. Every individual on the board went through rigorous rounds of assessment to prove their worth. After which they invested a large part of their time researching and compiling the most relevant data for our readers.

The editorial board has been involved in producing this book since its inception. They have spent rigorous hours researching and exploring the diverse topics which have resulted in the successful publishing of this book. They have passed on their knowledge of decades through this book. To expedite this challenging task, the publisher supported the team at every step. A small team of assistant editors was also appointed to further simplify the editing procedure and attain best results for the readers.

Apart from the editorial board, the designing team has also invested a significant amount of their time in understanding the subject and creating the most relevant covers. They scrutinized every image to scout for the most suitable representation of the subject and create an appropriate cover for the book.

The publishing team has been an ardent support to the editorial, designing and production team. Their endless efforts to recruit the best for this project, has resulted in the accomplishment of this book. They are a veteran in the field of academics and their pool of knowledge is as vast as their experience in printing. Their expertise and guidance has proved useful at every step. Their uncompromising quality standards have made this book an exceptional effort. Their encouragement from time to time has been an inspiration for everyone.

The publisher and the editorial board hope that this book will prove to be a valuable piece of knowledge for researchers, students, practitioners and scholars across the globe.

List of Contributors

Ajay Kumar Prajapati
Bharathiar University, Coimbatore, India

Barbara Kot
Department of Microbiology, Institute of Biology, Siedlce University of Natural Sciences and Humanities, Siedlce, Poland

Nashaat S. Hamza and Abdalla Khalil
The International Medical Center, Jeddah, KSA

Timothy Kudinha
Charles Sturt University, Orange, NSW, Australia

Zaitseva Elena Aleksandrovna and Komenkova Tatiana Sergeevna
Pacific State Medical University, Vladivostok, Russia

Melnikova Elena Aleksandrovna
Pacific State Medical University, Vladivostok, Russia
Regional Children's Clinical Hospital№1, Vladivostok, Russia

Shadrin Andrey Mikhailovich
G.K. Skryabin Institute of Biochemistry and Physiology of Microorganisms, Russian Academy of Sciences, Pushchino, Moscow Region, Russia
Pushchino State Institute of Life Sciences, Pushchino, Moscow Region, Russia

Luchaninova Valentina Nikolaevna
North-Western State Medical University named after I.I. Mechnikov, Saint-Petersburg, Russia

Ran Pang
Department of Urology, Guang An Men Hospital, China Academy of Chinese Medical Sciences, Beijing, P.R. China

Jianhua Deng
Department of Urology, Peking Union Medical College Hospital, Chinese Academy of Medical Sciences and Peking Union Medical College, Beijing, P.R. China

Xinyao Zhou
Department of Rumatology, Guang An Men Hospital, China Academy of Chinese Medical Sciences, Beijing, P.R. China

Lorenza Murgia, Ottavia Stalio, Paolo Visca and Alyexandra Arienzo
Department of Sciences, Roma Tre University, Rome, Italy

Valeria Ferrante and Valentina Cellitti
Interuniversity Consortium "Biostructures and Biosystems National Institute", Rome, Italy

Salvatore Di Somma
Emergency Medicine, Department of Medical-Surgery Sciences and Translational Medicine, Sapienza University of Rome, Sant'Andrea Hospital, Rome, Italy

Giovanni Antonini
Department of Sciences, Roma Tre University, Rome, Italy
Interuniversity Consortium "Biostructures and Biosystems National Institute", Rome, Italy

Sorwer Alam Parvez and Dolilur Rahman
Shahjalal University of Science and Technology, Sylhet, Bangladesh

Payam Behzadi
Department of Microbiology, College of Basic Sciences, Shahr-e-Qods Branch, Islamic Azad University, Tehran, Iran

Lovelesh Kumar Nigam, Aruna V. Vanikar, Rashmi D. Patel, Kamal V. Kanodia and Kamlesh S. Suthar
Department of Pathology, Lab Medicine, Transfusion Services and Immunohematology, Institute of Kidney Disease and Research Sciences, BJ Medical College Campus, Ahmedabad, Gujarat, India

Md. Mahabubul Islam Majumder, Tarek Ahmed, Saleh Ahmed and Ashiqur Rahman Khan
Department of Medicine, Comilla Medical College, Comilla, Bangladesh

Charalampos Konstantinidis
Urology and Neuro-Urology Unit, National Rehabilitation Center, Athens, Greece

Achilleas Karafotias
Urology Department, General Hospital "Asklepieio Voulas", Athens, Greece

Index

CPSIA information can be obtained
at www.ICGtesting.com
Printed in the USA
LVHW062009100122
708212LV00002B/130

9 781639 875627